PREFACE

The purpose of this text is to provide a clear, succinct guide to the fields of health education and health promotion. Its primary beneficiaries are students who are preparing themselves for a career as health educators or health promoters.

The discipline of health education and the profession of health educator have evolved as a result of a number of forces. These forces in many ways are the same influences that affect our health and our perception of it. The health educator, when entering the profession, should be aware of the many factors which influence our health. These factors include heredity, environment, health care services, and our own behavior.

Health education, while currently viewed as a unique discipline, has a history which is linked to that of health, the development of other disciplines, and the rise of health promotion. It is an outgrowth of other disciplines. The early chapters of this text establish the relationship of health education and health promotion to other disciplines and to health as a condition. This is done in pragmatic, philosophical, and historical contexts.

Health education and health promotion take place in an assortment of settings. Chapters 5, 6, and 7 present justifications for programs in different settings, examples of successful programs in a variety of milieus, and a thorough discussion of the comprehensive school health education program.

Since the product of a successful health education/promotion endeavor is either the development of behaviors conducive to well-being or a change in behavior to those conducive to health, it follows that the health educator must have a theoretical base from which to work. Three models of human development are presented in Chapter 8 with applications to health education. Chapter 9 presents several theories of learning and human behavior with applications to health education.

The competencies and skills required of health educators are addressed in chapters 10, 11, and 12. These competencies follow to some degree the Responsibilities and Competencies for Entry-Level Health Educators originally identified by the Role Delineation Project.

Chapter 13 is a discussion of issues identified by the United States government as priorities for health, including health education. It relates the recent history leading up to and including the Year 2000 Objectives for the Nation, especially those directed toward improving the health of young people.

Finally, we look at current and future issues which may affect the way health educators perform. Some of these issues, such as those surrounding credentialing and professional preparation, affect health educators in the present. Others are predicted to occur in the near future,

such as realignment of funding and the need to become more entrepreneurial in our profession.

The author wishes to acknowledge colleagues who have contributed to the preparation of this text. For their careful and thoughtful reading and comments on a preliminary draft, I am grateful to Steven Furney of Southwest Texas State University and to Stephen Bohnenblust of Mankato State University. In addition, I wish to express sincere appreciation to Tommy Frederick of Delaware State University for his support and encouragement.

J. Thomas Butler

For Lily and Charlene. Thanks for your love, support, patience, and sacrifice.

and

For those faculty members on the campuses of America's institutions of higher education who still believe that teaching their students is their highest calling.

Principles of Health Education and Health Promotion

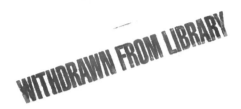

J. Thomas Butler
Delaware State University

Morton Publishing Company
925 W. Kenyon Avenue, Unit 12
Englewood, Colorado 80110

Printed in the United States of America

10   9   8   7   6   5   4   3   2

ISBN: 0-89582-263-6

TABLE OF CONTENTS

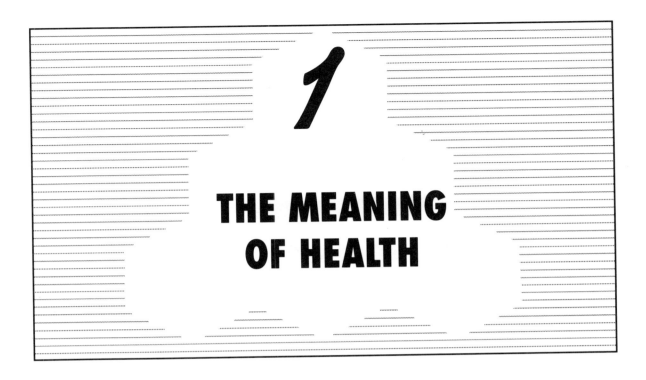

THE MEANING OF HEALTH

During the last generation health education emerged from being a poorly defined, unprofessional practice into a full-fledged discipline. Fully certified and appropriately educated workers in many states practice health education as a specialty. Health education once was viewed as a rainy-day activity conducted by physical education teachers (often gym teachers or coaches). Now health educators have degrees in health education equivalent to degrees in English, mathematics, and social studies, and they apply their specialty to the same extent.

WHAT IS "HEALTH"?

To understand the nature of health education, a definition of the word "health" is in order. It has nearly as many definitions as authors on the subject. Many experts have defined the term, a selected few of which are:

Health is a state of complete physical, mental, and social well-being and not merely the absence of disease or infirmity. (World Health Organization, 1947)

Health is the condition of the organism which measures the degree to which its aggregate powers are able to function. (Oberteuffer, 1960)

Health can be regarded as an expression of fitness to the environment, as a state of adaptation. (Dubos, 1965)

Health is the quality of life involving dynamic interaction and interdependence among the individual's physical well being, his mental and emotional reactions and the social complex in which he exists. (School Health Education Study, 1967)

An integrated method of functioning which is oriented toward maximizing the potential of which the individual is capable. It requires that the individual maintain a continuum of balance and purposeful direction with the environment where he is functioning. (Dunn, 1967)

Health is a state of well-being sufficient to perform at adequate levels of physical, mental and social activity, taking age into account. (Lalonde, 1974)

Health can be defined as the quality of people's physical, psychological, and sociological functioning that enables them to deal adequately with the self and others in a variety of personal and social situations. (Bedworth and Bedworth, 1992)

Health is the capacity to cope with or adapt to disruptions among the organic, social, and personal components of the individual's health system. (Bates and Winder, 1984)

A primary theme running through all of these definitions of health is that of a *positive force*. They make frequent reference to health as a state of well-being. They make no reference at all to bad health or the common description of ill people, "They are in poor health." Health is good; the lack of it is bad.

Terris (1975) stated:

Disease may occur without illness. Health and illness are mutually exclusive, but health and disease are not.... Since health and disease may coexist, one cannot construct a continuum to show their relationship.

Shirreffs (1984) modified this theme only slightly by asserting that health and illness are separate and can exist together. You can be ill and still be healthy. Illness in this context is the presentation of visible symptoms, whereas disease is the underlying defect or malfunction within the organism. According to this point of view, an ill person can be quite healthy. That person may be socially, mentally, and emotionally well, with a temporary physical malfunction to which the immune system has the ability to adapt.

Hoyman (1975) stated, "Health is a multidimensional unity, involving the whole person in his total environment." This reinforces the common theme of most definitions of the term "health," that physical well-being is only a part of the state. Physical illness may seriously affect the physical body, while the mental, social, spiritual, and emotional person may be less affected, equally affected, or even unaffected. The total person is a multidimensional creature, and his or her health also must be seen as having many dimensions.

How would you measure your own health? Would it be in terms of years in your life span? Would it be in terms of the quality of those years? These are questions for each individual to consider. Perhaps more important questions would be: How can you improve your own health? What are you willing to do to make yourself healthier? Do some factors affect your health over which you have no control?

DIMENSIONS OF HEALTH

The word "health" originally meant "wholeth," or "wholeness" (Dolfman, 1973). The state of being called health, as viewed through the origin of the word, then, implies involvement of the entire individual. This is what the World Health Organization meant in 1947 when it defined health as "complete physical, mental, and social well-being and not merely the absence of disease or infirmity." Many authors (e.g., Levy, Dignan, and Shirreffs, 1992) propose additional dimensions such as emotional and spiritual. With the emphasis currently placed upon recognition of one's cultural heritage and upon multicultural appreciation, an argument could be made that a cultural dimension is appropriate. Such arguments are countered by the contentions that the spiritual realm is inexorably linked to the emotional and mental dimensions and that the cultural development is part and parcel of the social dimension. In our discussion, we address the dimensions of physical, emotional, social, and mental health because these are most frequently targeted for development in health education programs.

No dimension of health functions in isolation. When an individual has a high level of health, all dimensions function in an integrated, coordinated way. The person's environment, including school, family, work, and community are in tune with one another to produce harmony. The way in which these aspects jointly contribute to the richness of a person's life helps determine that individual's uniqueness as well as his or her health (Hammerschlag, 1988).

Physical Health

The physical condition of the body is reflected in a number of ways. Measurements such as blood pressure, heart rate, body composition, flexibility, agility, vital capacity, and strength provide some insight into physical health. Responses to injuries and recovery from disease can be indicative of physical health. People can behave in ways that enhance physical health, such as exercising regularly and eating a balanced diet. It is equally important to avoid behaviors that decrease physical health, such as cigarette smoking and excessive alcohol consumption.

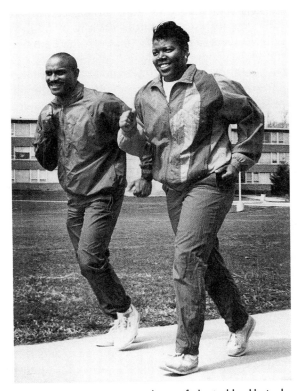

Regular exercise is an essential part of physical health. It also contributes to mental, emotional and social well-being.

Our bodies frequently send messages to us: "Please let me get a good night's sleep," "Allow my sprained ankle to heal," "Send down some vegetables tonight," "My muscles are tense." These and other messages can guide us toward physical health. Getting regular medical check-ups can head off medical problems before they become serious. Basic self-care skills can help people cope with minor health problems on their own (Levin, 1976).

Emotional Health

Emotional health requires understanding one's emotions and knowing how to cope with problems that arise in everyday life and the stress we all endure. It means being able to work, love and be loved, study, and pursue the activities that define our being. It also means enjoying those activities. The quality of a person's life is largely reflected in his or her emotions.

Emotions can affect our physical health. For example, people with good emotional health have low rates of stress-related diseases such as ulcers, migraine headaches, and asthma (Padus, 1986; Tucker, Cole, and Friedman, 1987). Long-term stress or emotional strife can lead to collapse of the immune system (Ornstein and Sobel, 1987; Squires, 1987), increasing the risk of developing other diseases. Considerable evidence suggests that long-term stress can increase the risk of heart disease. Beginning in the 1950s, cardiologists Friedman and Rosenman (Rosenman et al. 1966) conducted a series of investigations into the relationship between coronary heart disease and personal life stress. They identified a personality type, which they labeled Type A, that seemed to be a significant risk factor in coronary heart disease when found in combination with elevated blood pressure and blood fats. Type A behavior is described as an action-emotion complex observed in a person aggressively involved in a long-term, ceaseless struggle to achieve more and more in less and less time, even against opposition by other things or persons. Coronary-prone Type A individuals are supposedly hard-driving, competitive, subject to vocational deadlines, restless, impatient, frequently in a hurry, self-centered, perfectionistic, and oblivious to the environment (Friedman and Rosenman, 1974).

In recent years a personality trait called *hardiness* has been credited with strengthening the immune system against the destructive effects of stress (Kobasa, 1979). Hardiness is characterized as an optimistic and committed approach to life, viewing problems, including disease, as challenges that can be handled. Hardiness, or something akin to it, can be developed through stress management techniques and reassessing one's own goals and priorities. Many of the things that cause us stress also give us joy, such as our families and work. One of the keys to emotional health is to realize that we usually can manage stressful situations and can reduce the effects of stress on our bodies and minds.

Social Health

We all occupy roles in a number of groups or institutions. These roles include son or daughter, friend, student or teacher, neighbor, co-worker, and mate. Each role contains expectations. Social health refers to the ability to perform the expectations of our roles effectively, comfortably, with pleasure, without harming other people (Levy et al., 1992).

Performing role expectations sometimes means taking risks. It sometimes means having responsibilities. Frequently these responsibilities impact other people and involve meeting others' needs. These needs include love, intimacy, safety, companionship, and cooperation—all important factors in social health. Sometimes when people are deprived of these needs, they act in ways that

threaten their overall health and well-being (Moss, 1973; Gore, 1978).

Mental Health

Mental health probably is the most difficult dimension of health to describe. Certainly it encompasses intellectual processes. To this extent, it includes the ability to make sound decisions and to think critically. Emotional health sometimes is considered to be a part of mental health, as emotions can act to the detriment of intellectual decision making.

Many people misinterpret one's actions as a sign of deficient mental health. Conforming to social demands is not necessarily a mark of mental health. Questioning what goes on around you indeed may be a sign of mental health. Actions and reactions alone do not automatically classify us as mentally healthy or as mentally ill. A situation that may produce anxiety for some people may not cause anxiety for others because of basic personality differences. Showing no anxiety in a given circumstance may be a sign that the person is not facing a problem

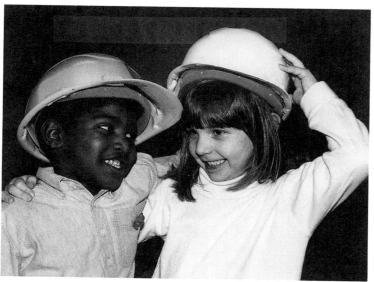

Well-planned educational experiences promote social health.

or trying to resolve it. In actuality, anxiety may lead to solving problems.

Looking at a group of people he thought had fulfilled a good measure of their potential, Abraham Maslow (1968) identified qualities in people whom he described as *self-actualized*. These qualities also may be applied to people who are mentally healthy. According to Maslow, these people:

◆ are able to deal with the world as it is and don't demand that it should be otherwise.

◆ are able to largely accept themselves, others, and nature.

◆ experience profound interpersonal relations.

◆ have a continuing fresh appreciation for what goes on around them.

◆ are able to direct themselves, rather independently of culture and environment.

◆ trust their own senses and feelings.

◆ are creative.

◆ are democratic in their attitudes.

MAJOR FACTORS INFLUENCING HEALTH

If you were to sit down with pencil and paper, you probably could list hundreds of factors that directly influence your health and the health of others. Most, if not all, of those factors could be grouped into four categories: heredity, environment, health care services, and behavior.

Heredity

A number of factors affecting our health are inherited via our genetic background and therefore are beyond our control. Some of these traits may contribute to effective functioning: others may interfere. Disorders such as Down syndrome, Marfon's syndrome, sickle cell anemia, thalassemia, and Tay-Sachs disease have their roots in heredity. Even alcoholism has been

demonstrated to have a strong genetic component. Tendencies toward disorders such as hypertension have been shown to be genetic and more likely to appear in certain ethnic groups.

Our gender and possibly our size can make us susceptible to certain influences on our health. Percentage of body fat, weight, and even obesity can be inherited. Just as a genetic propensity toward high levels of body fat may negatively influence an individual's health, the propensity toward low or moderate levels of body fat must be positive influences on health.

Environment

The environment is becoming more and more important to our health and the deterioration of health. As the ozone layer is being depleted, we humans are exposed to more ultraviolet radiation. The risk of eye damage and skin cancer is greater with exposure to the sun. Sunburn is really radiation burn, and skin cancer can develop even without sunburn.

Our water and food supplies are becoming more and more polluted. Agricultural runoff and profit-hungry industry have combined to make water unsafe in many American communities. Cases of cancer and even fetal damage traced to polluted water are becoming all too common. If water is contaminated, the food we eat also is likely to be contaminated.

The air we breathe is a health hazard to many of us. For years many large urban areas have exceeded acceptable levels of pollutants such as ozone and carbon monoxide. Winds, offending industries, and automobiles have spread dense pollutants to many rural areas as well. The resulting pollutants in the air may fall to the earth in the form of acid rain, further damaging the soil, water, and food. Governmental agencies such as the Environmental Protection Agency, as well as Congress, have wrestled for years with the problem of air pollution. Unfortunately, the lobbying power of big business has crippled the effectiveness of many proposals to clean up the air. Presently, stricter regulations mandated by the federal Clean Air Act are being implemented. It remains to be seen if any long-range positive environmental impact will occur. We already know that implementation of the regulations has tremendous financial burdens.

Many people are susceptible to allergic reactions to substances in their environments. The presence of these substances may be increased by climatic conditions.

Noise has been identified as an environmental hazard. Some sources of noise are voluntary, such as music played at high volume through headphones and at rock concerts. Many people, however, are exposed to high decibel levels in their workplace and at home. Besides the noise of appliances, televisions, and stereos, many Americans live close to airports, highways, highly congested areas, and construction sites. Indeed, areas of high population density are a source of almost constant exposure to excessive noise levels.

Many Americans consider themselves and their children subject to social and cultural pollution via television and radio. Certain depictions of sexuality are offensive to some people and certainly present an unhealthy and unrealistic picture of sex to children. Advertisements for foods and alcohol, and billboard and magazine advertisements for tobacco depict inaccurate and misleading situations regarding these products. Children may not be able to determine that the "part of this nutritious breakfast" touted in a commercial is really the least nutritious part.

Teens may not have the maturity to understand that using a harmful product will not enhance attractiveness and sex appeal as depicted in the advertisement. To say that parents can turn off the television or throw out the magazine is missing the point. Children cannot avoid these images in today's world.

The modern network of society may not provide an environment necessary for individual growth. Instead it may impinge on the individual's freedom to function adequately. Overcrowding is an example. Failures in the family, the school, and the church to provide opportunities

for children to develop self-esteem may contribute to experimentation with alcohol or other drugs (Butler, 1982).

Health Care Services

The cost and availability of health care services has an obvious effect on the health of every American. The rise in cost of health care over the past several years has far outdistanced inflation. An ever-increasing percentage of our gross national product is devoted to the delivery of health care. The cost of health care has exceeded the means of many Americans. Insurance companies have become more selective in the procedures they cover and the clients they will insure. All this has made health care too expensive for a huge number of Americans, including millions of children.

For those who can afford health care, whether it be through their own resources, private or group health insurance, or government-sponsored programs such as Medicaid, the primary emphasis of care traditionally has been on diagnosis and treatment. The emphasis on expensive treatment is, of course, a major cause of the higher costs and lack of availability. Even though we know how to prevent many illnesses and disorders, the medical community has not done its part in stressing prevention to its patients. The medical community cannot bear the full blame, though, as we, the consumer, must put prevention into practice by making decisions that affect our lifestyles and daily lives and thereby gain the full benefit of preventive medicine and avoid the costs of treatment.

In 1972 the Health Maintenance Organization Assistance Act was passed with the hope of setting up a new system for delivering health care. Although the HMO movement has not lived up to its potential, it at least established that health care costs can be reduced and that health education and prevention can be implemented successfully into the medical system. By definition, HMOs have a health education component, the effectiveness of which varies greatly.

Although individual HMOs differ widely in delivery of services, costs, and health education, the HMO concept offers a good deal of promise.

Regardless of the model for delivering services, effectiveness of the care frequently depends upon the quality of communication between practitioner and patient. Communication may be weakened by physicians who fail to bridge the gap between medical jargon and the patient's ability to understand and comprehend. Medical schools have a responsibility to develop in aspiring physicians the kind of communication skills necessary to bridge this gap. Physicians should consider each patient with his or her own strengths and weaknesses and try to overcome weaknesses that impede good communication.

On the other hand, patients may be reluctant to discuss or describe their symptoms and talk about issues that are embarrassing to them. Health educators can assume a role in this area. Students and clients should understand the importance of taking an active part in their own health and complying with physicians' advice. They cannot do this unless they make a special effort to provide all the information a physician needs to render an accurate diagnosis and unless they fully understand the advice they receive. Patients have to feel comfortable and be assertive enough to ask questions and to leave the appointment only after they have all the information necessary to comply with the physician's advice. Fostering assertiveness is part of the role of health education.

Ross and Mico (1980) identified several transitions in the field of health care that already have produced or have the potential to produce positive effects on the system in the coming few years. The first is a definite change in attitude in the United States regarding health care as a right rather than a privilege. With the advent of insurance companies, most Americans gained access to health care. In recent years, however, health care costs have driven insurance premiums beyond the reach of many citizens. Approximately 37 million Americans are without health insurance, which is totally unacceptable.

This situation is at least partially a result of another transition—from costs being determined by professionals to being determined by insurers. This gives an enormous amount of power to a third party in the delivery relationship, most apparent in the Medicaid system of establishing diagnosis-related groups (DRGs). DRGs establish payment schedules for specific diagnoses, which means that Medicaid will pay only so much for a medical procedure. It also means the insurer influences the choice to use that procedure or even to treat the patient at all. If this power is allowed to accrue in the hands of for-profit insurers, the implications for health care are frightening.

Health care costs are being influenced by other factors as well. We have seen a trend to prepare a large number of specialists. Even the family practitioner is now a specialist. Specialists' services generally are more expensive than those of generalists, the old "family doctors." More recently the number of specialists being trained in medical schools seems to be decreasing.

The traditional practice of a single physician's maintaining and operating an office is rapidly becoming a part of history in most areas. By grouping several physicians in one office, they can reduce overhead and staff salaries. An extreme example of this trend is the health maintenance organization (HMO), one form of which is a single company which employs physicians of many specialties and pays them a salary. This is a powerful contrast to individual physicians who charge each patient for each service.

The way health care is financed may be altered extensively in the next few years. The 1992 election ushered in an administration that promised to change the way health care is delivered and financed. Health policy historically has been fragmented and determined locally. Even the Medicaid system is subject to state policies. Many experts, looking into the future, see a federally managed system of health care reimbursement. This would place much control over the practice of medicine in the hands of federal bureaucrats. An even more drastic possibility is the adoption of a system similar to that of Canada, in which the federal government employs physicians and, in effect, renders health care to citizens.

The most powerful transition in health care stems from the patient. From being totally dependent on physicians, and passive recipients of health care, more people are becoming active in their own health care. They are forcing physicians to regard them as partners in the support of their own health. They realize that their greatest health ally is themselves.

Behavior

To maximize the health of the population, individuals must take responsibility for their own actions and the status of their own health. Although many causes of illness and deteriorating health are linked to heredity and environmental pollutants, lifestyle is a determining factor in the state of one's health. The individual is the ultimate decision maker in his or her own life. What we do is the major influence on our health. The implications for behavior change, habit formation, and lifestyle development form the basis for health education.

Consider that:

◆ cancer is the second leading cause of death in the United States, and lung cancer causes more deaths than any other form of cancer. The American Cancer Society (1992) estimated that cigarette smoking is responsible for 90% of the lung cancer deaths in men and 79% of the lung cancer deaths in women.

◆ a major risk factor for oral cancer is the use of smokeless tobacco (American Cancer Society, 1992).

◆ diet high in fat and/or low in fiber may be a significant causative factor in colon and rectum cancer (American Cancer Society, 1992.)

◆ diet, cigarette smoking, and lack of exercise are related closely to heart disease, the leading

cause of death in the United States (Levy et al., 1992).

◆ although many research studies indicate that the use of lap and shoulder safety belts in vehicles reduces the risk of death and serious injury by 60-70%, many adults fail to use the restraints (Insel and Roth, 1991).

◆ even though AIDS is not contracted readily, many people engage in the precise acts (unprotected sex and injectable drug use) that transmit the disease.

◆ the U. S. Surgeon General set forth as an objective for 1990 the immunization of 90% of all children for polio, measles, pertussis (whooping cough), tetanus, tuberculosis, and diphtheria. This indicates that, although the immunizations are inexpensive and have been available for decades, many parents are not having their children immunized (Green, 1990). American one-year-olds have lower immunization rates than one-year-olds in fourteen other countries. Polio immunization rates for nonwhite babies in the United States rank behind forty-eight other countries, including Botswana, Sri Lanka, Albania, Columbia, and Jamaica (Children's Defense Fund, 1990).

◆ although the U. S. Public Health Service identified cigarette smoking as "clearly the largest single preventable cause of illness and premature death in the United States" (U. S. Department of Health, Education, and Welfare, 1979), almost a third of the adult population continues to smoke.

The recognition that behavior is related to health is not new. Belloc and Breslow (1972) followed nearly 7,000 adults for five and a half years. The research showed that life expectancy and better health are significantly related to six simple health habits:

1. Eating three meals a day at regular times and no snacking.

2. Exercising moderately three times a week.

One Day in the Lives of American Children

17,051 women get pregnant.

2,795 of them are teenagers.

1,106 teenagers have abortions.

372 teenagers miscarry.

1,295 teenagers give birth, one every 67 seconds.

689 babies are born to women who have had inadequate prenatal care.

719 babies are born at low birthweight (less than 5 lb., 8 oz.)

129 babies are born at very low birthweight (less than 3 lb., 5 oz.).

105 babies die before their first birthday

67 babies die before one month of life.

27 children die in poverty; one every 53 minutes.

10 children die from gunshot injuries.

30 children are injured by guns.

6 children commit suicide.

135,000 children bring a gun to school

7,742 teens become sexually active.

623 teenagers get syphilis or gonorrhea.

211 children are arrested for drug abuse, one every 7 minutes.

437 children are arrested for drinking or for drunken driving.

1,512 teenagers drop out of school, one every 8 seconds of the school day.

1,849 children are neglected or abused, one every 47 seconds.

3,288 children run away from home, one every 26 seconds.

1,629 children are in adult jails.

2,556 children are born out of wedlock.

2,989 children see their parents divorced.

34,285 people lose their jobs.

100,000 children are homeless.

Source: Children's Defense Fund, *Children 1990: A Report Card, Briefing Book, and Action Primer.* Washington, DC: CDF 1990.

3. Getting adequate sleep (seven-eight hours each night).
4. Maintaining normal weight.
5. Drinking alcohol in moderation, if at all.
6. No smoking.

Among the findings were that 80% of deaths caused by cancer and cardiovascular disease are premature and can be prevented by practicing these six behaviors.

The Surgeon General (U. S. Department of Health, Education, and Welfare, 1979) pointed out that individuals can improve their health by taking actions for themselves, including:

1. Eliminating cigarette smoking.
2. Decreasing alcohol use.
3. Making moderate dietary changes, including reducing the intake of calories, fat, salt, and sugar.
4. Doing moderate regular exercise.
5. Periodically being screened for disorders such as high blood pressure and certain cancers.
6. Adhering to speed laws and using seat belts.

Kolbe (1993) stated that only six types of behaviors cause the major health problems that face the nation. If looked upon as behaviors that could be changed or eliminated, they bear remarkable resemblance to the Surgeon General's list of actions to improve individual health. They are:

1. Behaviors that result in unintentional and intentional injuries;
2. Drug and alcohol abuse;
3. Sexual behaviors that result in pregnancy and sexually transmitted diseases, including HIV infection;
4. Tobacco use;
5. Excessive consumption of fat and calories;
6. Insufficient physical activity.

Kolbe indicated that these behaviors are usually established in youth, are interrelated, persist into adulthood, contribute simultaneously to diminished levels of health, education, and social outcomes, and are preventable.

The obvious question becomes: If we know how to reduce health risks, why do so many people behave in ways that put them at greater risk? The answers to this question are not easy to come by. Regardless, let us postulate a few answers:

1. They do not value health.
2. They enjoy the thrill of risk-taking.
3. They are unable to balance the risk versus the benefits of the action.
4. The benefit gained from the action is worth the risk of shorter life span, disease, or injury.
5. They are unaware of the risks.
6. People take unnecessary risks because risk-taking behaviors, habits, and addictions are established early in life before the sufficient maturity is developed.

Whatever the reasons, they certainly must relate to either lack of *knowledge* or *attitudes* that are not conducive to health, or to both.

WHAT IS OPTIMAL HEALTH?

Everybody does not have the same capacity for health. Each person is defined by his or her own set of conditions which may affect health. *Optimal health* is the highest level of health possible under the current set of environmental conditions and capacity of the organism.

An individual's optimal level of health varies according to environmental constraints, capacity to deal with those constraints, and permanent or temporary disabilities. A person who adapts to environmental changes that have the potential for causing stress has a higher level of optimal health than a person who has little capacity to make adjustments. A person who labors under enormous environmental constraints has a lower level of optimal health than a person with fewer constraints. Certainly, people with severe physical or mental disabilities might be less able to adapt to their environments and have a lower optimal health level. Of course, many people with severe physical handicaps have attained extremely high levels of overall health despite their limitations.

The level of optimal health combines each of the dimensions of health—physical, emotional, social, mental. These four dimensions are interrelated. Although one or more components may be more prominent, none should be overlooked. Figure 1.1 depicts the shared contributions of the four components of optimal health.

The challenge for each individual is to gain the highest level of health possible or to attain as closely as possible. Health care deliverers have a role in helping the individual approach optimal health. Perhaps more important than any other group, health educators must assist others to attain optimal health. This is what health education is really all about.

SUMMARY

Health is a positive entity with four dimensions: physical health, emotional health, social health, and mental health. Heredity, environment, health care services, and behavior all affect health. To attain the highest level of health possible—the optimal level of health—each person has to make decisions resulting in a lifestyle that is conducive to health. This implies the presence of positive attitudes about health and the knowledge needed to make practical decisions.

REFERENCES

American Cancer Society. *Cancer Facts & Figures—1992*. Atlanta: ACS, 1992.

Bates, I. J. and A. E. Winder. *Introduction to Health Education*. Palo Alto, CA: Mayfield Publishing, 1984.

Belloc, N. B. and L. Breslow. Relationship of physical health status and health practices. *Preventive Medicine, 1* (August, 1972): 415-521.

Bedworth, D. A. and A. E. Bedworth. *The Profession and Practice of Health Education*. Dubuque, IA: Wm. C. Brown Publishers, 1992.

Butler, J. T. Early adolescent alcohol consumption and self-concept, social class and knowledge of alcohol. *Journal of Studies on Alcohol, 43* (May, 1982): 603-607.

Children's Defense Fund. *Children 1990: A Report Card, Briefing Book, and Action Primer*. Washington, DC: Children's Defense Fund, 1990.

Dolfman, M. L. The concept of health: An historic and analytic examination. *Journal of School Health, 43,* (October, 1973): 491-497.

Dubos, R. *Man Adapting*. New Haven, CT: Yale University Press, 1965.

Dunn, H. *High Level Wellness*. Arlington, VA: R.W. Beatty, 1967.

Friedman, M., and R. H. Rosenman. *Type A Behavior and Your Heart*. Greenwich, CT: Fawcett Publications, 1974.

Gore, S. The effect of social support in moderating health. *Journal of Personality and Social Behavior, 19* (1978): 157-165.

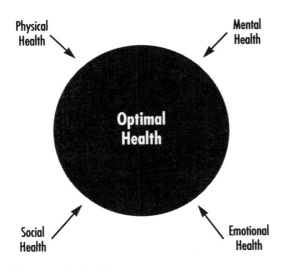

FIGURE 1.1.   Optimal Health

Green, L. W. *Community Health* (6th ed.). St. Louis: Times Mirror/Mosby College Publishing, 1990.

Hammerschlag, C. A. *The Dancing Healers: A Doctor's Journey of Healing with Native Americans.* San Francisco: Harper & Row, 1988.

Hoyman, H. Rethinking an ecologic system model of man's health, disease, aging, death. *Journal of School Health, 45* (November, 1975): 509-518.

Insel, P. M. and W. T. Roth. *Core Concepts in Health* (6th ed.). Mountain View, CA: Mayfield Publishing, 1991.

Kobasa, S. C. Stressful life events, personality, and health: An inquiry into hardiness. *Journal of Personality and Social Psychology, 37* (January, 1979): 1-11.

Kolbe, L. J. Developing a plan of action to institutionalize comprehensive school health education programs in the United States. *Journal of School Health, 63* (January, 1993): 12-13.

Lalonde, M. *A New Perspective on the Health of Canadians.* Ottawa: Information Canada, 1974.

Levin, L. S. The layperson as the primary care practitioner. *Public Health Reports, 91* (May-June, 1976): 206-210.

Levy, M. R., M. Dignan, and J. H. Shirreffs. *Life and Health: Targeting Wellness.* New York: McGraw-Hill, 1992.

Maslow, A. H. *Toward a Psychology of Being* (2d ed.). Princeton, NJ: Van Nostrand-Reinhold, 1968.

Moss, G. M. *Illness, Immunity and Social Interaction.* New York: John Wiley, 1973.

Oberteuffer, D. *School Health Education: A Textbook for Teachers, Nurses, and Other Professional Personnel.* New York: Harper and Brothers, 1960.

Ornstein, R., and D. Sobel. *The Healing Brain: A New Perspective on the Brain and Health.* New York: Simon & Schuster, 1987.

Padus, E. *The Complete Guide to Your Emotions and Your Health.* Emmaus, PA: Rodale Press, 1986.

Rosenman, R. H., M. Friedman, et al. Coronary heart disease in Western collaborative group study. *Journal of the American Medical Association, 195* (January 10, 1966).

Ross, H. S. and P. R. Mico. *Theory and Practice in Health Education.* Palo Alto, CA: Mayfield Publishing, 1980.

School Health Education Study. *Health Education: A Conceptual Approach to Curriculum Design.* St. Paul: 3M Education Press, 1967.

Shirreffs, J. The nature and meaning of health education. In Rubinson, L. and W. F. Alles, *Health Education: Foundations for the Future.* Prospect Heights, IL: Waveland Press, 1984.

Squires, S. The power of positive imagery: Visions to boost immunity. *American Health, 6* (July/August, 1987): 56-61.

Terris, M. Approach to an epidemiology of health. *American Journal of Public Health, 65* (October, 1975): 1037-1041.

Tucker, L. A., G. G. Cole, and G. M. Friedman. Stress and serum cholesterol: A study of 7,000 adult males. *Health Values, 11* (May/June, 1987): 34-39.

U. S. Department of Health, Education and Welfare. *Healthy People: The Surgeon General's Report on Health Promotion and Disease* (Publication No. 79-55071). Washington, DC: Public Health Service, 1979.

World Health Organization. Constitution of the World Health

Organization. *Chronicle of the World Health Organization, 1* (1947).

2

THE DEFINITION AND ROLE OF HEALTH EDUCATION

The term "health education" has long been misunderstood by school administrators and parents. In many cases those involved in the search and hiring process do not know what a health educator should be able to do in a given setting. This misunderstanding has led to allocating responsibility for health education to people who have little preparation in the field.

In schools the science teacher, the physical education teacher, or the school nurse frequently gets that duty. In hospitals, and even in health maintenance organizations, administrators are reluctant to trust health education to people who are not trained in medicine. Nurses and physicians often conduct health education—or "patient education," as hospitals term it—without aptitude, training, or motivation to do so. In some cases training in patient education is required for nurses. This ranges from superficial to extensive. Legal requirements may make patient education mandatory, but they cannot make it effective.

WHAT IS HEALTH EDUCATION?

As with the term "health," "health education" has a plethora of definitions. This term is not easy to define to the satisfaction of all professionals. Health education takes place in a number of settings. Most people believe they can do it well. Indeed, the actions of every parent, teacher, and role model communicate something about health. The message, however, may be far from satisfactory. Let us examine a few definitions of health education.

A process affecting intellectual, psychological, and social dimensions that increases our capacity to make informed health decisions affecting self, family and community well-being. (Bedworth and Bedworth, 1978)

The process through which individuals, social groups, and communities attend to and assimilate information about health and disease, and mobilize appropriate behavior for health-promotive ends. (Wilner, Walker, and Goerke, 1973)

Any combination of learning experiences designed to facilitate voluntary adaptations of behavior conducive to health. (Green, Kreuter, Deeds, and Partridge, 1980)

The process of providing learning experiences for the purpose of influencing knowledge, attitudes, or conduct relating to individual, community, or world health. (Joint Committee on Health Problems in Education, 1948)

A process with intellectual, psychological, and social dimensions relating to activities that increase the abilities of people to make informed decisions affecting their personal, family and community well-being. This process, based on scientific principles, facilitates learning and behavioral change in both health personnel and consumers, including children and youth. (Joint Committee on Health Education Terminology, 1973)

Planned learning experiences and supportive activities that help people develop their abilities to evaluate behavioral options and their probable consequences, and make informed decisions about their responsibilities and actions concerning:

1. Personal practices aimed at promoting vigorous well-being, preventing avoidable disability and premature death, and effectively handling minor diseases and discomforts;

2. Prompt, appropriate use of health services when needed;

3. Selection and carrying out of needed diagnostic, treatment, habilitation, rehabilitation, and maintenance procedures; and

4. Involvement in community efforts (at local, area, state, regional, national and/or international levels) to develop effective, efficient, and appropriate environmental programs, socioeconomic measures, and health services systems that facilitate health improvement. (Bureau of Health Planning and Resources Development, 1973)

Any activity with clear goals planned for the purpose of improving health-related knowledge, attitudes, or behavior. (Carlyon and Cook, 1981)

A deliberately planned, structured learning opportunity about health that occurs in a setting at a given point in time and involves interaction between an educator and a learner. (Bates and Winder, 1984)

Any health-related educational activities, whether in schools, community, clinical, or work settings. (Pollock and Middleton, 1989)

That continuum of learning which enables people, as individuals and as members of social structures, to voluntarily make decisions, modify behaviors, and change social conditions in ways which are health enhancing. (1990 Joint Committee on Health Education Terminology, 1991)

The process of assisting individuals, acting separately and collectively, to make informed decisions about matters affecting their personal health and that of others. (Henderson and McIntosh, 1981)

The Main Theme in Health Education

What do these definitions have in common? Clearly the thread running through these definitions is the notion that health education is a process. It is not a product but, rather, a series of planned activities directed toward goals. It includes an array of deliberate experiences that affect the way people think, feel, and act regarding their own health and the health of their communities. As Oberteuffer, Harrelson, and Pollock (1972) stated:

> The goal of health education is to help each person seek that pattern of behavior which moves him toward an optimal level of health rather than the reverse and to give him the ability to avoid many of the imbalances, diseases, and accidents of life.

Reaching for this worthy goal is the mission of health education and its practitioners.

Implied, though not consistently stated, in definitions of health education is that it is an applied science basic to the general education of all young people. Its body of knowledge represents a synthesis of facts, principles, and concepts drawn from biological, behavioral, sociological, and health sciences, interpreted in terms of human needs, human values, and human potential (Pollock and Hamburg, 1985).

Whatever definition you choose, one fundamental principle must guide the work of health educators: Individuals, families and communities can be taught to assume responsibility for their own health and, to some extent for the health of others, and this assumption of responsibility in turn brings about changes in their behaviors and lifestyles. The basic challenge is to find the most productive ways to influence voluntary individual and community behavior without violating individual freedoms guaranteed by the U. S. Constitution.

The process of health education includes:

◆ a planned opportunity to learn about health

◆ occurring in a given setting

◆ at a given point in time

◆ involving interaction between teacher and learner

Misconceptions of Health Education

Mistaken beliefs surround health education. For instance, many people believe, though they do not frequently verbalize this in public, that anyone can teach health well. During the 1980s one of the dominant themes in education was the "back to the basics" movement. This movement was based on the poor performance of American children on standardized tests and on the loss of U. S. technological supremacy in and dominance of world markets. In the meantime, health education had made significant gains despite the attitude that special training was not necessary to deliver it effectively. The back to the basics movement ignored the poor performance of American children on fitness tests and measures of general wellness. As a result, health education suffered in many school districts. Fortunately, many parents and administrators recognized that nothing is as basic as the health of their children. They realized that emphasis on mathematical, writing, and reading skills should not come at the expense of the child's health.

Another misconception about health education is that anyone can write an effective health education curriculum. Structuring learning experiences throughout an academic year or developing a kindergarten through high school program requires special expertise. Although little consensus may be found among health educators as

to acceptable standards for practice in health education, different practices may be justifiable when they are based upon a strong philosophical and academic background. Curricular needs frequently depend upon the needs, resources, and principles inherent in a given community. Just as specific expertise is essential to develop a science curriculum, expertise in health education is needed to create curricula in that area.

Health education frequently is equated with hygiene classes. The old hygiene class dealt mainly with practices like handwashing and teeth brushing. Though these are necessary activities, today's health education equips students to make decisions affecting their wellbeing throughout life. It helps them cope with the challenges of modern life. It imparts the knowledge necessary to reach one's optimal level of health and influences attitudes so students appreciate the importance of each decision that affects health.

A UNIQUE DISCIPLINE

Health education is rooted in other disciplines. Certainly the behavioral sciences, public health, and education are primary contributors to the

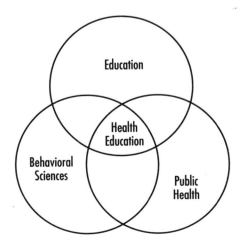

FIGURE 2.1. The Roots of Health Education

discipline of health education. Health science education also strengthens health education as a discipline. Although health education relies upon and utilizes other disciplines, it should be granted status equal to disciplines such as home economics, social studies, science, and physical education.

The behavioral sciences, incorporating psychology, sociology, and anthropology, are concerned with how people behave and why. The primary determinants of behavior are:

1. *Psychological predispositions*, including attitudes, knowledge, beliefs, skills, and experiences.

2. *Environmental reinforcement*, from family, friends, authority figures, and associates.

3. *The sociocultural context*—sustained societal norms about attitudes and behavior.

Because behavior change is the desired outcome of health education, these primary determinants as established by the behavioral sciences become crucial to the practice of health education.

Public health services are provided by government agencies and supported by taxation. Health education relies on public health for, among other things, health statistics for epidemiologic information. Determinants of health problems—environment, medical care, personal lifestyle—often are discovered in the public health realm. Indeed, the pathway of health education and behavior changes often begins in the public health realm.

Obviously education—the study and practice of teaching and learning—plays a role in the development of health education. In fact, health is one of the "seven cardinal principles of public education" (Commission on the Reorganization of Education, 1918/1928).

Health science education has a much narrower meaning than health education. The former refers basically to the acquisition of health facts, their relation to each other, and how these relationships can be the foundation for health principles or laws (Bedworth and Bedworth,

1992). Health education means imparting health science principles via the educational process by trained, competent individuals to meet certain objectives relating to knowledge, attitudes, and behavior.

Nixon (1967) summarized the criteria of a discipline:

1. A discipline has an identifiable domain; it asks vital questions; it deals with immensely significant themes, a specifiable scope of inquiry, a central core of interest; it has a definite beginning point; and it has stated goals.

2. A discipline is characterized by a substantial history and a publicly recognized tradition exemplified by time-tested works.

3. A discipline is rooted in an appropriate structure; it has its unique conceptual structure, and it employs a syntactical structure; the structure organizes a body of basic concepts; and it consists of conceptual relationships as well as appropriate relations between facts.

4. A discipline possesses a unique integrity and an arbitrary quality.

5. A discipline is recognized by the procedures and methods it employs; it utilizes intellectual and conceptual tools as well as technical and mechanical tools; it follows a relevant set of rules; it is recognized by its basic set of procedures, all of which lead to ways of learning and knowing in the domain of the discipline.

6. A discipline is recognized as a process as well as noted for its products (knowledge, principles, generalizations).

7. A discipline relies on accurate language, a participants' language, to provide precise careful communication both within its ranks and to outsiders.

Based upon these criteria, health education is certainly a discipline. In practice, however, many school districts do not treat health education as a discipline. Should physical education teachers be considered health educators? Should coaches be assigned to teach health education? What is the role of the school nurse in health education? As you think about these questions, remember that the academic preparation of health educators is unique. Most physical educators are educationally prepared to teach physical skills.

Most coaches are trained to win games. Nurses are primarily educated to deal with clinical problems of health. Unless they are trained additionally in health education, none of these practitioners is prepared to deal with health education.

CATEGORIZING HEALTH EDUCATION PRACTICE

Greene and Simons-Morton (1984) presented three broad categorizations of health education practice: *setting-specific, content-specific,* and *process-specific.**

Setting or target group-specific
   College and university health education
   School health education
   Occupational health education
   Consumer health education
   Patient education
   Community or public health education
   State or national health education

Content/area-specific
   Nutrition education
   Death and dying education
   Sex education
   Drug and alcohol abuse prevention education
   Cancer education
   Health promotion
   Disease prevention

Process/responsibility-specific
   Health education consultant
   Health education planner
   Health education teacher
   Health education trainer
   Health education specialist: media, evaluation
   Health counselor
   Community organizer

The setting-specific category refers to either the institutional base or the prime target group. The content-specific category denotes the subject matter or the health problem the program

addresses through the program. The process-specific categorization encompasses direct health education services such as teaching, counseling, and organizing. Greene and Simons-Morton point out that practitioners who call themselves content specialists—such as sex educator, alcohol and drug abuse specialist, and nutrition educator—underscore the rivalry that sometimes develops between people professionally trained as health educators who work in special content areas and those trained in content areas who also practice health education. It also leaves open to question the practice of universities' advertising for and employing specialists in a specific content area in departments of health education.

The Society for Public Health Education (SOPHE) (Cleary, 1978) identified three types of health educators: (a) those who teach in schools; (b) those who plan, coordinate, and evaluate health education programs; and (c) those with a professional identity other than "health educator" who conduct health education. In reality, at the local level the first two types often merge because frequently those who teach also lead or participate in curriculum development and evaluation. As mentioned, professionals in other areas, such as nursing, social work, home economics, and physical education, often have the role of health educator in schools.

Responsibilities associated with the health educator can be categorized as program planner, implementer of program components, deliverer of services, administrator of programs, and evaluator. Each of these responsibilities requires a unique set of skills, but in the real world a health educator usually is called upon to take on multiple responsibilities.

1. *Program planning* is at least a two-part process. First, the planner must assess the needs of the population. This step allows for justification of the program's direction and eventual evaluation. Program planning should not be done by one person but, rather, by a team of interested parties including consumers, parents, and students. It involves examining data on problems,

Source: Greene, W. H. and Simons-Morton, B. G. Introduction to Health Education. Prospect Heights, IL: Waveland Press, 1984. Reprinted by permission of the publisher.

concerns, and behaviors related to the population at risk. It may be done by data collection or by perusal of existing data. Needs assessment should result in a prioritized list of behaviors and the determinants of these behaviors.

The second step is to develop the program components. It begins by tying the identified problems and concerns to specific goals and objectives addressing those concerns. Objectives should be stated in behavioral, measurable terms to facilitate evaluation. The program components should be organized into a progressive entity consisting of strategies, interventions, and activities.

2. The actual *implementation* of program components may include acquiring funding for staff selection and training, and procuring facilities and materials. It also may require recruiting and attracting the target group (students or consumers). Frequently the health educator must train other health professionals and volunteers for duties associated with the program.

3. *Delivery of services* may consist of selecting and conducting learning activities, counseling, consulting, and community organizing. In this context counseling means helping people learn how to achieve. Although this is not by definition a part of health education, health educators often are called upon to help people attain personal growth, resolve their problems, and improve their interpersonal relationships. As consultants, health educators serve in an advisory capacity or as resource persons. They also may prepare resource materials for programs. Health educators sometimes serve as community organizers, helping groups of individuals to help themselves or to use the resources available to them.

4. *Program administration* may be the health educator's province as well. This might entail selecting and placing personnel, preparing budgets, scheduling, and allocating resources especially in programs funded by grants. Coordinating activities and facilitating staff activities are examples of administrative duties.

5. *Evaluation* is critical to the success and continued support of any program, and certainly to health education. Carefully designed programs provide measurable outcomes for evaluation. This allows for justification of continued funding and administrative support and for program revision. Although evaluation is done most effectively by those without a vested interest in the program, the health educator frequently is called upon to provide data for use in evaluation.

WHAT HEALTH EDUCATION IS NOT

Perhaps understanding what health education is not is as important as grasping what it is. Much misunderstanding is based upon bad experiences and misconceptions. The following statements are commonly held untruths, along with explanations of the origin or perpetuation of the misconceptions and reasons for their being untrue.

Health education is hygiene education. Although hygiene education once dominated health instruction, this is no longer the case. Hygiene classes typically considered each of the body systems in terms of maintaining and protecting the body from disease and infirmity. Standard hygiene classes emphasized cleanliness, grooming, and in some cases nutrition.

Health education is physical education. Health education was first established as part of physical education in many schools. Administrators and state legislators sometimes still think of health and physical education as a single entity. Laws spoke, and in some cases still speak, of the two as if they are one. The assumption has been that because physical education is intended to promote health, physical educators are well-qualified to teach health. Although much of the professional preparation of physical educators is shifting toward the promotion of wellness, their preparation does not fully engender the skills and competencies necessary for delivering comprehensive health education. The acquisition of physical skills remains the primary thrust of physical education.

Health education is primarily concerned with disease. Health educators are concerned with promoting and maintaining health. Implicit in this concern is to establish behaviors that are conducive to health, which requires the acquisition of certain knowledge and attitudes as the basis for these healthy behaviors. In-depth knowledge of pathology and treatment of disease is appropriate for medical training but not for the elementary or secondary school classroom.

Health education is primarily a study of human anatomy and physiology. Detailed knowledge of human anatomy and physiology is not necessary for making intelligent decisions regarding health. Although some knowledge of the structure and function of the body may be helpful in understanding certain health issues, this is not the main emphasis in health education. The study of anatomy and physiology should never become a central part of the health education course of study (Bedworth and Bedworth, 1978).

Anyone can teach health. Unfortunately, administrators have assigned virtually anyone to teach health in many schools, perpetuating this misconception. The task often falls to anyone who has an incomplete teaching load. This might be the science teacher, the driver education teacher, the physical education teacher, or the coach. We know of one example of a drama teacher's being assigned the "Family Life Education" course, a unit within the health education curriculum that begs for a qualified, sensitive health educator. Just as mathematics instructors, English instructors, and science teachers have studied their own unique fields, health educators have learned their distinctive discipline. To substitute an unqualified individual for "the real thing" is an insult and disservice to our children.

Memorizing facts assures a healthy life. Memorizing facts relating to health does not guarantee healthy behavior and quality living. A qualified health educator with competencies in developing all the variables important to healthy lives is needed. Health education is not about memorizing facts.

Information alone leads to change in attitude and then to a change in behavior. In evaluating drug informational curricula, Schaps (1981), reported some changes in students' knowledge about drugs and their effects but no significant attitudinal and behavioral changes. This suggests that a number of other factors should be addressed, as the problem of drug use among young people is complex.

The same can be said for other behaviors. Knowledge is only one factor in the choice of foods, for example. Perception of self, peer influence, ability to think critically when analyzing conflicting and frequently misleading messages presented in advertisements and packaging are just a few of the factors. The decision to participate in regular exercise can be influenced by a number of factors such as perception of one's own body, reluctance to undress and shower among peers, previous experiences, and a belief that the effort will or will not have future benefits.

WHY HEALTH EDUCATION?
The Sad State of Health Affairs

At the turn of the century, a vast majority of deaths was from contagious diseases, including influenza. Widespread understanding of the germ theory, development of immunizations, improvements in sanitation and water treatment, and development of treatments such as antibiotics have greatly reduced the risk that humans will succumb to infectious disease. The leading causes of death are now heart disease, cancer, stroke, accidents, cirrhosis of the liver, and others related to lifestyle. Even the rapid spread of AIDS stems in large part from lifestyle and personal choices. The consequences of high-risk behavior such as smoking, drinking, and unprotected sexual intercourse—often initiated in adolescence—can have lasting impact. A staggering 70% of the mortality of young people can be attributed to four causes: motor vehicle crashes (35%), other unintentional injuries (15%), homicide (10%), and suicide (10%) (Lavin, Shapiro, and Weill, 1992).

We are killing ourselves with our unhealthy habits and lifestyles. Health professionals are aware of the effects of smoking, being overweight, lacking exercise, making poor nutrition choices, using psychoactive substances, and dangerous driving habits on the length of life. Perhaps more important, they also are aware of the effects of choices in these areas on the quality of life. Although many of these lifestyle choices and habits are established early in life, the overt consequences frequently are not manifested until much later. Research indicates that school health education can make a difference in health knowledge, attitudes, and behavior (Gilbert, Gold, and Dambert, 1985). This finding alone makes a good case for implementing school-based health education.

Death and illness are not the only consequences of unhealthy choices. More than 50% of young people first engage in sexual intercourse during their teenage years (Moore, 1990). Complicating the problem, teens on the average wait more than a year after they first have intercourse before they seek contraceptive providers, placing themselves at great risk for becoming pregnant or contracting sexually transmissible diseases (Bar-Cohen, Lia-Hoagberg, and Edwards, 1990). One million teenage girls—nearly one in 10—get pregnant each year (U.S. Department of Health and Human Services, 1987). Of those who get pregnant before age 16, most will become pregnant again before age 18. In 1988 unwed teens accounted for 322,406 births, or 8.2% of all births (Center for the Study of Social Policy, 1991). Few pregnant teenage girls receive early prenatal care. One of the results was an infant mortality rate in 1988 that lagged behind 18 other nations and the highest teen pregnancy rates of six industrialized nations—including France, England and Wales, Canada, the Netherlands, and Sweden (Children's Defense Fund, 1990). The lives of these young mothers are forever changed, and the unfortunate legacy to their children is immeasurable.

Accidents are the leading cause of death of young children. In addition, many injured children suffer needlessly or become permanently handicapped because of injuries that could have been prevented.

Child abuse and neglect has become a national disgrace. Every year almost 2.5 million children and adolescents are reported to suffer physical, sexual, or emotional abuse or neglect (District of Columbia Rape Crisis Center, 1990). These are only reported cases.

Violence and suicide ravage our society. The teen death rate from violence increased 12% between 1984 and 1988, to a rate of 69.7 per 100,000 teenagers aged 15-19 (Center for the Study of Social Policy, 1991). The leading cause of death in 15-19 year-old minority youth is homicide (National Commission on the Role of the School and the Community in Improving Adolescent Health, 1990). Suicide in the teen population is escalating annually. In a study of middle and high school students, 36% reported having nothing to look forward to; 34% considered suicide; and 14% attempted suicide (American School Health Association, 1989). Every year, approximately 5,000 young people take their lives— three times the rate of 20 years ago (Schubiner, 1989). Suicide is the second leading cause of death among young people ages 15-24 (U.S. Department of Health and Human Services, 1989).

The mental health status of adolescents is troubling. According to the report *Healthy People 2000* (U. S. Department of Health and Services, 1990), an estimated 7.5 million, or about 12% of our nation's children suffer from mental disorders severe enough to warrant treatment. In national surveys of middle school and high school students, 61% had feelings of depression and hopelessness and 45% admitted difficulty in coping with stressful home and school situations (American School Health Association, 1989).

The effects of substance abuse on individuals and on society range from the intolerable to the unthinkable. Approximately 4.6 million teens use alcohol (National Institute on Drug Abuse, 1988). In a National Commission on the Role of the School and the Community in Improving Adolescent Health (1990) survey, 39% of high school seniors reported they had gotten drunk within the previous two weeks. Roughly four to six elementary school-age children of 25 live in a family in which a member abuses alcohol or other drugs. Studies show these children are prone to learning disabilities, eating disorders, delinquency, truency, and teen pregnancy (School Board of Manattee County, Florida, 1988).

About 30% of adolescents smoke cigarettes regularly (Centers for Disease Control, 1989), despite the fact that virtually all know it is harmful. Most of these children tried cigarettes before age 11 (U.S. Department of Health and Human Services, 1987). About 35% of the teens surveyed have tried marijuana and about 8% have tried cocaine (Centers for Disease Control, 1989).

Obesity is a problem for at least one in five teenagers, and excess weight troubles one in four (Gans, 1990). Eating disorders harm an increasing number of young people. Over the last 20 years the incidence of anorexia nervosa has doubled (American School Health Association, 1989).

Lack of exercise in children threatens their long-term health. Half of girls ages 6 to 17 and 30% of boys in the same age range cannot run a mile in less than 10 minutes, a standard of acceptable fitness set by the President's Council on Physical Fitness (Trusell, 1988). Sedentary habits carry over into adulthood. Couch sprouts become couch potatoes who become operating table spuds.

Although we have been able to reduce mortality related to infectious diseases, one group of diseases still afflicts the population in high numbers. Sexually transmissible diseases (STDs) strike an estimated 2.5 million teenagers each year (Gans, 1990). The risk of contracting an STD is directly linked to the number of sex partners a person has. Therefore, even though they are caused by microorganisms, STDs clearly are related to lifestyle choices.

The human suffering that poor health decisions and lifestyles impose on American youth is enough in itself to justify health education in the school, community, clinics, and other settings. The economic effect of health education serves as another incentive.

Health Education and Economics

The cost per student of school health education is relatively low. Even if school health programs were to lead to a modest 10% reduction in costs associated with certain risk-taking behaviors, the cost savings would equal billions of dollars. Medical costs make up a sizable portion of the financial costs of risk-taking behavior. Indirect costs such as lost wages, lower productivity, more absenteeism, high job turnover, and disability payments account for huge expenditures. For example, employees with alcoholism cost the United States an estimated $20 billion annually in lost productivity (Green, 1990).

Seven of the 10 leading causes of death in the United States could be reduced significantly if people at risk were to address five behaviors: improper diet, smoking, lack of exercise, alcohol abuse, and use of antihypertensive medication. Health education is a good investment in addressing these behaviors. Even if health education programs resulted in a modest reduction in risk behaviors, the programs would be cost effective. The Committee for Economic Development (1987) reported that every dollar spent on immunization programs saves $10 in later medical costs; one dollar invested in quality preschool programs pays back $4.75 in terms of lower costs for special education, public assistance, and crime. This type of program planning requires decision makers with foresight. We know that the economic savings from a successful tobacco education program could reach several billion dollars annually (Lewitt, 1984), but these savings may take years to be realized.

Finally, one has only to look at industry for an economic perspective. Many large American corporations, as well as several of the most successful industrial giants in Japan, provide health promotion programs for employees; these consist of health education, fitness programs, stop smoking programs, nutrition counseling, and weight control programs. Companies have found these programs to be cost-effective. If profit-motivated corporations see the benefit of health education, it certainly follows that we should apply this sort of thinking to our schools.

Learning and Health

Health and learning have a reciprocal relationship. Children learn to make decisions about their health, and acquiring and maintaining health is related to academic success. Most authorities have recognized the relationships between health and education. As the National Health/Education Consortium (1990) concluded:

> *Education affects health.* . . . Health professionals know that education can promote good health. . . . The reverse is also true: ignorance can put even a healthy child at risk. . . . *Health affects education.* Teachers know that learning comes easier to a healthy child. . . . Any health problem can interfere with learning.

In its landmark work, *Code Blue,* the National Commission on the Role of the School and the Community in Improving Adolescent Health (1990) reinforced this idea by saying:

> Efforts to improve school performance that ignore health are ill-conceived, as are health improvement efforts that ignore education. This means that increasing academic achievement will require attending to health in the broadest sense. The Commission finds that education and health are inextricably intertwined.

The Council of Chief State School Officers (1991) determined:

> Good health is prerequisite to a good education. Effective education complements and supports the health and social services needed to overcome the conditions that put a young person at educational risk.

OBSTACLES TO HEALTH EDUCATION

Estimates concerning the number of comprehensive school health instructional programs in U. S. schools vary from 5% to 14%. A survey of state mandates for school health programs revealed that 32 states required health education at some time during K-12; 13 additional states required a combination of physical education and health education. Eleven states required a specific time requirement for health education as a separate subject at the elementary level, but only five required more than 50 hours. At the secondary level, 31 states had a time requirement but none required that health be taught as a separate subject for more than 50 hours each year (Lovato et al. 1989). Why isn't health education universally accepted? Why doesn't every school district and every school have a quality comprehensive health education program?

A number of obstacles stand in the way of successful health education programs. Although each district and even each school has its own individual characteristics, a few obstacles to health education seem to appear frequently.

1. *The already packed curriculum.* The states require specific amounts of instruction in mathematics, science, language, and social studies. Other subjects, such as home economics, demand a place in the curriculum. In addition, continual burdens are placed upon the school system to meet the special needs of certain children and to solve more and more societal problems. It all results in competition for time and resources. School board members, frequently have their own priorities, which may hinder

school efforts to provide the resources necessary to develop and implement health education. Pollock and Hamburg (1985) summed up the problem:

> The resulting competition for funds, faculty, and facilities is not likely to favor health teaching. While schools are criticized for their graduates' lack of basic skills because this keeps them from finding jobs, when those same graduates lack ability to handle stress or other health problems, few consider that these skills could have been learned, too. Their lack is just as apparent, as reflected in high rates of absenteeism, poor job performance, alcoholism, and other preventable health problems . . .

2. *The directives concerning health education.* School health programs often are planned at national and state levels and then are prescribed to local school systems for implementation. Although most directives have strong philosophical bases and are well-intentioned, these programs are not always accompanied by the resources needed to execute them. In principle, the farther removed a recommendation is, the less influence it has in motivating action. People have less fear of a new program if it is initiated and planned locally, allowing for a community base of support and participation in the planning process. Local needs provide fuel to run local programs. The makeup of existing social and economic factors, community beliefs and standards, and the salient health concerns of the community members are vital considerations. In addition, in times of financial crisis, school health programs must be coordinated with the many health professionals and agencies already established in the community (National School Board Association, 1991).

3. *Inattention of administrators.* The assumption that administrators, even school board members, are fully aware of the health problems of students is unrealistic. To expect administrators to understand the value of health education in reducing children's health problems is even more unrealistic. That kind of information never trickles down quickly enough to have much impact on local administrative decisions except

in cases of epidemic or crisis. The scant information that does come to the administrator's attention is filtered by misconceptions, assumptions, and countering arguments from various pressure groups.

4. *Lack of community support for health instruction.* A number of misconceptions and outright fallacies frequently underlie this lack of support. At other times opposition stems from unpleasant experiences in one's own health instruction. Perhaps the most dangerous opposition comes from organized groups, often instigated from outside the community. These ultraconservative organizations often distort the nature of health education, accusing the programs of destroying values developed at home, encouraging promiscuity, and undermining religious training. Even though the claims of these groups may be ludicrous, their organization and dedication make them formidable adversaries.

5. *A "Catch 22" situation.* In the absence of a health educator or health teaching specialist in the school, developing a vigorous comprehensive health education program is difficult. Even an administrator who is convinced of the need for health education has a dilemma. How to provide an effective health education program without depriving other basic curricula of funding or time is a difficult proposition.

6. *Lack of certification requirement.* Although most states mandate health instruction, many do not require certification in health education. This leads to health instruction by those who are unqualified to do so, typically physical education teachers or coaches who may not be motivated or properly skilled to deliver health instruction well. In other situations teachers can teach one period per day outside of their own discipline. Unfortunately, this period often is health education. Even if the teacher is committed to the task, he or she lacks the training to carry it out. The students are short-changed; the taxpayers are cheated; the reputation of health education is tarnished. When these situations prevail, justification for health education becomes even more difficult. School board

members who were subjected to programs such as this are not likely to respect health education.

7. *Perception of health education as a frill.* As a goal, health is elusive. As a subject in school, it is complex. Traditional tests of knowledge, even those that test application, do not lend themselves to demonstrating the effectiveness of health education. The success of health education depends on what people do, or sometimes what they do not do, in the days, weeks, and years ahead. It can be demonstrated only after years of behavior. Answers on a test do not fully reveal the benefits to the student. Parents, teachers, students, and principals are not comfortable with this ambiguity. Because it cannot be instantly measured and evaluated, some people reason, it must not be important; it must be a frill.

SUMMARY

Health education is a unique discipline that embodies the process of assisting individuals to change undesirable behavior or to continue behavior that is conducive to health. By gaining knowledge and acquiring attitudes that make health a high priority, behavior congruent with a lifestyle leading to a high level of health and wellness is established.

Health education occurs in a variety of settings and targets individuals in various stages of their lives. It addresses several content areas. Health education requires competence in planning, program implementation, delivery of services, administration, and evaluation. It may include counseling, teaching, consulting, and other responsibilities.

Although the United States is the richest nation in the world, we are staggering beneath the weight of our health problems—the very problems addressed by well-designed and adequately staffed health education programs. Comprehensive health education programs have the potential to reduce our nation's health problems and associated human and economic costs. Although misunderstanding of health education abounds and many obstacles arise in opposition, the discipline is gaining in respect and acceptance.

Despite formidable barriers, many states have legislation mandating health instruction in schools. Public concern for health problems related to alcohol, teenage suicide, eating disorders, teen pregnancies, and others has lifted health education into the curricula of many school districts. The Surgeon General's report (U. S. Department of Health and Human Services, 1979) emphasized the critical need for a public health revolution based on health promotion and disease prevention. Worksite health education is now a common practice. Medical patient education is a legal requirement. Public health and voluntary health organizations are heavily involved in health education. The process has begun; it must be continued and improved upon for the good of our nation and its children.

REFERENCES

American School Health Association, Association for the Advancement of Health Education, and Society for Public Health Education. *The National Adolescent Student Health Survey Report on the Health of America's Youth.* Oakland, CA: Third Party Publishing, 1989.

Bar-Cohen, A., B. Lia-Hoagberg, and L. Edwards. First family planning visit in school-based clinics. *Journal of School Health, 60* (October, 1990): 419-422.

Bates, I. J. and A. E. Winder. *Introduction to Health Education.* Palo Alto, CA: Mayfield Publishing, 1984.

Bedworth, D. A. and A. E. Bedworth. *Health Education: A Process for Human Effectiveness.* New York: Harper and Row, 1978.

Bedworth, D. A. and A. E. Bedworth. *The Profession and Practice of Health Education.* Dubuque, IA: Wm C. Brown, Publishers, 1992.

Bureau of Health Planning and Resources Development. *Educating the Public About Health: A Planning Guide* (DHEW Pub. No. 78-14004). Washington, DC: DHEW, 1973.

Carlyon, W., and D. Cook. Science education and health instruction. *BSCS, 4,* 1981.

Center for the Study of Social Policy and Annie E. Casey Foundation. *Kids Count Data Book.* Washington, DC: Center, 1991.

Centers for Disease Control. Results from the national adolescent health survey. *Morbidity and Mortality Weekly Report, 38* (1989): 147-150.

Children's Defense Fund. *Children 1990: A Report Card, Briefing Book, and Primer.* Washington, DC: Children's Defense Fund, 1990.

Cleary H. Health Education, state-of-the-art, parameters of the profession. Proceedings of the Workshop on Commonalities and Differences in the Preparation and Practice of Health Education. Bethesda, MD, 1978.

Commission on the Reorganization of Education. *Cardinal Principles of Secondary Education.* (Department of Interior, Bureau of Education, Bulletin no. 35, 1918). Washington DC: U. S. Printing Office, 1928.

Committee for Economic Development, Research and Policy Committee. *Children in Need: Investment Strategies for the Educationally Disadvantaged.* New York: CED, 1987.

Council of Chief State School Officers. *Beyond the Health Room.* Washington, DC: U.S. Government Printing Office, 1991.

District of Columbia Rape Crisis Center. *Fact Sheet: Child Sexual Abuse.* Washington, DC: D.C. Rape Crisis Center, 1990.

Gans, J. E. *America's Adolescents: How Healthy Are They?* Chicago: American Medical Association, 1990.

Gilbert, G. G., R. S. Gold, and C. L. Dambert. Why school health education? The federal point of view. *Health Education, 16* (April/May, 1985): 125-127.

Green, L. W. *Community Health* (6th ed). St. Louis: C. V. Mosby, 1990.

Green, L. W., M. W. Kreuter, S. G. Deeds, and K. B. Partridge. *Health Education Planning: A Diagnostic Approach.* Palo Alto, CA: Mayfield Publishing, 1980.

Greene, W. H. and B. G. Simons-Morton. *Introduction to Health Education.* Prospect Heights, IL: Waveland Press, 1984.

Henderson, A. C. and D. V. McIntosh. *Role Refinement and Verification for Entry-Level Health Educators: Final Report.* San Francisco: National Center for Health Education, 1981.

Joint Committee on Health Education Terminology. *Health Education Monographs,* 33 (1973): 63-70.

Joint Committee on Health Problems in Education of the National Education Association and the American Medical Association, *Health Education.* Washington, DC: National Education Association, 1948.

Lavin, A. T., G. R. Shapiro, and K. S. Weill. *Creating an Agenda for School-Based Health Promotion: A Review of Selected Reports.* Boston: Harvard School of Public Health, 1992.

Lewitt, E. Costs to American economy for cigarette-induced major illnesses: 1964-1983. *Smoking and Health, 1* (1984).

Lovato, C., D. Allensworth, and M. Chan. *School Health in America* (5th ed.). Kent, OH: American School Health Association, 1989.

Moore, K. *Facts at a Glance.* Washington, DC: Child Trends, 1990.

National Commission on the Role of the School and the Community in Improving Adolescent Health. *Code Blue: Uniting for Healthier Youth.* Alexandria, VA: National Association of State Boards of Education; Chicago: American Medical Association, 1990.

National Health/Education Consortium. *Crossing the Boundaries Between Health and Education.* Washington, DC: National Commission to Prevent Infant Mortality, 1990.

National Institute on Drug Abuse. National household survey on drug abuse: Population estimates. Washington, DC: NIDA, 1988.

National School Board Association. *School Health: Helping Children Learn.* Alexandria, VA: National School Board Association, 1991.

1990 Joint Committee on Health Education Terminology. Report of the 1990 Joint Committee on Health Education Terminology. *Journal of School Health, 61* (August, 1991): 251-254.

Nixon, J. E. The criteria of a discipline. *Quest, 9* (Winter, 1967): 42-48. (Monograph)

Oberteuffer, D., O. A. Harrelson, and M. B. Pollock. *School Health Education* (5th ed.). New York: Harper and Row, 1972.

Pollock, M. B. and M. V. Hamburg. Health education: The basic of the basics. *Health Education, 16* (April/May, 1985): 105-109.

Pollock, M. B. and K. Middleton. *Elementary School Health Instruction* (2d ed.). St. Louis: Times Mirror/ Mosby, 1989.

Schaps, E. A review of 127 drug abuse prevention program evaluations. *Journal of Drug Issues, 11* (Winter, 1981): 17-43.

School Board of Manattee County. *Curriculum Guide for Children with Chemically Dependent Family Systems.* Bradenton, FL: 1988.

Schubiner, H. Preventive health screenings in adolescent patients. *Primary Care, 16* (January, 1989): 211-230.

Trussell, J. Teenage pregnancy in the U.S. *Family Planning Perspectives, 20* (November/December, 1988).

U. S. Department of Health and Human Services. *Objectives for the Nation.* Washington, DC: U.S. Government Printing Office, 1979.

U. S. Department of Health and Human Services, Public Health Service, National Institutes of Health. *School-Based Opportunities for Tobacco Use Interventions.* Washington, DC: U.S. Government Printing Office, 1987.

U. S. Department of Health and Human Services. *AIDS Prevention Guide: For Parents and Other Adults Concerned About Youth.* Atlanta: Public Health Service, Centers for Disease Control.

U. S. Department of Health and Human Services. *Healthy People 2000: National Health Promotion and Disease Prevention Objectives.* Washington, DC: U. S. Government Printing Office, 1990.

Wilner, D. M., R. P. Walker, and L. S. Goerke. *Introduction to Public Health* (6th ed.). New York: Macmillan, 1973.

Wilson, C. C., Editor. *School Health Services.* Washington, DC: National Education Association, 1971.

3

HISTORY OF
HEALTH EDUCATION

The history of health education naturally follows, to some extent, the history of health and efforts to promote it. The words and works of the great prophets, philosophers, scientists, teachers, and thinkers of the world who glorified the mind, body, and their oneness have contributed mightily to the status of health education of today. Though we are concerned particularly with the history of health education in the United States, events in other countries and on other continents have greatly affected the development of health practices and health education in the United States. To appreciate the development of the discipline, we view it in this chapter from an historical perspective of health in general, as well as the times at which events occurred. Means (1962, 1975) is a good source for detailed narrative on the development of health education up until 1975.

ANCIENT SOCIETIES

Almost every society has had some organized set of practices regarding health and social issues. The earliest of these practices to be recorded was the Code of Hammurabi. The great king of Babylon contrived and left a set of laws that had wide implications for understanding the value placed on health at the time, around 1900 B.C. Embodied in the Code is a code of conduct for physicians as well as regulations concerning marriage, social relations, and other important issues of the period. Although the Babylonians had no idea of the "germ theory," the code illustrates that they did take steps to prevent the spread of disease.

Ancient writings, records, and cave drawings provide some insight into the health practices and regulations of primitive times. Archeologic evidence reveals that the Minoans of 3000–1430 B.C. and the Myceneans of 1430–1150 B.C. built drainage systems, toilets, and water-flushing systems.

The Egyptians, circa 1000 B.C., are considered today to be among the healthiest of ancient societies. The records of Herodotus described many customs indicating the importance the Egyptians placed on health. They practiced cleanliness by taking frequent baths. They had toilets and constructed public drainage pipes. The ancient Egyptians had the first written records of community health planning aimed at preventing public health problems by way of irrigation canals and granaries for proper storage of foods (Benson and McDevitt, 1980). They also practiced medicine, using many pharmaceutical products. The Egyptians generally are given credit for inventing beer. One of the oldest temperance tracts, advocating moderation, was written in Egypt in 1000 B.C., tolerating alcohol but denouncing excessive drinking and drunkenness (Green, 1990).

The Hebrews' Mosaic law was an extension of Egyptian hygienic practices. It is considered the first formal hygienic code. Included in the Mosaic law were regulations applicable to personal and community responsibilities, including cleanliness, protections against the spread of infectious diseases, disinfection of dwellings following illness, sanitation of campsites, disposal of excreta and garbage, protection of the food and water supply, and isolation of people with leprosy. The segregation of lepers, as recorded in the book of Leviticus, was an early community practice of preventive medicine.

The roots of Eastern mysticism began in India with Hinduism. The ancient Hindus saw the body and spirit as inseparable. They practiced meditation and relaxation as means to promote health in the total person. This is particularly compelling in light of the modern interest in holistic health and the emphasis on meditation and relaxation to reduce stress.

The Greek era in history stretched over several centuries, although the Classic period of Greek history is considered to be from 460 B.C. to 136 B.C. The Greeks advocated the same primary constituents of health as we recognize today, including the emphasis on the individual. This was evidenced through the teaching of Socrates, Plato, Aristotle, Plutarch, and Hippocrates, the father of medicine. Hippocrates stressed the natural causes of disease as well as the role of environment in the spread of disease. Hippocrates understood the roles of climate, soil, water, way of life, and nutrition as aspects of disease prevention. He stated that only when one's mind and body are in harmony can a state of health exist (Ellis and Hartley, 1984). Galen, the successor to Hippocrates, wrote a manuscript on hygiene that was in use for more than 1000 years. It taught that exercise, especially in the forms of games and gymnastics, developed strength, endurance, coordination, and grace.

Personal cleanliness, disease control, and diet also were important to the Greeks. The emphasis on individual well-being among the Athenians applied only to the minority of nobles. The infirm and ill often were ignored and sometimes even killed. Environmental sanitation was of much lesser concern than individual health during the Classic period.

With the decline of the Greek society and the rise of the Roman Empire, the Romans adopted Greek ideas about health and health practices. The primary difference between the Greek and Roman philosophies of health was that instead of featuring individual health, the Romans were more concerned with the general health of the population. The Romans believed the individual existed only to serve the State. The influence of Greek hygiene soon diminished. Community health, including administrative and engineering measures, was an important part of Roman civilization. Examples are regulation of sewage disposal, drainage networks, houses of prostitution, public baths, and building construction to ensure adequate ventilation and heating. The Romans provided for water protection and transported water great distances through a series of aqueducts, some of which are still in use. Many ancient-Roman paved and guttered streets are still in service.

THE MIDDLE AGES

The decay of the Roman Empire led to its ultimate overthrow. The decadence of the time led to the period known as the Middle Ages. During the period A.D. 476–1000, the period commonly referred to as the Dark Ages, an attitude developed that should be considered totally illogical today. Disease was considered to be punishment for sin. In a cruel irony, for some diseases, such as acquired immune deficiency syndrome (AIDS), some people still harbor this medieval idea. Because of this notion, interest in and knowledge of physical health were generally lacking, especially in Europe. The self was devalued. Only the spiritual dimension of the person was recognized.

Regulation, strict discipline, and spirituality were so pervasive that observing one's own nude body was considered immoral. As a result, bathing was infrequent. In fact, the more the people neglected and even abused their bodies, the more social acceptance they gained. Refuse and body wastes accumulated around dwellings. Filth and misery were the norm. No attention was paid to ways of preventing suffering and illness.

Other parts of the world also suffered from widespread lack of health. During the sixth and seventh centuries, followers of Mohammed established and strengthened their religious faith. Islam attracted followers from Africa, the Near East, Asia, and the Iberian peninsula. After the death of Mohammed, pilgrimages to Mecca, in present-day Saudi Arabia, began. Each pilgrimage, or hajj, delivered a cholera epidemic to the homeland (Pickett and Hanlon, 1990). This was not to be the last time that travel for religious purposes would lead to disaster.

Leprosy, perhaps the most dreaded disease of the time, spread from Egypt to Asia Minor to Europe. Lepers were deprived of civil rights, forced to wear clothing to identify themselves as lepers and carry a horn or bell to warn others of their approach. Although we may consider these measures inhumane, they contributed to the virtual elimination of leprosy in Europe.

The later medieval period, from about A.D. 1000 to about 1453, was one of epidemics and pandemics. An epidemic currently is defined as an occurrence of a disease in numbers above those that normally would be expected. Pandemics are widespread epidemics, frequently affecting more than one nation. With the Age of Chivalry came new emphasis on health. Training for knighthood took precedence over religious training and led to the need to be physically strong and well for battle. Unfortunately, the general population did not reap the benefits of this change. The health and well-being of only one small segment of the population—those who would do battle—was considered important. Six great crusades to the Holy Land took place between 1096 and 1248. The crusaders who left their homes in such excellent health frequently were killed not by battle but by cholera. In fact, the disease was brought to Europe, where it killed huge numbers of people.

In 1348, bubonic plague, dubbed the Black Death, cut a path from Asia to Africa, Turkey, Greece, Italy, and north through Europe. During the 1340s, more than 13 million people died from bubonic plague in China alone. India was almost depopulated. At its worst, the city of Cairo, Egypt, lost 10,000 to 15,000 people each day. Cyprus was depopulated, and ships drifted in the Mediterranean and in the North Sea, all crew members dead. From 1348 to 1350, 20% of the population of Europe died from bubonic plague or pulmonary anthrax or a combination of the two. In England, two million people died, approximately half of the population of the country. The total mortality from the Black Death is estimated to be more than 60 million, with 25 million deaths in Europe. As many as 200,000 small towns and villages in Europe may have lost all of their inhabitants (Hecker, 1839).

Recognizing that spread of the disease might be related to overcrowding, poor sanitation, and migration, the community of Ragusa, present day Dubrovnik, in 1377 decreed that travelers from plague-infested areas must stop at designated places and remain there two months before entering the city. In 1383, Marseille, France, enduring 16,000 deaths in one month from the Black Death, passed the first quarantine law and constructed the first quarantine station.

THE RENAISSANCE

The Renaissance, from A.D. 1453 to 1600, marked a change in thinking. Doubt that disease was punishment for sin slowly crept into the beliefs of the time. Thinkers of the day became concerned with life and all of its manifestations, a philosophy called humanism. They ushered in the rise of nationalism; interest in the arts, literature, and philosophy; education for health; and realism. Individual scientific interest, shunned and persecuted during the Middle Ages, heralded a spirit of inquiry that eventually would lead to the understanding of infectious diseases.

Contributing greatly to the interest in health was the invention of the printing press in 1438, which allowed for wide consumption of information on health and science. Vittorino Da Feltre, Guarino Da Verona, Hieronymus Mercuialis, Sir Thomas Elyot, and Francis Bacon all wrote about health and healthful living. John Comenius recommended proper exercise, adequate sleep, nutrition, and other health habits. His school of realism laid the foundation for many educational practices still in use. The English poet John Milton wrote that youth "should divide their day's work into three parts as it lies orderly; their Studies, their Exercises, and their Diet" (Rice, Hutchinson, and Lee, 1958). John Locke expressed concern in his writings for nutrition, sleep, and exercise.

By the middle of the 16th century, influenza, smallpox, tuberculosis, bubonic plague, leprosy, anthrax, and impetigo were identified as different diseases with different causes. Diphtheria and scarlet fever were recognized as being different from all other diseases. Fracastoro became aware that syphilis was transmitted by way of sexual relations and theorized in 1546 that microorganisms caused disease. This was an astounding theory in light of the fact that the microscope had not yet been invented.

Even with all the progress in the identification of the causes of disease, health care workers held no prestige. From the sixteenth through the nineteenth centuries, those caring for the sick were drawn from the social outcasts of society because of the low status delegated to this work (Benson and McDevitt, 1980).

EUROPE AND THE COLONIES IN THE 1600s AND 1700s

Just as war and religious pilgrimages had profound effects on health during ancient and medieval times, overcrowding affected the well-being of millions in the 1600s and 1700s. In Europe the development of industry and nationalism invited heavy population concentrations in the cities. This led to fresh attacks of diseases. Between 1600 and 1665, Europeans suffered through three severe pandemics of bubonic plague. The populations of many cities were decimated.

To compound the health problems of the times, apprentice slavery was legally condoned in England, allowing exploitation of pauper children. These children, with no defense from the government, were indentured to owners of mines and factories. The most vulnerable and precious resource of any society, its children, were treated as chattel, making their lives often miserable and usually unfit. Even the churches set up parish workhouses that were concerned largely with instilling the ideals of obedience, labor, and religion.

A number of significant beneficial events were taking place in Europe. Thomas Sydenham, an Englishman generally regarded as the first distinguished epidemiologist, made a differential diagnosis of scarlet fever, malaria, dysentery, and cholera in 1658, establishing these diseases as separate and distinct. Athanasius Kircher instituted a new method of the study of disease by examining the blood of plague victims with a primitive microscope. Anton van Leeuvenhoek, a Dutch janitor given credit for discovering the microscope, first observed bacteria and found in 1676 that they could be killed by vinegar. British physician Edward Jenner demonstrated in 1796 the effectiveness of smallpox vaccine. These developments were significant in the eventual treatment and prevention of life-threatening diseases.

Meanwhile, in North America health information was passed on from generation to generation among the Native American tribes. Group concern for health was evidenced in the selection and preparation of food, recognition of the need for pure water, and burial of the dead. Most tribes had regulations relating to family responsibilities. Europeans considered the practice of Native American "medicine" primitive because it frequently was based upon religion and what the explorers considered to be superstition. Nonetheless, European explorers found a generally healthy population in North America. With the white European settlers, however, came disease and epidemics. Native Americans possessed none of the immunity that comes from generations of exposure to microorganisms, and they were unprepared to take protective measures. To compound the problem, the settlers had little interest in the health of the people with whom they came in contact in the New World. By the time the Pilgrims landed at Plymouth, the Native Americans of the surrounding countryside had been all but eliminated, apparently by smallpox introduced by the Cabot and Gosnold expeditions. Similar effects were found in Central America and the Caribbean. The pattern of travel and conquest as a means of spreading disease continued.

The early colonists in North America found life frought with many hardships. They faced the necessity of clearing land and building homes, securing food and transportation, as well as problems brought by the weather and the people they referred to as Indians. Many starved, died violent deaths, or expired from infectious diseases, which often were of epidemic proportions. In fact, many of the early settlements were eliminated completely by diseases, most notably smallpox.

Community health action in the colonies was taken only during epidemics and consisted of isolation and quarantine. Smallpox was a deadly enemy, producing several pandemics, conspicuously those in the Massachusetts Bay colonies in 1633, New Netherlands (New York) in 1663, and Boston in 1752. During the Boston attack, only 174 of the city's 15,000 residents completely escaped smallpox. During the life of George Washington, 90% of the people age 21 and older had had smallpox. Epidemics brought by the colonists came close to eliminating the threat posed by Native Americans as disease spread through the tribes.

Measures to protect community health were feeble and mostly ineffective. As a way of keeping track of the population, causes of death, and maintaining property rights, the Massachusetts colony passed an act in 1639 requiring that each birth and death be recorded. The Plymouth colony followed suit. In 1701 Massachusetts passed legislation providing for the isolation of smallpox victims and for ship quarantine. In 1746 the Massachusetts Bay colonies passed regulations to prevent the pollution of Boston Harbor. Local boards of health were established in several cities in the late 1790s. Some of these, most notably those in New York and Massachusetts in 1797, came as a result of yellow fever. It had become a worse pestilence than smallpox during the 18th century and would continue during the 19th century. At one time, Philadelphia, the capital of the nation, was virtually abandoned because of yellow fever.

THE 1800s

During the 19th century, the brutality of the French Revolution helped to spawn the eventual seeds of humanitarianism and innovation. Ideals changed tremendously to more modern educational, social, and political thought. Although the 19th century was the Age of Enlightenment, epidemics continued in Europe, fed by the filth and overcrowding of the cities. The incidence of smallpox, cholera, typhoid, tuberculosis, and other diseases was extremely high.

The 1800s saw physicians still practicing the medicine of the ancient Greeks by starving, bleeding, and purging their patients. Surgery was conducted without anesthesia. Often physicians went from one surgery to another without washing their hands. Only a few effective drugs were available, among them digitalis for heart failure and quinine for malaria. The 19th century, however, brought major advances in medicine and health, sometimes from unexpected sources. In 1815, during the Napoleonic wars, Delpech was able to observe the patterns of development of gangrene in injured men. He theorized that "animal-like matter jumps from one object to another." Fifty years passed before this observation was put to preventive use, but it marked a major stage in the comprehension of disease and gangrene.

Legislation relating to community sanitation was passed in England in 1837. With that legislation, public health was recognized officially for the first time. Soon thereafter, the Factory Commission was appointed to study the health conditions of the laboring population of the nation. Child employment conditions were of particular interest to the commission. Edwin Chadwick was made secretary of the commission. In 1842, the "Report on the Inquiry into the Sanitary Condition of the Laboring Population of Great Britain" was published. The report pointed out that half of the children of the working classes died before age 5. Chadwick's distinctive descriptions of the wretched conditions of the working class kindled a resolve in compassionate people to address the problems of the laboring class and their children. The Factory Commission's report led to establishment of the board of health in 1848, and John Simon was appointed the first medical health officer of London. Although the board of health lasted only four years, Chadwick's report remains a milestone in public health history.

In 1867 Joseph Lister described antisepsis, the process that prevents transmission of disease through routine medical procedures as well as everyday tasks such as food preparation. In the 1870s Louis Pasteur discovered how microorganisms reproduce. He also developed the first scientific approach to immunization. It is a matter of monumental frustration that 120 years later, children are crippled and killed because they are not adequately immunized. Also in the 1870s, Rudolf Virchow, a German physician, developed the science of pathology, which led to an understanding of disease processes. Although we have yet to completely take advantage of these discoveries, they have contributed greatly to society's ability to prevent and treat disease.

Between 1800 and 1850, the United States was swept by epidemics of smallpox, typhus, yellow fever, cholera, and typhoid. Tuberculosis also took thousands of lives. Shattuck (1850/1948) reported that the average age at death in Boston decreased from 27.85 years in 1820–1825 to 21.43 in 1840–1845. In New York, the average age at death decreased from 26.15 to 19.69 during the same period. Medical problems were met by physicians with poor training and sometimes questionable motives. Superstition, misconception, and reliance on the supernatural ruled much of the treatment of disease.

Community health promotion in the United States saw its first significant development in the mid-19th century. This event, publication of the *Report of the Sanitary Commission of Massachusetts* (Shattuck, 1850/1948) served as a guide in the health field for a century. Although technically a layperson, Shattuck was intelligent and highly interested in sanitation. Some of the recommendations of the Shattuck report were to:

◆ establish state and local boards of health;

◆ collect and analyze vital statistics;

◆ exchange health information;

◆ initiate sanitation programs for towns and buildings;

◆ maintain a system of sanitary inspections;

◆ study the health of school children;

◆ research tuberculosis;

◆ study and supervise the health conditions of immigrants;

◆ supervise mental disease;

◆ control alcoholism;

◆ control food adulteration;

◆ control exposure to nostrums;

◆ control smoke nuisances;

◆ construct model tenements;

◆ construct standard public bathing and wash houses;

◆ preach health from the pulpit;

◆ teach the science of sanitation in medical schools;

◆ introduce prevention as a phase of all medical practice;

◆ sponsor routine health examinations.

Shattuck's report even had direct implications for health education in the statement:

> Every child should be taught early in life, that, to preserve his own life and his own health and the lives and health of others, is one of the most important and constantly abiding duties: . . . Everything connected with wealth, happiness and long life depend on health.

THE MODERN ERA OF HEALTH

Shattuck's report signaled the beginning of the modern era of health. Society began to attack health problems in a disciplined way, even though this attack at first was based upon untrue assumptions. The modern era of health can be divided into five phases: the miasma phase (1850–1880), the bacteriology phase (1880–1910), the health resources phase (1920–1960), the social engineering phase (1960–1975), and the health promotion phase (late 1970s until the present).

Miasma Phase (1850–1880)

During the miasma phase, disease was thought to be caused by noxious vapors. This is understandable when considering the smells that must have been present in the streets and surrounding the sick. An early, extreme example of this thinking was the conclusion that people who ventured about at dusk were doomed to contract malaria because of the bad air present at dusk. Disease control efforts were directed entirely toward general cleanliness. Communities began to institute street cleaning and garbage and refuse disposal. Despite this misconception as to the real cause of disease, quarantine, especially at ports, was being practiced more frequently.

In an effort to reduce the outbreaks of yellow fever introduced through the port of New Orleans, the state of Louisiana established a commission to deal with quarantine issues. Though this often is referred to as the first state board of health, it did not function in terms of the usual concept of a state board of health. The first true state health department or board of health was established in 1869 in Massachusetts, with Dr. Henry I. Bowdich as the first head. The board concerned itself with public and professional education in hygiene, various aspects of housing investigation and prevention of various diseases, methods of slaughtering, sale of poisons, and conditions of the poor.

Florence Nightingale, a true pioneer in health care and health promotion, was the first nurse to define the laws of nursing and the concept of nursing as a profession. She was well known for her hospital reform during the Crimean War (1854–1856) and for advocacy regarding nursing education for hospital nurses. She established a school at St. Thomas Hospital, which had quite high standards for the time. Nightingale also is known as a social reformer and as an initiator of public health nursing (Monteiro, 1985). In her book *Notes on Nursing*, Nightingale (1959/1946) established the concept that nursing the well was even more important than nursing the sick and that preventive hygiene superseded curative care.

The American Public Health Association was founded in 1872. The association, still a leader today in the arena of public health, proposed to go far beyond the quarantine mentality of the day. It projected the interests of hospital hygiene, sanitation, prevention of disease transmission, and other concerns of the public.

Bacteriology Phase (1880–1910)

Bacteriologists such as Louis Pasteur and Robert Koch demonstrated that specific microorganisms cause specific diseases, ushering in the bacteriology phase. This knowledge made it possible to use more specific means to prevent the transmission of disease. These means included protection of water, milk, and food supplies; inoculations; sewage disposal; and insect control. Significant discoveries of the period include:

◆ The development of inoculation against rabies;

◆ Discovery of the tubercle bacillus and streptococcus;

◆ Demonstration that the cholera vibrio was transmitted by water and food;

◆ Establishment of the relationship of the *Anopheles* mosquito to malaria and the *Aedes aegypti* mosquito to yellow fever;

◆ Practical use of phenol as an antiseptic;

◆ Passage of the Pure Food and Drug Act.

Even given these momentous discoveries, old methodologies, such as isolation, quarantine, and placarding, were still the rule of disease prevention, and health education as we know it was virtually nonexistent.

Health Resources Phase (1910–1960)

World War I provided the first large-scale measure of the health status of Americans. The induction examination of men into the armed forces produced dismal results. Approximately 34% of the men examined were rejected because of physical or mental disabilities. This finding led to a change of course in public health in the United States. The results of the pre-induction physical exams clearly demonstrated that health problems other than infectious diseases were now the enemy. This introduced Americans to the fact that chronic diseases such as heart disease, cancer, and cirrhosis were the major enemies in the battle for well-being. Many of these health problems could have been prevented and many of these disabilities could have been corrected.

Preventing and controlling communicable diseases clearly was not enough. Providing for its citizens the highest level of the health resources the nation could muster was to be the new direction. Health departments began to direct programs toward personal health services such as those for mothers, infants, and children. Most important, the seeds of the idea of individual behavior and responsibility were planted in the American consciousness.

Medically, tremendous advances took place during this period. For example, insulin treatment of diabetes mellitus was demonstrated in 1922, penicillin was discovered in 1928, the Pap smear for cervical cancer detection was developed in 1941, successful field testing of the Salk poliomyelitis vaccine was completed in 1952, and the Sabin poliomyelitis vaccine was field-tested in 1956. The discovery of DNA's double helix began an even more exciting page in our attack on disease. By finding the stuff genes are made of and cracking the code used to convey its instructions, we opened the door to understanding the diseases that come from the genes inside our own cells.

World War II produced fantastic changes in society and health care. New drug treatments and improved medical technology led to better care of soldiers on the battlefield. New life support systems, prosthetic devices, and other advances had enormous impact on the management of chronic medical conditions. Scientific inquiry and development literally exploded with new therapies, surgical techniques, and medical discoveries.

The largest investment during this phase was in hospitals, health manpower, and biomedical research. In 1946 the Hill-Burton Act passed the U. S. Congress, providing for huge expenditures to construct facilities for medical care. Medical, nursing, and dental schools increased in number and quality. The National Institutes of Health was established, creating a central research unit in government for developing methods, drugs, diagnostic tests, and preventive vaccines. Voluntary health agencies became more involved in health promotion, particularly through health education.

A milestone in international health occurred in 1948 with the founding of the World Health Organization. The WHO has been a world leader in providing health services to the disadvantaged of the world and in stimulating and conducting medical research.

Social Engineering Phase (1960–1975)

With the obvious realization that health advances brought about by technology and resources were not distributed evenly throughout the population, provision of equal access to health services was given priority in legislation and policy in the social engineering phase. Economically, educationally, and socially disadvantaged people frequently missed the benefits of community health programs. "Outreach"

programs designed to deliver services to the doorstep of those in need became the mainstay of local health departments.

By this time, the insurance industry was an integral part of the health care delivery system. Those who could afford insurance usually received medical care. Often, those who could not afford it went without or received inadequate medical care. Much legislation was passed that was designed to funnel federal monies through state and county agencies to provide medical and social services to those previously deprived of these services. This was characterized by the "New Frontier" legislation of the Kennedy administration and the "War on Poverty" legislation of the Johnson administration. Perhaps the most significant legislation in the history of providing medical care was Medicare and Medicaid, passed in 1965. The two groups most likely to be without health insurance, the elderly and the poor, were to be covered by Medicare and Medicaid. As a result of these progressive laws, much of the gap in the utilization of medical services that had existed between high-income and low-income people had been closed by the end of the 1960s. Of course, the differences in death and disease rates between rich and poor, white and black, urban and rural populations lingered.

At the outset of the 1970s, a different issue unfolded. The search for ways to contain costs of medical care became critical. The late 1960s and early 1970s saw a round of health planning acts, peer review requirements for quality control, and new forms of medical care delivery. The health maintenance organization (HMO), pushed by the Health Maintenance Organization Assistance Act of 1973, was the most noticeable new form of medical care delivery. The attention to fine-tuning the medical care system resulted in neglect of the health care system. State and local health departments lost much of their financial and political base.

The social engineering phase is differentiated from other phases by characteristics such as the large expenditures of federal and state money for health care and the design of a "system" of health care built around federal and state financing (Medicare and Medicaid), regional planning, sophisticated delivery of services, and improved quality control. Virtually ignored in the legislative scheme was prevention. Health education and preventive behaviors were far down the list of federal priorities. Rather than build fences to stop people from falling off the cliff, the federal government chose to build hospitals at the bottom of the hill. Partially as a result of this line of thinking, health care costs have continued to exceed the rate of inflation for years and have become an ever larger percentage of the gross national product.

Health Promotion Phase (1974–present)

Statistics available from 1960–1978 indicate that of the $192 billion our nation spent on health care, only $1 billion was spent on wellness efforts (Cunningham, 1982). Rather than viewing this as negative, it really represented a fairly good start when put in perspective. Almost simultaneously with the passage of legislation regarding health planning and health care delivery, renewed interest in disease prevention and health promotion arose in Great Britain, Canada, and the United States. In 1974, the Lalonde report brought renewed attention to health issues in Canada. The landmark document *Healthy People* (U. S. Department of Health, Education, and Welfare, 1979), followed a year later by publication of *Objectives for the Nation* for 1990 (U. S. Department of Health and Human Services, 1980), were indications that some in federal government recognized the importance of preventive behavior. Subsequent publication of *Healthy People 2000* (U. S. Department of Health and Human Services, 1991) set the stage for health promotion work in the 1990s.

During the late 1970s, a new epidemic struck that appeared to kill all of its victims. Acquired immune deficiency syndrome (AIDS) was first reported in the news as a disease concentrated in homosexual males. By the early 1980s, medical people understood that AIDS was caused by the human immunodeficiency virus (HIV), which was transmitted by exchange of body fluids. When some AIDS cases were discovered to have been contracted through blood transfusions, steps were taken quickly to increase the security of the blood supply. The general population in the United States was slow to accept the danger of contracting AIDS through heterosexual relations, and fear and prejudice toward homosexuals grew. Many Americans failed to appreciate that in many parts of Africa, AIDS was decimating a large portion of the heterosexual population. By the mid–1980s, the facts were clear: HIV is transmitted by sexual relations with someone who harbors the virus, by using needles used previously by someone carrying the virus, and by receiving the blood of someone who has the virus, either through a transfusion or through a break in the skin. In short, the method of HIV transmission is through exchange of body fluids.

Massive education campaigns were implemented in every phase of society, from within the homosexual community to the public schools to television. These campaigns are based largely upon the concept that preventive behavior can reduce the risk of acquiring HIV. Some conservatives have opposed public school education efforts directed toward AIDS prevention because of the values often perceived in the process and the frankness necessary for successful communication. At this time AIDS has no cure or immunization, and it still is considered universally fatal.

Finally, the discovery of DNA and the exploration of individual genes during the health promotion phase has allowed medical science to study the causes of inherited disorders and genetic anomalies that make up a large portion of the unconquered maladies of humanity. This relatively new branch of science opens up the possibility that diseases such as cancer, AIDS, malaria, schizophrenia, and Alzheimer's will at last be subdued.

It is easy to interpret the present as a transition to another phase of the modern era of health. The Clinton administration has promised serious changes in the health care delivery system. Talk of "managed care" and "socialized medicine" are commonplace. It will take time to evaluate the impact of any changes on costs, services, quality of life, and research.

It is important that politicians, citizens, and health care professionals maintain the positive momentum of the health promotion movement. We should see the health care delivery system as a partner in the maintenance and improvement of the health of individuals. Health education should also be considered an integral member of the partnership to promote the well being of our citizens.

HISTORICAL OVERVIEW OF HEALTH EDUCATION

The evolution of health education in the United States is tied inexorably to the evolution of education in general and must be considered in relation to trends and events in history. Europeans have had particular influence on American education. The many educational theorists who conceived of the mind and body as dependent and inseparable entities have contributed indirectly to health education. In addition, many series of events or movements have influenced the state of the profession.

Emile, by Jacques Rousseau, is one of the most widely read documents on education. Rousseau's ideas about health and physical activity were outlawed earlier in France but later contributed to practical reform in educational thought and practice throughout the world. Among other European giants in education were Friedrich Hoffman, who wrote many essays on health; Johann Bernard Basedow, originator of physical education in the *Philanthropinum* at Dessau, Germany; Johann Heinrich Pestalozzi, the father of elementary education; and Friedrich Froebel, originator of the kindergarten.

Early American Schooling

It is interesting that an institution of higher education was founded in the United States before compulsory schooling for children was installed. Harvard College was founded in 1636, almost 200 hundred years before the first American high school came into being. Harvard was the only college in the country for 50 years. It holds special importance to health educators because it was home to the first required course in hygiene in American higher education. The course consisted of only five lectures.

Massachusetts was the first of the colonies to establish a law requiring all children to read and write. Passed in 1642, this law was meant mainly to force the population to understand religion and law. In 1647, the "Old Deluder" law was passed in Massachusetts, requiring towns with at least 50 families to have an elementary school

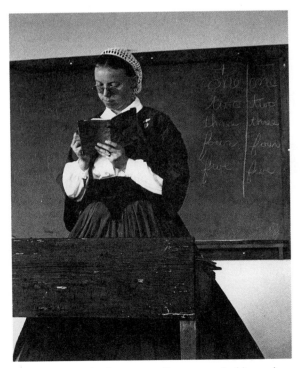

Early American schools were usually one-room buildings where only boys attended. Teaching was mostly a female profession.

and those with at least 100 households to have a Latin grammar secondary school.

In 1751, one of Benjamin Franklin's lifelong dreams came to pass with the founding of the Academy. Located in Philadelphia, the Academy was the first institution of secondary education in America. It, as Franklin himself, advocated "healthful situation" and physical exercise. In 1821, the American high school was founded.

In the early days of American education, only boys went to school. Days and terms were short. Individual needs received little attention. Literacy and religion were the major subjects taught in school. Oral recitation was the primary means of instruction, as few printed materials were available. The schools frequently had no sanitary facilities, used wood stoves, and were poorly built, ventilated, and lighted. Health and hygiene were not emphasized in the colonial or early American school.

William A. Alcott, the "father of school health education" in the United States, wrote a prize-winning book in 1829 on the healthful construction of schoolhouses. He was the first to write a health book suitable for children.

Horace Mann, the first secretary of the first state board of education in the United States, and probably the most influential educator of his day, discussed the problem of school hygiene in his *First Annual Report of the Secretary of the Board of Education* (Massachusetts) in 1837. He made powerful recommendations for including physiology and hygiene in the curriculum of the common (elementary) school in all six of his annual reports between 1837 and 1843. Subsequently, in 1850, Massachusetts became the first state to require mandatory physiology and hygiene by law in all public schools (Pollock, 1987). Mann also wrote, in several ensuing works, about the value of physical strength and health and education for health.

The 1800s

Between 1800 and 1850, the United States was undergoing great changes. Land acquisitions

expanded the size of the country. Inventions and the growth of industry changed American life. Political and social changes led to changes in education. The provisions for education varied a great deal among the states. In 1840, Rhode Island passed a law making education mandatory. Other states soon followed suit, although conditions, facilities, and methods remained shoddy. At the same time, teaching as a profession gained attention as new ideas, including those from abroad, influenced the schools. The principles and policies upon which health education would be built were starting to form. By 1880, there were more than 35 textbooks written specifically for the study of health.

The period between 1850 and 1900 saw further change in America. Westward population drift led to the taming of the Wild West. The Civil War divided, bloodied, and scarred the country. The Spanish-American War was the last

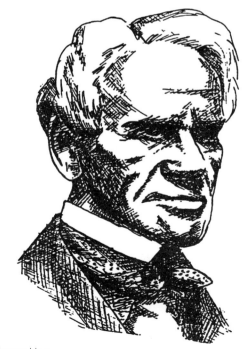

Horace Mann

Source: R. K. Means, *Historical Perspectives on Health Education* (Thorofare, NJ: Charles B. Slack, 1975). Reprinted by permission of the publisher.

large violent event of the century. In the field of education, functional learning was the rule, aimed at preparation for life. In Oswego, New York, Pestalozzianism formed the foundation of the "Oswego movement" promoting elementary school education. William T. Harris founded the first public kindergarten. The Morrill Act of 1862 provided financial support for agricultural and vocational schools. In 1874, the Kalamazoo case established the right of the community to tax its citizens to support public schools. The present system of credits was initiated in education in 1892, based on the recommendation of the Committee of Ten appointed by the National Educational Association. The compulsory, tax-supported education system that exists today was coalescing.

The Temperance Movement

The *scientific temperance movement* began with the founding of the Women's Crusade in 1874 by Dr. Dio Lewis. The Women's Christian Temperance Union, as it later was called, became one of the most important pressure organizations in

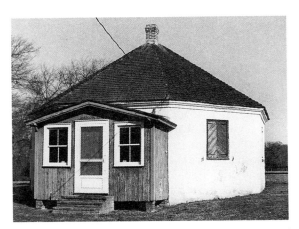

Octagonal school buildings such as this one in central Delaware were considered quite sufficient. Each of the eight grades sat on one of the eight walls facing the teacher. The teacher and the wood stove usually occupied the center of the room. This school was in continuous use from 1836 to 1930.

history. It preached of the evil effects of alcohol, tobacco, and narcotics, using every medium, including the schools. As a result of the work of the WCTU, led by Mary Hanchett Hunt, 38 states and territories passed laws between 1880 and 1890, requiring the teaching of hygiene and physiology, and in 16 states the subjects were required in all grades of all pupils (Rogers, 1933). Every state passed legislation requiring instruction on the effects of alcohol and narcotics, and Congress established a comparable law for the territories (Rogers, 1930). Many of these laws remained in effect even after the temperance movement became less influential. The curricula on alcohol often contained myths and fallacious information (Payne and Schroeder, 1925), but it focused attention on health and hygiene education.

The Physical Education Movement

The roots of the *physical education movement* can be traced to 1892 in Ohio and 1899 in North Dakota, when those states passed laws making physical education a mandatory part of public school curricula. The concept of physical education before 1900 included health instruction. During the next 30 years, virtually all states passed legislation similar to that of Ohio and North Dakota. One of the early crusaders for health and a leader of the physical education movement was Catherine Esther Beecher. According to Rice and Hutchinson (1958), Beecher often is referred to as the "originator of the first American system of gymnastics and as the first woman physical education leader in America." At age 22, she opened the Hartford (Connecticut) Female Seminary and developed a system of physical education that incorporated calisthenics and work in physiology. Her textbook, *Physiology and Calisthenics for Schools and Families* (Beecher, 1856) included 26 lessons on physiology for schools, families, and health establishments. Among Beecher's recommendations were the daily teaching of physical education and physiology, a coordinator or head of the school health program, and instruction beyond the simple dissemination of information.

Another pioneer in the physical education movement was Thomas Denison Wood. In 1891, at age 26, Wood developed the Department of Physical Training at Stanford University. The Stanford program was far advanced for its time. Wood also initiated graduate and undergraduate programs in health education at Columbia University that became the national standard. He was one of the originators of the Joint Committee on Health Problems in Education of the National Education Association and the American Medical Association and served as chairman of the committee from 1911 to 1938. He also was chairman of the International Conference on Health Education of the World Education Congress. Wood was a founder and officer of the American Child Health Association for many years. In 1930, he was chairman of the Committee on the School and the Child of the White House Conference on Child Health and Protection. Wood was renowned for (LaSalle and Wood, 1960):

> his crusade to have school administrators accept their responsibility for the promotion of child health; his labors to help physicians and educators identify and interpret problems of school health; his concept of the school health program as embracing health services, healthful environment (including hygiene instruction), and health instruction, all of which must be coordinated; his concept of improved behavior, rather than mere knowledge, as the ultimate goal in health instruction; his definition of health as "an abundance of life rather than freedom from disease"; his viewpoint that health is a means which enables humans to move toward their goals, and that it is never an end in itself; his realization that the school, the home, and the community must work together if the health of the child is to improve.

The Child Study Movement

The *child study movement* emerged in American education before the turn of the century. Flowing from ideas and practices of European educators, the movement was based upon new ideas of the psychology of learning and grounded in the notion that children's needs and interests are significant motivators in the learning process. Thus, for the first time, concern for the pupil as an individual began to affect American education on a large scale. John Dewey's work in his laboratory school at the University of Chicago helped teachers realize the importance of knowing the individual pupil and opened the door for more experimental institutions. Health education benefited from this movement because of the recognition of individual differences and the total behavior of the child as significant to the educational process (Means, 1975).

The years 1900–1920 were tumultuous times in the United States and the world. At home, women gained the right to vote, the federal income tax was instituted, and prohibition was tried and failed. World War I ravaged much of the world. At home, many young men failed the induction examinations, shocking the nation into the realization that the country was sadly lacking healthwise. This led to enactment of

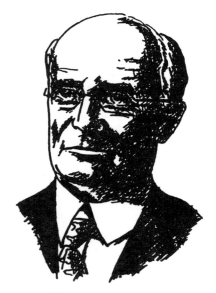

Thomas Denison Wood

Source: R. K. Means, *Historical Perspectives on Health Education* (Thorofare, NJ: Charles B. Slack, 1975). Reprinted by permission of the publisher.

laws concerning health and physical education in the school. Influenced by war, colleges
became the training ground for the military.

The Era of Medical Inspection

The *era of medical inspection* actually had its
genesis before 1900 because of the prevalence of
communicable diseases in children and the
recognition that the schools could be useful in
reducing the transmission of disease. In several
cities, physicians and public health workers
examined children and teachers in the schools.
In 1899, Connecticut required teachers to conduct visual examinations of school children. In
1902, New York City required routine inspections of pupils to detect contagious eye and
skin diseases. Connecticut and Vermont began
similar programs. In 1902, New York City
employed school nurses, and by 1911 more than
100 cities had school nurses. In 1906, Massachusetts made medical inspections compulsory
in public schools. Although the medical inspection movement made some progress, it was
hampered by a number of problems, not the
least of which was inadequate funding. The
evaluation of many potential military inductees
as unfit to serve contributed to medical examinations becoming a conspicuous part of school
programs.

Around 1900, curricula began to have a new
emphasis. Education for marriage, sometimes
called "sex hygiene," began to appear as a
theme in health education. Boys and girls usually were separated for this instruction. Even in
the late 1920s, however, courses in physiology
and hygiene still frequently omitted any mention
of sex.

Open-air Classrooms

Shortly after the turn of the century, the nation
became infatuated with *open-air classrooms* and
schools. These outdoor classrooms often had no
walls. The practice originally was intended to
promote the care and instruction of children
whose state of health was below normal. The
first open-air classroom in the United States was
in the Sea Breeze Hospital on Coney Island in
1904 (Brannon, 1911). Sea Breeze specialized in
treating of children with tuberculosis. Open-air
classrooms later were found in other types of
hospitals. Following the lead of Providence,
Rhode Island, many cities provided open-air
classrooms in regular schools, including some
mandated by local law. The Report of the Joint
Committee on Health Problems in Education of
the National Education Association and the
American Medical Association (1937) indicated
that as late as 1930, 1,105 open air schools
existed in the United States, caring for 31,386
pupils with health needs. Early in the history of
open-air schools and classrooms, health education was integrated into the overall educational
plan, including emphasis on the development of
attitudes.

Differentiating Health Education and Physical Education in the Early 1900s

Anderson (1972) suggested that health education and physical education were considered
synonymous until 1910. Then the American
Physical Education Association recognized a distinction between the two fields by making
"School Hygiene and Physical Education" the
theme for its 17th annual meeting.

Health education still was not fully established in American schools. According to the
Report of the Committee on the Status of Physical Education in Public Normal Schools and
Public High Schools (1910), 16% of high
schools gave regular instruction in hygiene, 11%
prescribed such instruction, and 8% granted
credit for these courses.

School Health Demonstrations and Organizations

The Locust Point demonstration, beginning in
1914 and continuing for three years, was one of

the earliest school health demonstrations. It gained extensive national and international attention. The demonstration was carried out in a school of 900 pupils in a lower-class section of Baltimore. It had one part-time physician, assigned by the Department of Health, and a full-time nurse. The objective of the project was to increase the level of health of the community. Teachers disseminated information about various aspects of health, such as balanced diet, importance of sufficient rest and sleep, and the benefits of outdoor exercise. Three facts emerged from the demonstration. In Jean's (1946) words:

> The interest of the teacher in promoting health can be secured; that the interest of the child himself is an essential in influencing his health behavior; and that the child does influence the health behavior of the family.

The *modern health crusade* of the National Tuberculosis Association was a massive organized effort at improving the health behavior of school children. It was supported financially by donations and by funds appropriated from the Visiting Nurse Association. Simple health rules were printed and distributed to children. Prizes, buttons, and toothbrushes were awarded to children. In 1914, these Open Air Crusaders organized in southern Illinois and were encouraged to practice four rules: Sleep with your window open; have fresh air where you work or play; breathe through your nose with your mouth closed; and get the rest of your family to do the same (Means, 1975).

The movement soon was taken up by other states and then spread to the national level. The Christmas Seal Campaign was initiated in Wilmington, Delaware, in 1907 and was adopted nationally the following year as an effort to raise funds to fight tuberculosis. The Christmas Seals effort was first an American Red Cross campaign and later was adopted by the National Tuberculosis Association. Beginning in 1915, children buying or selling 10 cents worth of seals each enrolled as a Modern Health

Crusader and were given certificates with the following health rules (Strachan, 1932):

1. Always breathe fresh air. Never sleep, study, work, or play in a room without a window open.

2. Eat nourishing food and drink plenty of pure water. Avoid food that is hard to digest, like heavy pastries. Never eat or drink anything that weakens the body, like alcoholic drinks.

3. Make sure that everything you put in your mouth is clean. Wash your hands always before eating and bathe your whole body often. Clean your teeth every day. Do not smoke before you grow up.

4. Exercise every day in the open air. Keep your shoulders straight. Take ten deep breaths everyday.

The Record for Health Chores became the basis for the National Health Crusaders. Children were encouraged to perform several health chores each day, with various levels of achievement recognized. The program soon became international in membership. In 1924, the Joint Committee on Health Problems in Education published *Health Education–A Program for Public Schools and Teacher Training Institutions*, which outlined responsibilities and facets of a comprehensive school health program. At this time, the National Tuberculosis Association stopped promotion of the Modern Health Crusade, although the chore cards remained available until 1930. The crusade owns a particular place in history, however, for through it the National Tuberculosis Association brought health education based upon behavioral aspects of learning into the school—an approach for the future.

According to the Report of the Committee on the Status of Physical Education in American Colleges (1916), 80% of institutions of higher education offered hygiene instruction and 80 of them gave credit toward the bachelor's degree for those courses. Georgia Normal and Industrial College was the first institution to grant an undergraduate degree in health education. In 1917, under the direction of Kathleen W. Wooten, the Health Department of that college offered courses in

"Personal Hygiene and Mothercraft," later titled "Health of the Family." In 1918, the course "Health Education for Teachers" was added to the curriculum. Soon thereafter, Teachers College of Columbia University and the Harvard University-MIT combined program began to award degrees in health education.

One of the most important education documents ever published was the *Cardinal Principles of Secondary Education* (National Education Association, 1918). It marked a significant turning point in secondary education in the United States. The seven principal objectives, as identified by the Commission on the Reorganization of Secondary Education of the National Education Association, were health, command of fundamental processes, worthy home membership, vocation, citizenship, worthy use of leisure, and ethical character. The cardinal principles provided direction for secondary education, further legitimized health education, and influenced the course of health education.

The Health Education Movement

The Child Health Organization of America was formed in 1918 as the Modern Health Crusade was waning. Founding of the CHO often is considered the beginning of the *health education movement*. The CHO was founded on the recommendation of the Committee on War Time Problems of Childhood of the Pediatrics Section of the New York Academy of Medicine. The committee itself, chaired by L. Emmett Holt, was created as a result of concern over childhood malnutrition. The CHO was founded to proliferate the ideal that knowledge is not always enough to result in practice, and that teachers are the logical source to provide the kind of health instruction that will be effective in establishing acceptable practices.

In 1919, the CHO conducted a national campaign to better the health of American children. The program emphasized the positive rather than the negative. The Rules of the Game

became the basis for further development of health education programs. The rules were (Reaney, 1922):

1. a full bath more than once a week;
2. brushing the teeth at least once every day;
3. sleeping long hours with windows open;
4. drinking as much milk as possible, but no coffee or tea;
5. eating some vegetables or fruit every day;
6. drinking at least four glasses of water a day;
7. playing part of every day out of doors; and
8. a bowel movement every day

The campaign's approach was summed up by Van Ingen (1935):

> Health education was considered an essential part of the school curriculum and recognition was given both to the possibility and to the necessity of coordinating physical education, home economics,

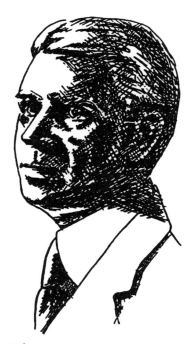

L. Emmett Holt

Source: R. K. Means, *Historical Perspectives on Health Education* (Thorofare, NJ: Charles B. Slack, 1975). Reprinted by permission of the publisher.

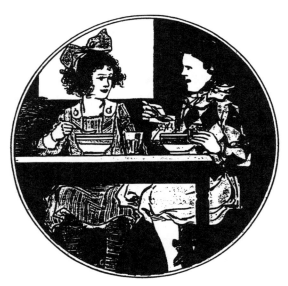

CHO CHO'S LUNCH

Now Cho Cho lives a good way off
And though at distance he would scoff
Because his legs and lungs are strong,
You know that twelve to one's not long
And school o'clock comes very soon.
But children need hot food at noon.

Rhyme of Cho Cho's lunch — Child Health Organization
activity from *Rhymes of Cho Cho's Grandma* by Mrs. Frederick Peterson, Macmillan, 1922.

Source: R. K. Means, *Historical Perspectives on Health Education* (Thorofare, NJ: Charles B. Slack, 1975). Reprinted by
permission of the publisher.

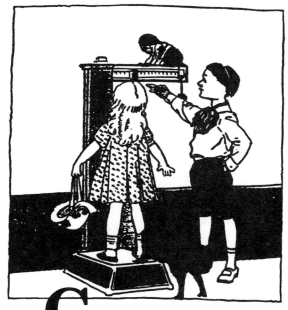

G is for *Gaining,*
as every Child could;
A half pound a Month
is the least that he should.

Health alphabet rhyme — Child Health Organization activity
from *Child Health Alphabet* by Mrs. Frederick Peterson, New
York: Child Health Organization, 1921.

Source: R. K. Means, *Historical Perspectives on Health Education* (Thorofare, NJ: Charles B. Slack, 1975). Reprinted by
permission of the publisher.

school lunches and other subjects and activities to
this important end. Instead of supplying a definite
program for teachers to follow, the aim was to
develop interest, initiative, and originality on the
part of the teacher.

The innovative program used clowns, health
dramas, health fairies, and health ventriloquists,
and produced many materials for health education. In its five years, the popular campaign had
extraordinary influence on the transformation
of information into impact, the promotion of
health in schools, and teacher education.

This era marked a turning point in school
health programming, for this was the point at

which an approach was derived based on motivational psychology and the understanding of
behavior. The term "health education," which
replaced "hygiene," was first proposed at a
New York conference of the Child Health
Organization in 1919. The word "hygiene" had
become unpopular in schools, and it was
believed that a new, more definitive term would
be helpful in popularizing health practices (Jean,
1946).

In 1920, the National Education Association's Committee on Standards for Use in the
Reorganization of Secondary School Curricula

selected health as the first of four objectives. This was an indication of the priority the most powerful education organization in the United States placed on health.

Technological advances between 1920 and 1940 were rapid. Development of the automobile and the airplane improved transportation immeasurably. The telephone, radio, rapid printing press, and motion picture changed the way the nation did business and communicated. Electric power came of age. Despite these advances, the Great Depression wrecked the economy. Program and personnel reductions were the rule in business. Effects of the depression on education were almost lethal, with drastic cuts in personnel and in program offerings. Many schools, especially rural schools, were closed. Salaries were cut, and curricula were revised to fit scaled-down budgets. According to Means (1975), "National problems in the 1930s facilitated a renewed look at education from all angles and provided a more realistic and scientific basis for the years ahead."

Reconstruction

Education underwent a kind of reconstruction, trying new ideas, plans, and fads. Educational research began to flourish. Though somewhat controversial, most states had established compulsory education. The lean times of the depression focused attention on children's health needs. Concern shifted to the individual child, recognizing the needs of the gifted child as well as the slow learner and the child with a handicap. Junior high schools and junior colleges both developed rapidly. The vocational rehabilitation school movement also began to unfold.

Safety Education

After World War I, the United States offered little safety education. The evolution of safety education after that time, however, was closely aligned to that of health education. The driving force behind safety education was Herbert J. Stack, Director of the Center of Safety Education at New York University. For his pioneering work, Stack has been dubbed the father of safety education. During the 1920s, much legislation was passed regarding education on specific safety topics such as fire prevention and traffic safety. Most of this legislation was weak and ineffective. During the 1930s, however, safety received more attention, usually as a part of health education. The National Safety Council brought safety to the public eye with numerous safety demonstrations. As boating and motor vehicle accidents increased, so did safety education, particularly driver's education. By the 1950s, safety education had gained an obvious place in school curricula and in teacher preparation.

Public Health Education

In the early 1920s, public health education was mostly propaganda, pamphlets, and publicity, with little systematic planning of programs. However, in 1922 the American Public Health Association formed a section on Health Education. The schools were much more systematic in their approach to health education. Public health workers eventually began to adopt the schools' more successful organized approaches and gradually eliminated the propagandizing.

Curricula and Research

The temperance movement, which provided the impetus for so much early health education, was still evident in health education curricula throughout the 1920s. Its influence was lessening, though, as other topics gained attention.

The Report of the Joint Committee on Health Problems in Education of the NEA and the AMA (1924), in *Health Education—A Program for Public Schools and Teacher Training Institutions*, clearly demonstrated a change in emphasis in health education with its statement of purpose for health education. According to the committee, the broad aims of health education were:

1. To instruct children and youth so that they may conserve and improve their own health.
2. To establish in them habits and principles of living which throughout their school life, and in later years, will assure that abundant vigor and vitality which provide the basis for the greatest possible happiness and service in personal, family, and community life.
3. To influence parents and other adults, through the health education program for children, to better habits and attitudes, so that the school may become an effective agency for the promotion of the social aspects of health education in the family and community as well as the school itself.
4. To improve the individual and community life of the future; to insure a better second generation and a still better third generation; a healthier and fitter nation and race.

One of the most far-reaching research projects of the 1920s, the Malden Study directed by Clair Turner, was a longitudinal study under the direction of the Harvard-Massachusetts Institute of Technology School of Public Health. The study used a control group, matched by age, economic characteristics, and other factors. Instruction in the experimental group was "habit-centered" and utilized height and weight tables to measure growth. Turner (1928) reported, "The health education program proved to be a sound, practicable and acceptable public school procedure. Definite improvement in health habits was shown." This emphasis on habits nurtured the embryonic notion that behavior is the critical variable in well-being. The study yielded the Malden Health Series, the first series with a separate book for each grade.

A Health Survey of 86 Cities, begun in 1923 (American Child Health Association, 1925), was done to determine what organized activities private and public agencies, including schools,

were conducting to improve the health of school children. Health education was judged to be mostly a hit-or-miss proposition. The study did lead communities to analyze the efficiency of their own work. In 1925, the researchers launched a follow-up study involving 70 cities to provide data for administrators to use in evaluating local school health activities. Results of the second study were published as five School Health Research Monographs from 1929–1932.

Commercial Efforts

During the 1920s, several commercial companies became interested in health education. They naturally looked upon education largely as a means to augment their sales. Many efforts of commercial companies, however, have benefited the health education of children. Many industries, such as dairy groups, food manufacturers, and insurance companies, became interested in the work of Sally Lucas Jean, president of the American Child Health Association. When she retired, she became consultant-at-large for health education for the ACHA and was able to influence many companies to invest in health education.

A group of soap and glycerin manufacturers formed the Cleanliness Institute and published materials on cleanliness for school use. These firms also took the opportunity to promote their products. The National Dairy Council, while centering its activities on the need for milk, has produced volumes of instructional materials on nutrition and remains active in this endeavor.

The Metropolitan Life Insurance Company was one of the first commercial organizations to become interested in health education. As early as 1871, MetLife published *Health Hints* for its policyholders. Under the direction of Miss Jean and Dr. Lee Frankel, the company expanded its work in health education, producing many worthwhile materials including teaching guides. In 1934, MetLife prepared an exhibit for the Smithsonian Institution giving health rules for children and protraying the progress of public health over the years. Among the company's services to schools and universities are Healthy Me grants, begun in 1985 as a $5 million initiative, to support health education; Healthy Networks, a 1991 meeting funded by a grant from MetLife and carried out by the Association for the Advancement of Health Education to facilitate communication and establish networks among the states to enhance health education; and the MetLife Pavilion in the EPCOT Center in Walt Disney World.

Companies have provided a great deal of support for health education over the years. These efforts should not be confused, however, with those of non-profit general interest groups such as the American Heart Association, American Cancer Society, American Lung Association, and March of Dimes.

The Proliferate Thirties

By 1929, 36 states had laws dealing with health and physical education in schools; 33 states had mandatory health and physical education. Regarding health and physical education, 27 states had standards for time allotment, 30 had published courses of study, 27 had standards for teacher training, 18 had standards for teacher certification, and 20 had general standards for the school program (Meredith, 1933).

One of the true giants in health education, Delbert Oberteuffer, produced one of the most significant early investigations in health education in this country. The Ohio Research Study (Oberteuffer, 1932) was a byproduct of Oberteuffer's doctoral dissertation. The study represented the first attempt to discover students' health needs and interests and use them as a basis for curriculum development. Begun in 1929 and completed three years later, the purpose of the secondary school Ohio Research Study was to determine what to teach in health in secondary schools and where to teach it, and to supply Ohio secondary schools with a practical course of study based on the findings. Using

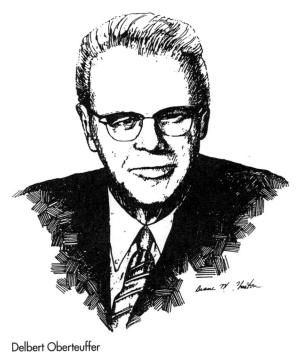

Delbert Oberteuffer

24 junior and senior high schools, Oberteuffer gathered student health questions, and questions from several health texts and popular books on health. He also analyzed data from health examinations, vital statistics, and judgments from an expert panel to provide information for curricular decisions. The study provided a graded health education curriculum for grades 7–12 free of charge to teachers and schools in Ohio and eventually all over the United States. The Ohio Research Study served as a model for other research into curriculum for many years.

Among a series of White House conferences on health issues, the 1930 White House Conference on Child Health and Protection stands out as one of the most significant. Its purpose was to study the status of the health and well-being of children, to report what was being done, and to recommend what ought to be done and how to do it (Means, 1975). The 1930 conference produced the most comprehensive list of statements regarding children's needs ever derived from a single conference. It pointed to the teacher's responsibility in guiding the child toward healthy living, selecting materials for health teaching and health education curriculum; school health services, including health examinations, immunizations, dental care, school lunch, and adequate guidance; and healthful school living, including fire safety, drinking water, ventilation, heating, shower facilities, and gymnasia.

The Cattaragus County (New York) Studies, sponsored by the Milbank Memorial Fund, was another important research project. The 5-year study began in 1931 under the direction of Ruth Grout. The first phase demonstrated the superiority of health instruction in improving health practices and knowledge of health. It also showed that older pupils exposed to health education for a longer time showed greater changes in health habits than younger pupils (Grout and Pickup, 1938). The second phase of the project demonstrated the positive influence of a well-planned and organized health education program on the physical conditions in the school environment. This was especially true of sanitary and hygienic conditions in the year that special emphasis was given in the teaching program to problems of the environment (Greenleaf and Grout, 1938). The third phase of the Cattaragus County project showed the value of inservice education for teachers (Strang, Grout, and Wiehl, 1937). Taken together, the Cattaragus County Studies, through the techniques they utilized and their results, added immensely to knowledge in school health education.

The University of Michigan in 1935 separated the two fields of concentration: school health education and adult health education. This seems to be the first such separation in higher education. The adult health education concentration was soon renamed public health education (Rugen, 1972).

Under the direction of Dorothy Nyswander, the Astoria Study ran from 1936 through 1940. It dealt primarily with school health services in the Astoria Health District of New York City. The study led to significant advancements in cooperation and interaction among school screening methods, health instruction, and curriculum; school health personnel ratios; staff training; and cooperation of health counselors (Nyswander, 1942).

The Progressive Education Association concluded in 1938, after an 8 year study, that health should be the first of 11 educational goals. In the same year, the Educational Policies Commission of the NEA included personal and community health as objectives under one of the four purposes of education in American democracy (Johnson et al., 1969). These recognitions of the importance of health education were important to the reputation of the fledgling profession.

The War Years

The School Community Health Project, sponsored by the W. K. Kellogg Foundation, began in 1942. A teacher in a Battle Creek, Michigan, suburb organized a class to teach girls to be nurses' aides. Through the cooperation of community agencies, including hospitals, the class became highly successful. As word of the idea spread, the Michigan Department of Public Instruction solicited the Kellogg Foundation for support. By the 1943–44 school year, 150 Michigan high schools taught the program. Later, 24 additional states received grants from the foundation to start similar projects. The project demonstrated that effective health education is best accomplished through cooperative services of professional personnel of schools and agencies and that this cooperation can be achieved through a health council. It also demonstrated the importance of community understanding and support of health education to its effectiveness (W. K. Kellogg Foundation, 1950).

The nation struggled through World War II and emerged a victor only to find itself engaged in a cold war. Once again, a war demonstrated through military pre-induction examinations the need for health and fitness of the population. After the war, a period of temporary inflation was followed by a booming economy. The Korean conflict and the Vietnam conflict marred the good times. Autopsies of cadavers from the Korean conflict demonstrated a high rate of atherosclerosis in presumably healthy young men. The birth rate rose, and the space race shifted into high gear. The Salk and Sabin vaccines saved countless children from the devastation of poliomyelitis.

During World War II, high school and college enrollments dropped dramatically, accompanied by decreased financial support for education. The war did, however, stimulate interest in the health of high school students (Strachan and Jordan, 1947). A number of significant events in 1940 contributed to align health education with other fields of education. The Office of Education initiated the Physical Fitness program in 1941, with the aid of the Army, Navy, Public Health Service, and U. S. Children's Bureau. The Victory Corps, launched in 1942, emphasized fitness and vocational studies in high schools. The committee on Wartime Health Education for High School Students was appointed and a program titled "High School Victory Corps" was developed. Materials and resources were developed for health education. Health programs in schools and colleges enlarged, providing a wider variety of content, new activities and services, and an emphasis on healthful school living. General education recognized and supported health education as an essential part of the curriculum during these troubled times.

Throughout the 1940s, Oberteuffer and others vigorously proposed stronger teacher preparation in health education. He also acted to dispel the idea many still hold that only physicians should give health instruction.

Post-War Health Education

By 1945, the nation tended toward expanded class time for health education. Compulsory education in health, first aid, social hygiene, and occupational health problems was becoming the norm. By 1950, health education was generally considered to be emerging as an integral part of elementary, secondary, and collegiate curricula (Means, 1975).

The United Nations Conference of 1945 in San Francisco led to the founding of the World Health Organization in 1948. At the urging of Clair Turner, a Health Education section was established. Most of the early health education work of that organization was in the area of public health education. It also did some work in school health in cooperation with the United Nations Educational, Scientific, and Cultural Organization (UNESCO). UNESCO was created at the same time as the WHO to promote the three areas identified in its title.

After the war, as the G.I. Bill sent young war veterans back to school, the schools became laboratories of social experiment. In 1954, the Supreme Court ruled that racial segregation in public schools was unconstitutional, setting the stage for confrontations in many schools, especially in the South. In 1955, the White House Conference on Education made significant recommendations regarding state and local school organization, education salaries, federal aid for building construction, and evaluation of teacher preparation programs. The military threat posed by the Soviet Union prompted passage of the National Defense Education Act of 1958, increasing funding for math and science education.

During the 1950s a number of studies were conducted to evaluate the role of school health services and health service personnel, particularly the school nurse. The Committee on School Nurse Policies and Practices of the American School Health Association (1956) published a paper entitled "Recommended Policies and Practices for School Nursing," which has been a

Ten Conceptual Statements from the School Health Education Study

1. Growth and development influences and is influenced by the structure and functioning of the individual.

2. Growing and developing follows a predictable sequence, yet is unique for each individual.

3. Protection and promotion of health is an individual, community, and international responsibility.

4. The potential for hazards and accidents exists, whatever the environment.

5. There are reciprocal relationships involving man, disease, and environment.

6. The family serves to perpetuate man and to fulfill certain health needs.

7. Personal health practices are affected by a complexity of forces, often conflicting.

8. Utilization of health information, products, and services is guided by values and perceptions.

9. Use of substances that modify mood and behavior arises from a variety of motivations.

10. Food selection and eating patterns are determined by physical, social, mental, economic, and cultural forces.

Source: Sliepcevich, E. M. Health Education: A Conceptual Approach to Curriculum Design. *School Health Education Study*. St. Paul, MN: 3M Education Press, 1967.

useful guide over the years. Bland (1956), Netcher (1956), and Poe and Irwin (1959) all conducted important research on the functions and evaluation of the school nurse.

The President's Conference on the Fitness of American Youth in 1956 was the first of several President's Conferences on Fitness. The initial conference, held in Annapolis, Maryland, explored fitness issues, including the role of schools and health education. One of the outcomes of this conference was the establishment of the President's Council on Youth Fitness. The Council promotes fitness programs in schools, initiates new programs, and coordinates the efforts of individuals and groups interested in fitness.

In 1960, the White House Conference on Education specified health as one of the 14 areas about which American youth should have

education (Johnson et al., 1969). In the same year, the Golden Anniversary White House Conference on Children and Youth had as its purpose "to promote opportunities for children and youth to realize their full potential for a creative life in freedom and dignity" (Brown, 1959). Among the 1,400 recommendations, a good deal of attention was given to all aspects of school health education programs, especially school health services and healthful school living.

The Concept Approach

The concept approach to health education, introduced in the mid-1960s, stemmed from the School Health Education Study (1962). From its beginning as an idea at a luncheon conversation in New York Governor Nelson A. Rockefeller's office, involving Dr. Granville Larimore, First

Deputy Commissioner, New York State Department of Health, and Mr. Samuel Bronfman of the Samuel Bronfman Foundation, the SHES was the first real foundation toward comprehensive school health education as we now know it. The SHES was funded by the Bronfman Foundation and Minnesota Mining and Manufacturing (3M) and directed by Elena M. Sliepcevich. It was the first attempt to scientifically develop a health education curriculum that followed the basic principles used for all other educational curricula. Taking part in the study were 135 school systems, 1,460 schools, and more than 840,000 students from 38 states. The first phase of the study involved a survey of health education in the nation's schools, evaluation of instructional practices, and testing of student health behavior.

The findings revealed dreadful conditions. Practices more applicable to physical education were applied to the organization of health education, grouping of students, number of periods allotted for health education, preparation of those assigned to teach, and titles given to courses (Means, 1975). In some cases state requirements for certification of elementary school teachers did not require any preparation in health education. The SHES demonstrated obvious inadequacies in instructional materials, as well as lack of time in the curriculum and unqualified staff. The findings indicated problems and weaknesses so huge that immediate action was crucial.

In its second phase, the SHES dealt with development of curriculum materials. The result was a concept approach that has become a model for health education curriculum development. The conceptual approach is predicated on three key concepts: (a) *growing and developing*, (b) *decision making*, and (c) *interaction*. The 10 concepts in the accompanying box define the body of knowledge important to health education. Part of the beauty of the SHES format is that the conceptual statements represent major ideas under which health subject matter could "fit." The framework need not be revised with each new health problem or crisis (Cortese, 1993). It also produced a cycle plan delineating the scope and sequence of health education for K-12 curriculum development. Many teaching materials and publications flowed from the SHES. The legacy of this important endeavor survives in modern health education and probably will for years to come.

Teach Us What We Want To Know

In 1967, the Connecticut State Board of Education initiated a study to determine the health interests and concerns of school children in all grades. The report, called *Teach Us What We Want to Know* (Byler, 1969), quantified in detail the health areas of interest or concern to students of various ages. The study continues to influence curriculum development in health education. Student input in curriculum development has become an accepted principle.

The Seventies

During the decade of the 1970s, the nation continued to mature educationally and new ideas were tried. The open classroom experiment met with some success but little popularity. That decade also saw tremendous growth in community colleges. Higher education became less a refuge for the elite and more of a training ground for the general population. Educational research flourished. In 1977, smallpox became the first infectious disease to be totally eradicated by public health efforts.

The nation had not approached the real potential of health education. After more than a year of study, the President's Committee on Health Education identified serious shortcomings in health education. The committee reported the following (U. S. Department of Health, Education, and Welfare, 1973):

Although many of the major causes of illness and death can be affected by individual behavior, health education is a neglected, under-financed, fragmented activity with no agency inside or outside of government responsible for establishing short- or long-term goals.

Virtually no component of society makes full use of health education. That includes the health care delivery system, the educational system, voluntary health agencies...

School health education in most primary and secondary schools either is not provided at all, or loses its proper emphasis because of the way it is tacked onto another subject such as physical education or biology, assigned to teachers whose interests and qualifications lie elsewhere.

There has been little effort to bring together the fields of health education, parent education and early childhood education for planning and evaluation.

Sadly, more than two decades later these words still apply in many parts of the country.

The 1970s produced a number of significant events in health education. It was a period of promoting legislation by state and local governments to mandate improved delivery of health education. A national task force developed a handbook for state policymakers on planning and implementing Comprehensive School Health Education. In 1974, the Bureau of Health Education (now the Center for Health Promotion and Education) was established in the Centers for Disease Control, U. S. Public Health Service. The Bureau of Health Education contracted with the National Parent-Teacher Association Comprehensive School/Community Health Education Project for the years 1975–80 to increase community awareness and understanding of health education needs and to develop support for more effective health education. The National Center for Health Education, a nongovernmental agency, was established in 1975 to promote health education.

In 1975–1976 the U. S. Congress considered passage of the Comprehensive School Health Education Act. Although the bill did not pass, it focused attention and provided visibility to health education. That visibility probably contributed to passage of amendments to the Elementary and

Secondary Education Act of 1965, Title III, authorizing funds for states and local districts to develop and implement comprehensive school health education programs. Block grants were provided for health education programs for the states to be utilized by individual school districts. The new U. S. Department of Education established the Office of Comprehensive School Health in 1978. Unfortunately, the office was eliminated in the subsequent administration. *Healthy People: The Surgeon General's Report on Health Promotion and Disease Prevention* was published by the U. S. Department of Health, Education, and Welfare (1979). (See Chapter 13 for a discussion of this publication.)

The Eighties

The 1980s, though economically prosperous in the early years, saw a good deal of retrenchment in education. Many colleges and universities reduced faculty and eliminated departments. During the last part of the decade, this trend intensified as recession took a heavy toll on education in many states.

While the face of higher education was getting a makeover in the 1980s, the entire world was being terrified and altered by AIDS. It is the most feared infectious disease since the plagues of Europe. Although AIDS is a worldwide tragedy, it also has provided the opportunity for health educators to demonstrate their skill and expertise. The epidemic has led to the most exhaustive education efforts ever mustered against any single health entity. The message that AIDS usually is contracted as a result of chosen behaviors such as sexual activity and injectable drug use and is, therefore, mostly preventable, bombarded much of the population. From federal government publications to elementary classrooms, from churches to community action groups, the range of organizations that have attempted some form of education related to AIDS prevention is enormous. These prevention and education efforts have not been well-coordinated. The power of conservative groups who have fought against any form of sex education in schools and have particularly battled against AIDS education has driven home a remarkable point: Some people in America would rather risk the lives of their children than educate them to the lessons of life. As a profession, we still may not have established the confidence we need to meet our goals. At present, rates of HIV infection continue to increase in most segments of the population.

During the 1980s, health education saw its share of bright moments. The U. S. Department of Health and Human Services (1980) published *Promoting Health/Preventing Disease: Objectives for the Nation*, prompting action on the part of the health education establishment (See Chapter 13 for a discussion of this publication.) The PRECEDE model (Green et al., 1980), perhaps the most comprehensive framework for health planning, was published. The Office of the Surgeon General, U. S. Department of Health and Human Services (1981) expressed strong support for school health education.

In 1982, the Centers for Disease Control (CDC) reorganized and included a School Health Section, demonstrating further federal resolve. In the same year, the National School Health Education Coalition (NaSHEC) was formed to enhance networking and cooperation among health agencies for the improvement of health education. The Office of Disease Prevention and Health Promotion (ODPHP) entered into an agreement in 1985 with the American School Health Association (ASHA) to develop model strategies to relate the 1990 health education objectives for the nation to the school population. ODPHP, ASHA, Association for the Advancement of Health Education (AAHE), and the Society for Public Health Education (SOPHE) entered into a cooperative agreement for an ongoing national survey of knowledge, attitudes, and practices in school health. In 1987 CDC established cooperative agreements with 15 organizations for AIDS education. The landmark *Healthy People 2000: National Health Promotion and Disease Prevention Objectives* (U. S. Department of Health and Human Services, 1991) was released. This publication is discussed in Chapter 13.

THE ROAD TO CREDENTIALING

The qualifications necessary to become a health educator have long been debated. As programs developed in institutions of higher education to prepare professionals, many saw the need to establish some sort of uniformity. Perhaps this need also reflected a desire for means of comparing one program to another. Over several years, issuing formal credentials became the favored method of evaluating professionals. This, of course, led to the later establishment of certain criteria for professional preparation programs.

The actual process of formal credentialing was initiated in 1948 (Cleary, 1986). In that year, the American Public Health Association issued a report that actually was a follow-up to its 1943 publication, which contained a statement on qualifications and standards for health educators. The 1948 report's primary emphasis was information dissemination (Creswell, 1986).

Also in 1948, the National Conference on Undergraduate Professional Preparation in Health Education, Physical Education and Recreation was held at Jackson's Mill in Reston, Virginia. The conference was co-sponsored by nine educational organizations (Patterson, 1992). The Jackson's Mill Conference, as it came to be called, focused on improving professional preparation programs and recognizing professional competencies needed by teachers and leaders in health education, physical education, and recreation (Athletic Institute, 1948). This conference was followed by several others, including the Conference of the Undergraduate Professional Preparation of Students Majoring in Health Education in December 1949, and the National Conference on Graduate Study in Health Education, Physical Education and Recreation, in January 1950.

The American Public Health Association's Committee on Professional Education, chaired by Dr. Clair Turner, released a report in 1957 that recommended adding standards for educational evaluation, adding at least one year of graduate education in public health for qualification as a public health educator, and recognizing that the need for health educators was six to seven times greater than the supply. Furthermore, the report recommended that health educators' preparation emphasize social, biological, and health sciences as well as education and educational psychology (Creswell, 1986).

In 1962, the American Association for Health, Physical Education, and Recreation (AAHPER) sponsored a national conference titled "Professional Preparation in Health Education, Physical Education and Recreation Education." Objectives were derived from 13 basic beliefs underlying professional preparation. These objectives were the basis of a professional preparation philosophy that was functional and measurable. Seven areas were identified, on which principles and standards were centered:

1. Philosophy and objectives of professional preparation.

2. Organization and administration.

3. Student personnel.

4. Faculty.

5. Curricula.

6. Professional laboratory experiences.

7. Facilities and instructional materials.

Professional competencies were defined for each of these seven areas (Patterson, 1992).

During the decade of the 1960s, a number of significant reports were issued on the subject of professional preparation of health educators. These reports came principally from the Society for Public Health Education (SOPHE) and AAHPER. In 1967, professional standards were being developed for community health educators. Community health leaders were considering having their programs accredited. This would be helpful in placing graduates in the workforce and would allow accredited programs to be eligible for public health traineeship funds. To provide a mechanism for accrediting programs, the Public Health Service subcontracted with the National Commission on Accrediting to develop accreditation criteria and guidelines. Based on the result of this action, the American Public Health Association in 1969 issued its criteria and guidelines for accrediting graduate programs in community health education (Creswell, 1986).

In 1973, AAHPER sponsored a conference to improve professional preparation by identifying guidelines for undergraduate teacher preparation programs. The conference also produced recommended competencies and personal qualifications of health teachers (American Association for Health, Physical Education, and Recreation, 1974).

The process took a significant turn in February, 1978, establishing a direction that led more directly to the birth of a true credentialing process. Government support was provided for a workshop that has come to be known as the First Bethesda Conference, which involved a representative group of health educators. The purpose was to discuss the "commonalities and differences in preparation and practice of community, patient, and school health educators" (Hoover, 1980). The result of this workshop was a major recommendation that the roles and competencies of entry-level health educators be defined as the initial step in a credentialing process. The Division of Associated Health Professions of the Health Resources Administration and the National Center for Health Education entered into a contract in September 1978, which resulted in the Role Delineation Project. The National Task Force on Preparation and Practice of Health Educators was an outgrowth of the First Bethesda Conference. The task force, consisting of representatives of eight professional organizations, was to be given the responsibility of developing a credentialing system for health educators (Patterson, 1992).

Developing a credentialing system involved delineation of the roles of health educator and verification of those roles. This was done as the Role Delineation Project. At a 1981 meeting, information on curriculum content utilized in institutions that prepare health educators formed the basis for a resource document titled, *A Guide for the Development of Competency-Based Curricula for Entry Level Health Educators*. The guide subsequently was revised and retitled, *A Competency Based Curriculum Framework for the Professional Preparation of Entry-Level Health Educators*. Competencies and skills the Role Delineation Project deemed to be essential to entry-level health educators are defined in this document.

The Second Bethesda Conference met to decide future directions and goals of the Task Force (National Task Force on the Preparation and Practice of Health Educators, 1986). It was decided that the Task Force should proceed toward developing a plan of action for establishing a credentialing process for health educators, including raising money, developing self-assessment instruments, identifying the most appropriate structure to carry out credentialing in health education, and bringing together the organizations involved in credentialing for health education.

In June 1988, the National Commission for Health Education Credentialing (NCHEC) was established. NCHEC grants the credential titled "Certified Health Education Specialist" (CHES). The Role Delineation Project is the basis for the examination which leads to the CHES designation. (See Chapter 14 for a discussion of this and other issues relating to this subject.) The examination is administered by the Professional Examination Service, a national testing service. The first examination for CHES was given in 1990.

SUMMARY

Throughout history, people have struggled to maintain quality of life. Beyond mere infections, humankind has striven to overcome ignorance, overcrowding, war, and our own indifference. These struggles have led to momentous medical advances. Inexorably tied to medical progress is the enrichment of life that comes with education. As general education has progressed, so has education designed to promote the health of the individual. Countless individuals and organizations have contributed to this progress.

Professional health educators have worked diligently to gain recognition for their profession. They have worked tirelessly to provide curriculum standards and standards of professional competence. Through this effort has come the light of a dynamic profession, dedicated to the well-being of children and adults alike.

REFERENCES

American Child Health Association. *A Health Survey of 86 Cities*. New York: ACHA, 1925.

American Association for Health, Physical Education, and Recreation. *Report of the National Conference on Undergraduate Professional Preparation in Dance, Physical Education, Recreation Education, Safety Education and School Health Education*. Washington, DC: National Education Association, 1974.

American School Health Association. Recommended policies and practices for school nursing, ASHA Committee on School Nurse Policies and Practices. *Journal of School Health*, 26 (January 1956): 13-26.

Anderson, C. L. *School Health Practices*. St. Louis: C. V. Mosby Co., 1972.

Athletic Institute. *Report on the National Conference on Undergraduate Professional Preparation in Physical Education, Health Education and Recreation*. Chicago: Athletic Institute, 1948.

Beecher, C. E. *Physiology and Calisthenics for Schools and Families*. New York: Harper and Brothers, 1856.

Benson, E. and J. Q. McDevitt. *Community Health and Nursing Practice* (2d ed.). Englewood Cliffs, NJ: Prentice-Hall, 1980.

Bland, H. B. *An Analysis of the Activities of Indiana School Nurses Employed by Boards of Education.* Doctoral dissertation, Indiana University, Bloomington, 1956.

Brannon, J. W. Open-air schools in the United States. *Proceedings of the Fifth Congress of the American School Health Association.* Springfield, MA: AHSA, 1911.

Brown E. G. The 1960 White House Conference on Children and Youth. *National Parent-Teacher, 54* (October 1959): 16-18.

Byler, R. V. *Teach Us What We Want To Know.* New York: Mental Health Materials Center, 1969.

Cleary, H. Issues in the credentialing of health education specialists: A review of the state of the art. *Advances in Health Education and Promotion: A Research Manual, 1* Part A (1986): 129-154.

Cortese, P. A. Accomplishments in comprehensive school health education. *Journal of School Health, 63* (January 1993): 21-23.

Creswell, W. Professional preparation: A historical perspective. In U. S. Department of Health and Human Services, editor, *National Conference for Institutions Preparing Health Educators.* Washington, DC: Department of Health and Human Services, 1986.

Cunningham, R. *Wellness at Work.* Chicago: Inquiry, 1982.

Education Commission of the States. *Recommendations for School Health Education: A Handbook for State Policymakers.* Denver: ECS, 1981.

Ellis, J. and C. Hartley. *Nursing in Today's World* (2d ed.). New York: J. B. Lippincott, 1984.

Green, L. W. *Community Health* (6th ed.). St. Louis: Times Mirror/Mosby College Publishing, 1990.

Green, L. W., M. W. Kreuter, S. G. Deeds, and K. B. Partridge. *Health Planning: A Diagnostic Approach.* Palo Alto, CA: Mayfield Publishing, 1980.

Greenleaf, C. A., and R. E. Grout. A study of the effectiveness of a rural school health program in improving the school environment. *Milbank Memorial Fund Quarterly, 16* (April 1938): 1-17.

Grout, R. E. and E. G. Pickup. A study of pupil health practices. *Milbank Memorial Fund Quarterly, 16* (October 1938): 1-21.

Hecker, J. F. C. *The Epidemics of the Middle Ages.* London: Tribner & Co., 1839.

Hoover, D. B. Forword. *The Initial Role Delineation for Health Education: Final Report.* Bethesda, MD: U. S. Department of Health and Human Services, 1980.

Jean, S. L. Health education—some factors in its development. *News Letter,* School of Public Health, University of Michigan, *5* (June 1946): 1-4.

Johnson, J. A., H. W. Collins, V. L. Dupuis, and J. H. Johansen. *Introduction to the Foundations of American Education.* Boston: Allyn and Bacon, 1969.

Lalonde, M. *A New Perspective on the Health of Canadians: A Working Document.* Ottawa: Government of Canada, 1974.

LaSalle, D. and T. D. Wood. *Journal of Health, Physical Education, and Recreation, 31* (April 1960): 118+.

Means, R. K. *A History of Health Education in the United States.* Philadelphia: Lea & Febiger, 1962.

Means, R. K. *Historical Perspectives on School Health.* Thorofare, NJ: Charles B. Slack, 1975.

Meredith, W. F. Some trends in acceptance of credits in health and physical education for college entrance. *Research Quarterly, 4* (March 1933): 68-77.

Monteiro, L. A. Florence Nightingale on public health nursing. *American Journal of Public Health, 75* (February 1985): 181-186.

National Education Association, Commission on the Reorganization of Secondary Education. *Cardinal Principles of Secondary Education* (U. S. Department of the Interior, Bureau of Education, Bulletin No. 35). Washington, DC: Government Printing Office, 1918.

National Task Force on the Preparation and Practice of Health Educators. *Proceedings of the Second Bethesda Conference: Quality Assurance in Health Education.* New York: National Task Force, 1986.

Netcher, J. R. *Recommended Activities of Public School Nurses Employed by Boards of Education in Indiana.* Doctoral dissertation, Indiana University, Bloomington, 1956.

Nightingale, F. *Notes on Nursing: What It Is, and What It Is Not.* Philadelphia: J. B. Lippincott, 1946. (Originally published 1859)

Nyswander, D. B. *Solving School Health Problems: The Astoria Demonstration Project.* New York: Commonwealth Fund, 1942.

Oberteuffer, D. *A Program for Ohio Secondary Schools.* Columbus, OH: F. J. Heer Printing Co., 1932.

Patterson, S. M. A historical perspective of selected professional preparation conferences that have influenced credentialing for health education specialists. *Journal of Health Education, 23* (March 1992): 101-108.

Payne, E. G. and L. C. Schroeder. *Health and Safety in the New Curriculum.* New York: American Viewpoint Society, 1925.

Pickett, G., and J. J. Hanlon. *Public Health: Administration and Practice* (9th ed.). St. Louis: Times Mirror/Mosby College Publishing, 1990.

Poe, N. M. and L. W. Irwin. Functions of a school nurse. *Research Quarterly of the American Association of Health and Physical Education, 30* (December 1959): 452-464.

Pollock, M. *Planning and Implementing Health Education in Schools.* Palo Alto, CA: Mayfield Publishing, 1987.

Reaney, B. C. *Milk and Our School (Health Education No. 11).* Washington, DC: U. S. Department of the Interior, Bureau of Education, Health Education, 1922.

Report of the Committee on the Status of Physical Education in American Colleges. *American Physical Education Review, 21* (March 1916): 155-157.

Report of the Committee on the Status of Physical Education in Public Normal Schools and Public High Schools. *American Physical Education Review, 15* (June 1910): 453-454.

Report of the Joint Committee on Health Problems in Education of the NEA and the AMA. *Health Education—A Program for Public Schools and Teacher Training Institutions.* New York: National Education Association, 1924.

Report of the Joint Committee on Health Problems in Education of the National Education Association and the American Medical Association. *Open-Air Classrooms.* New York: National Tuberculosis Association, 1937.

Rice, E. A., J. L. Hutchinson, and M. Lee. *A Brief History of Physical Education* (4th ed.). New York: Ronald Press, 1958.

Rogers, J. F. *State-Wide Trends in School Hygiene and Physical Education.* U. S. Department of the Interior, Office of Education, Pamphlet #5, (rev.). Washington, DC: Government Printing Office, 1930.

Rogers, J. F. *Health Instruction in Hygiene in Grades IX-XIII* (U. S. Department of the Interior, Office of Education, Pamphlet #43). Washington, DC: Government Printing Office, 1933.

Rugen, M. *History of the Public Health Education Section.* Washington, DC: American Public Health Association, 1972.

School Health Education Study, 1961-62. *Journal of Health, Physical Education, and Recreation, 33* (January 1962): 28-29.

Shattuck, L. *Report of the Sanitary Commission of Massachusetts, 1850.* New York: Cambridge University Press, 1948.

Sliepcevich, E. M. Health Education: A Conceptual Approach to Curriculum Design. *School Health Education Study.* St. Paul, MN: 1967.

Strachan, M. L. *Fifteen Years of Child Health Education.* New York: National Tuberculosis Association, 1932.

Strachan, M. L. and E. F. Jordan. *From Pioneer to Partner.* New York: National Tuberculosis Association, 1947.

Strang, R. M., R. E. Grout and D. G. Wiehl. Evaluation of teachers' work in health education. *Milbank Memorial Fund Quarterly, 15* (October 1937): 355-370.

Turner, C. E. Malden studies on health education and growth. *American Journal of Public Health, 18* (October 1928): 1217-1230.

U. S. Department of Health, Education, and Welfare. *The Report of the President's Committee on Health Education.* Washington, DC: Government Printing Office, 1973.

U. S. Department of Health, Education, and Welfare. *Healthy People: The Surgeon General's Report on Health Promotion and Disease Prevention* (PHS Publication No. 79-55071). Washington, DC: Public Health Service, 1979.

U. S. Department of Health and Human Services. *Better Health for Our Children: A National Strategy*: Vol. 1. Major Findings and Recommendations. Washington, DC: Superintendent of Documents, 1981.

U. S. Department of Health and Human Services. *Healthy People 2000: National Health Promotion and Disease Prevention Objectives* (PHS Publication No. 91-50212). Washington, DC: Public Health Service, 1991.

U. S. Department of Health and Human Services. *Promoting Health/Preventing Disease: Objectives for the Nation*. Washington, DC: Public Health Service, 1980.

Van Ingen, P. *The Story of the American Child Health Association*. New York: American Child Health Association, 1935.

W. K. Kellogg Foundation. *An Experience in Health Education*. Battle Creek, MI: W. K. Kellogg Foundation, 1950.

4

PREVENTION AND HEALTH PROMOTION

The terms *health promotion* and *injury and illness prevention* are frequently misunderstood, even by the health educators whose responsibilities include carrying out related programs. Although they are different, they have a lot in common. Both denote the recognition of threats to health and the identification of those threats. A good deal of modern prevention education and health promotion is based on the relatively recent shift in causes of death from infectious diseases to causes more closely associated with lifestyle.

As Alles, Rubinson, and Monismith (1984) pointed out, in the context of health, prevention requires action to reduce or eliminate specific risk factors. Promotion requires effort by those who are seemingly healthy to enhance their health status beyond its present level. The distinction admittedly is a narrow one—so narrow, in fact, that the 1990 Joint Committee on Health Education Terminology (1991) chose to define the collective term "health promotion and disease prevention" as:

> . . . the aggregate of all purposeful activities designed to improve personal and public health through a combination of strategies, including the competent implementation of behavioral change strategies, health education, health protection measures, risk factor detection, health enhancement, and health maintenance.

LEVELS OF PREVENTION

A clear understanding of prevention seems to be a good starting place. Prevention occurs on three levels—primary, secondary, and tertiary. Each of the three levels has different implications for health educators, and each requires a different set of objectives and interventions.

Primary Prevention

Primary prevention emphasizes interventions to avert disease, illness, or deterioration of health before it occurs. These strategies usually incorporate health promotion, in medical, societal, and educational arenas.

Medical examples of primary prevention include scheduled immunizations and regular dental check-ups. Even though the medical care system offers some preventive services through its technology and medications, it can do little in primary prevention. The individual, together with the collective society, can do the most to improve health and longevity.

Societal interventions are exemplified by the fluoridation of water and mosquito surveillance and eradication. Indeed, primary prevention embodies a societal principle that exhorts individuals to adopt a healthy lifestyle.

Educational examples are: promoting skills that enable young people to cope with peer pressure; imparting knowledge of the relationships between weight control and heart disease; establishing nutrition programs based on a variety of healthy foods; and encouraging sexual abstinence or monogamous relationships to prevent transmission of AIDS.

The more directly a health behavior is linked to a health problem as a risk factor, the more its alteration contributes to primary prevention efforts (Greene and Simons-Morton, 1984). For example, people who are overweight and smoke cigarettes have a greater risk for diseases of the cardiovascular system. These individuals are excellent candidates for primary prevention activities aimed at reducing these risk factors.

Cardiovascular disease is the leading cause of death in the United States. Individuals can consciously decide to lower risk of cardiovascular disease by not smoking, by eating nutritious foods with low saturated fat, by learning how to deal with stress, and by exercising regularly.

The second leading cause of death in the United States is cancer. People can reduce risk of developing cancer by not smoking cigarettes, by adhering to a diet high in fiber and low in fat, and by avoiding excessive exposure to ultraviolet rays.

We all can practice primary prevention to reduce the risk of accidental injury or death. People can wear seat belts and shoulder harnesses each time they ride in a motor vehicle, forego alcohol when driving an automobile, wear safety equipment when working with machinery, and avoid three-wheeled, all-terrain vehicles.

Secondary Prevention

Secondary prevention is undertaken by identifying diseases at their earliest stages and applying appropriate treatments to limit the consequences and severity of the disease, as well as its prevalence. Secondary prevention thus entails early detection and treatment; it is curative. Medicine has long focused mainly on secondary prevention. It attempts to limit the course and destruction of conditions that already have occurred.

Medical examples of secondary prevention are numerous. Women are encouraged to have regular mammograms to detect breast cancers and Pap tests to detect cervical cancers while they are treatable. Men are advised to examine their testicles regularly to expedite treatment of testicular cancer by its early detection. People with high blood pressure are advised to take their medication as prescribed. All of us should have our cholesterol level measured periodically and make sensible decisions regarding diet and exercise to reduce high levels.

In the sphere of *education*, the health educator, or frequently the patient educator, has a crucial role in secondary prevention. Education may be the key to scheduling mammograms or to doing testicular self-examination. Educators with good communication and teaching skills often can spell the difference between minor consequences of a health problem and its development into a debilitating or life-threatening occurrence.

Schools sometimes are agents of secondary prevention. For instance, although parents seldom are aware of this, school children are inspected regularly for the telltale nits that signal the presence of headlice. Another example is the periodic vision screening of school children that most states require.

Unfortunately, medicine and most individuals have relied too heavily upon secondary prevention. Preventing a disease is obviously more cost-effective than treating it. Gradually, Americans are beginning to realize that primary prevention is more desirable than secondary prevention. In this context, the opportunity arises for developing comprehensive health education programs in the schools and broad programs of primary prevention at other sites.

Tertiary Prevention

Tertiary prevention prescribes specific interventions to assist diseased or disabled people in limiting the effects of their illness or disability. Tertiary prevention also may include activities to prevent recurrence of a disease.

This level of prevention relies heavily upon the *medical* care system. Rehabilitation and physical therapy are crucial components of tertiary prevention. It may include surgery and administering medications and counseling in lifestyle changes for patients such as those recovering from cardiac events.

Patient *education* plays an important role in tertiary prevention. Too often patients fail to follow through on their physicians' recommendations. Noncompliance is one of the main reasons for relapses. Thorough patient education can help the patients understand why making lifestyle changes or following a consistent program of rehabilitation is beneficial and can help them keep track of their own compliance and progress.

HEALTH PROMOTION

Closely related to primary prevention is health promotion, drawing from the concepts of holistic health, self-care, and disease prevention (Teague, 1987). As Greene and Simons-Morton (1984) explained:

> Health promotion begins with people who are basically healthy and seeks to develop community and individual measures which can help them adopt lifestyles which maintain and enhance the state of well-being.

In this context, "health promotion" can be defined as:

> A combination of educational, organizational, political, social, and economic interventions that have as their purpose adaptations and adjustments that will improve or protect the health of individuals who are already at a high level of health.

These adaptations and adjustments may be attitudinal, environmental, or behavioral. Health-promoting behaviors are directed toward sustaining or increasing the level of well-being, self-actualization, and fulfillment (Teague, 1987). Health education is only one strategy, though an important one, in health promotion.

The relationship between health promotion and primary prevention is clear. Both begin with healthy individuals. Both occur before the identification of health problems and are designed to help the individual maintain health and avoid injury or disease.

Leadership in the area of health promotion came, interestingly enough, from Canada. *A New Perspective on the Health of Canadians*, published in 1974 by the government of Canada under the direction of Marc Lalonde, Minister of National Health and Welfare, introduced into public policy the concept that all death and disease has four contributing elements:

1. Inadequacies in the existing health care system.
2. Behavioral factors or unhealthy lifestyles.

3. Environmental·hazards.
4. Human biological factors.

The primary theme of the document is that improvements in the environment and in individuals' lifestyles are the most effective means of averting death and disease. As a result of this report, the Canadian government began "Operation Lifestyle," which shifted the emphasis of its public policies from treatment to prevention of illness, or to "health promotion" (Bates and Winder, 1984).

The U. S. Department of Health, Education, and Welfare (1979) (now Health and Human Services) Task Force on Prevention identified 12 categories of behavior as targets of health promotion activities:

1. Smoking.
2. Nutrition.
3. Alcohol use.
4. Habituating drug use.
5. Driving.
6. Exercise.
7. Human sexuality/contraception.
8. Family development.
9. Risk management.
10. Stress management.
11. Coping/adaptation.
12. Enhanced self-esteem.

Others philosophically group the categories of smoking, alcohol use, and habituating drug use into one, because alcohol and nicotine (the active drug in tobacco) are habituating drugs. Most health promotion programs, however, treat them as separate entities because of their different etiologies, different views society takes of them, legal issues, and administrative considerations. Certainly all of these categories of health and health behavior are so integral to the American lifestyle that attempts to improve or maintain the health of large groups of people warrant their inclusion.

Emphasis on behavior, lifestyle, and personal choices is critical to health promotion. It is so crucial that Secretary of Health and Human Services Joseph Califano (1979) asserted, "You, the individual, can do more for your own health and well-being than any doctor, any hospital, any drug, any exotic medical device."

At the very least, health promotion should:

1. Enhance *self-efficacy* (Bandura, 1977), the perception of having the skills necessary to accomplish tasks necessary to affect one's own health.
2. Enhance *self-esteem* (Clark, 1978), the perception of self-worth.
3. Promote psychological *hardiness* (Kobasa, Maddi, and Kahn, 1982), the perception of control over one's life and decisions, commitment to something worthwhile, and the capacity to view change as a challenge.
4. Encourage *empowerment* (Rappaport, 1987), the development of perceptual skills associated with affecting one's environment or social system.
5. Strengthen families (Kumpfer, DeMarsh, and Child, 1988).

Health promotion can take place in a variety of settings—home, school, church, worksite, health care facility, voluntary health agencies, health maintenance organizations, prisons, private clubs, self-help groups. In fact, any milieu that can organize and plan activities has the potential to become a health promotion site.

Likewise, an assortment of professionals can engage in health promotion. In fact, it is best applied through a multidisciplinary approach. Practitioners of health promotion include physicians, nurses, exercise scientists, nutritionists, social workers, physical therapists, and health educators, among others.

Health promotion utilizes a variety of techniques. It can entail stress management, aerobic fitness, risk management and safety, environmental controls, mass media presentations, and, of course, health education. Because they have unique knowledge of content, skills in facilitating behavior change and maintenance, and abilities to plan, organize, and evaluate outcomes of programs, health educators are the cornerstone of health promotion programs. Promoting health involves advocating awareness of personal and community health, changing attitudes so behavior change is possible, and searching for alternatives to improve health (Squyres, 1985). "Increasing awareness," "changing attitudes," and "searching for alternatives" describe the essence of health education.

Over the last 75 years causes of death and suffering have shifted dramatically from infectious diseases to factors directly involved with lifestyle. This point is illustrated by the fact that today's top three causes of death in the United States—heart disease, cancer and stroke—are all frequently precipitated by poor diets, lack of exercise, and/or cigarette smoking.

Pelletier (1981) concluded that medical science is under attack because it has sought the means to health and ignored the ends. It is no doubt true that medicine has concentrated its resources on secondary and tertiary prevention. Its long history of concentration on treatment has been at the expense of real preventive medicine. Medicine deals with disease while at the same time having the tools and skills to deal with health. Only gradually and grudgingly has medicine entered the realm of health promotion and lifestyle change.

Even as acquired immune deficiency syndrome (AIDS), an infectious disease, claims more and more lives, its chief modes of transmission in the United States so far have been directly linked to lifestyle. Lifestyles that place people at greatest risk involve injectable drug use and unprotected sexual activity, especially anal sex. As most experts consider AIDS universally fatal, health promotion has become the main tool in eliminating the effects of AIDS in the uninfected individual. There is obviously a greater need to enhance and preserve the health of uninfected individuals than to wait and treat the disease.

Herein lies the role of health promotion. Many lives have been saved as the result of successful education programs directed to at-risk populations such as injectable drug users and homosexual males. Health promotion regarding AIDS should be expanded to the population at large, as everyone who is sexually active may be at risk. The AIDS epidemic has led a number of communities to change their school curricula, incorporating more frank discussions regarding sexual relations and the use of condoms. It also has contributed to more candid discussions between parents and children and in school and church. These efforts to avert the transmission of a deadly disease are the embodiment of health promotion.

Another example of a health promotion program is often carried out at wellness centers. Families and individuals are recruited

Health promotion, using a variety of techniques, can enhance and maintain health by changing attitudes and improving behavior. Age is no barrier to creative health promotion activities. Photo courtesy of Johnson & Johnson from the community and tested to determine percentage of body fat, blood pressure, and other relevant measures of fitness. Individuals are questioned regarding lifestyle factors such as exercise, diet, and smoking. A program, developed specifically for each person, may include an aerobic exercise prescription, weight control and nutrition advice, a smoking cessation program (if necessary), stress management training, and efforts to address any other obstacles to total fitness. A team of specialists, including a physician or nurse and a health educator, typically designs the program.

More examples of *educational interventions* are:

◆ stress management classes for middle management employees in a corporation;

◆ mailouts to the public, describing positive steps a person can take to reduce exposure to AIDS;

◆ health education classes for elementary school children to develop skills necessary to cope with peer pressure.

Examples of *organizational interventions* include:

◆ annual hearing screening in schools;

◆ identification of designated smoking areas and development of a smoking policy in a worksite;

◆ official recognition by business management of alcoholism as a disease and not a weakness in character;

◆ development of support groups by organizations that provide services to people with epilepsy, muscular dystrophy, cancer, and other chronic diseases and disorders.

Examples of *political/legislative interventions* include:

◆ passage of laws requiring use of seat belts in automobiles;

◆ requirement by the state Board of Education to implement a comprehensive family life curriculum in grades K-12;

◆ legislation requiring environmental polluters to measure their pollution and implement effective plans to reduce the pollution;

◆ requirement that all restaurants provide a section free from tobacco smoking.

Examples of *community and social interventions* include:

◆ organization and training of college students to avoid situations that contribute to vulnerability to sex crimes;

◆ neighborhood walking clubs;

◆ formation of wellness centers in health maintenance organizations, hospitals, and colleges, employing health educators to encourage positive health behaviors through programs that appeal to the community;

◆ establishment of a school health council made up of members of the community to encourage healthy lifestyles in children and a healthy environment in the school;

◆ health fairs at the neighborhood mall.

Examples of *economic interventions* include:

◆ insurance companies' offering incentives to those who practice healthy lifestyles;

◆ incentives from employers to those who stay healthy and do not miss work.

ROLE OF THE HEALTH EDUCATOR

Health education can play an important role in all three levels of disease and injury prevention and health promotion. Although we must keep in mind that the individual must maintain the right to make most decisions regarding practices and lifestyle, health educators often establish in the minds of participants the reason for their participation and behavior change. The health educator has the skills to assist clients in developing attainable objectives and to organize activities around those objectives.

On the most basic level, health education is the transmission of knowledge. Knowledge may help each health care professional do his or her job more effectively, and it may help each client behave in ways that are more beneficial to his or her health. Health educators are masters at getting health facts accepted and put to practical use. In addition, the professional health educator is a resource person, directing the client or student to sources of information necessary for transforming desires for health into action.

Facts, however, are not usually the determining factor in decisions about behavior. A multitude of determinants affect decisions regarding health practices. Self-concept, religious beliefs, peer pressure, cultural variables, personal values, and family models are only a few of these factors. The role of the health educator is to identify the factors that affect behavior and plan a program that will utilize various communication modes and the individual's own environment to elicit behavior that is conducive to a high level of health.

Health educators should have expertise in many different forms of communication and in many different technologies for communication. Not only do they have knowledge in different media of communication, but they also have insight into which methology to use in different situations. The range of problems, the three levels of prevention and health promotion, the size of the client group (from one to thousands), and the sensitivity of the issue demand sensible choices in methods and approaches.

Frequently health educators assist health care providers in planning the delivery of services. Health care providers may need to be informed about the community and how individuals feel about health and about certain practices and treatments. The two vignettes make this point.

Women in the Amish community are not comfortable displaying their bodies. They are not likely to take routine secondary prevention measures such as mammography, Pap tests, and breast self-examination, even though they may be at greater risk than the rest of the population for certain cancers because of diet. The health care system frequently has failed to reach the Amish community because of the provider's lack of understanding of the Amish culture. Health educators can serve as liaisons, educating Amish women in the need for these prevention steps and the health care providers in the need for sensitivity to Amish culture and sense of modesty. Once a bridge has been established between the two, a program can be established. One solution might be to conduct examinations and education programs in a neighbor's home. Because the Amish traditionally do not have electricity in their homes, a neighbor who is trusted by the Amish elders could provide a place in his home for this program.

In the fictional but nonetheless realistic example provided by the television program Northern Exposure, the young Dr. Fleishman is ignorant of the culture of the native Americans of Alaska. His only experience has been in New York City. Therefore, he is stunned by native practices regarding medicine and health. Equally amazed are some older residents of the area surrounding the community of Cicely. Only with great difficulty do they communicate health problems and remedies. If the writers of this series had invited a health educator to coach Dr. Fleishman on the customs of the native Americans of the region and to begin an education program in primary prevention in the community, the situation would have been greatly improved. It would, however, destroy much of the humor of the series.

Ware, Burt, et al. (1978) summarized the prevalent assumptions about the role of the health educator and the practice of health education in six major points:

1. Health educators have knowledge of behavioral determinants and of strategies to deal with these for any specified element of health-related behavior.

2. Health educators carry out evaluation of behavioral determinants and strategies to affirm whether they lead to or produce specific behaviors.

3. Health educators have a body of knowledge and skills to be able to assist people in their own self-care.

4. Health educators have the skills to help people evaluate possible alternatives for actions that may or may not result in any subsequent health-related behavior change.
5. Health educators have the responsibility for helping people not just to be healthy but to have something to be healthy for, whether this does or does not relate to health status.
6. Health educators facilitate, coordinate, or carry out some or all of the above.

These points are directly applicable to the role of the health educator in prevention and health promotion. Inherent in these assumptions is the health educator's knowledge of behaviors that affect health and the knowledge of what determines behavior. Health education as a discipline encompasses the knowledge and skills to assist individuals in taking control over their own lives and actions. To put this knowledge and skill to work, the health educator implements strategies dealing with any feature of health-related behavior. The health educator then must be able to evaluate the effectiveness of the strategy, including its planning and implementation, in an unbiased way. Further, health educators must aim for more than just the "absence of disease or infirmity" mentioned in the World Health Organization definition of health. They must aim for growth of the individual as a whole, self-esteem, and self-actualization. Adequately prepared health educators can carry out these objectives at all three levels of prevention.

SUMMARY

Prevention activities take place at three levels. Primary prevention consists of actions to prevent disease, illness, or deterioration of health before it occurs. Secondary prevention entails activities to identify diseases at their earliest stages and treatment to limit the consequences of the disease. Tertiary prevention is action to

assist ill or disabled people in reducing the effects of their illness or disability.

Health promotion is closely related to primary prevention. It begins with people who are basically healthy and applies creative measures to increase the likelihood that they will remain in good health. A good number of studies provides information about behaviors that contribute to health. Health promotion encourages these behaviors. Health promotion can take place in a variety of settings. An integral part of a good health promotion program is health education. Well qualified health educators frequently practice health promotion and can play an important role at all three levels of prevention.

REFERENCES

Alles, W. F., L. Rubinson, & S. Monismith. Health promotion. In L. Rubinson and W. F. Alles, *Health Education: Foundations for the Future*. Prospect Heights, IL: Waveland Press, 1984.

Bandura, A. Self-efficacy: Toward a unifying theory of behavior change. *Psychological Review, 84* (March, 1977): 191-215.

Bates, I. J., & Winder, A. E. *Introduction to Health Education*. Palo Alto, CA: Mayfield Publishing, 1984.

Califano, J. A., Jr. *Healthy People: The Surgeon General's Report on Health Promotion and Disease Prevention* (Publication No. 79-55074), Washington, DC: Public Health Service, 1979.

Clark, J. I. *Self Esteem: A Family Affair*. San Francisco: Harper and Row, 1978.

Greene, W. H. and B. G. Simons-Morton. *Introduction to Health Education*. Prospect Heights, IL: Waveland Press, 1984.

Kobasa, S. C., S. R. Maddi, and S. Kahn. Hardiness and health: A prospective study. *Journal of Personality and Social Psychology, 42* (January 1982): 168-177.

Kumpfer, K., J. DeMarsh, and W. P. Child. *Strengthening Family Program Parenting Handbook*. Salt Lake City: University of Utah, 1988.

Lalonde, M. *A New Perspective on the Health of Canadians: A Working Document* (Catalog No. H31-1374). Ottawa: Government of Canada, 1974.

1990 Joint Committee on Health Education Terminology. Report of the 1990 Joint Committee on Health Education. *Journal of School Health, 61* (August 1991): 251-254.

Pelletier, R. *Longevity: Fulfilling Our Biological Potential*. New York: Delacort Press/Seymour Lawrence, 1981.

Rappaport, J. Terms of empowerment/exemplars of prevention: Toward a theory for community psychology. *American Journal of Community Psychology, 15* (April 1987): 121-148.

Squyres, W. D. *Patient Education and Health Promotion in Medical Care*. Palo Alto, CA: Mayfield Publishing, 1985.

Teague, M. L. *Health Promotion Programs: Achieving High-Level Wellness in the Later Years*. Iowa City, IA: Benchmark Press, 1987.

U. S. Department of Health, Education and Welfare. *Healthy People: The Surgeon General's Report on Health Promotion and Disease Prevention: Background Papers*. Washington, DC: Public Health Service, 1979.

Ware, B. G., J. J. Burt, et al. *A new and accurate mappe of the world of health education drawne according to the latest discoveries—1978*. Unpublished background paper of Conference on Preparation and Practice of Health Education, Bethesda, MD, Feb. 15-17, 1978.

5

COMPREHENSIVE SCHOOL HEALTH EDUCATION

Health education takes place in a multitude of settings—hospitals, clinics, voluntary health agencies, and worksites, among others. The most appropriate place for health education to take place, however, is the school. School health instruction within a complete school health program is a basic part of the overall mission of education, for a number of specific reasons:

1. Pupils spend a major part of their young lives in school. We owe it to our children to safeguard their health and help them make decisions that will enhance their health.

2. Compared to other settings, schools offer the best opportunity to provide high-quality health instruction.

3. In many cases we can influence healthy living habits and attitudes in children before they establish habits that are detrimental to health.

4. Health is a "basic," addressed in the *Cardinal Principles of Secondary Education* (Commission on the Reorganization of Education, 1918/1928) equally as basic as the development of fundamental mathematics or language skills. Actually, the objectives of comprehensive health education are related closely to other cardinal principles: worthy home membership, citizenship, worthy use of leisure time, and ethical character (Seffrin, 1990).

School health education should not be haphazard, as many efforts have been in the past but, rather, a well-planned curricular endeavor practiced and evaluated realistically by trained professionals. It should be a comprehensive program from kindergarten through high school graduation. It must cover a variety of appropriate learning experiences suitable to the grade level. Effective health education is based upon a realistic assessment of pupil needs, interests, and capabilities. Community and parental values and interests also should be implicit to health education programs.

All of these issues form the concept of what has come to be called comprehensive school health education. As stated by the National Professional School Health Education Organizations (1984), comprehensive school health education is:

> . . . health education in a school setting that is planned and carried out with the purpose of maintaining, reinforcing, or enhancing the health, health-related skills, and health attitudes and practices of children and youth that are conducive to their health.

More recently, the 1990 Joint Committee on Health Education Terminology (1991) defined comprehensive school health program:

> A comprehensive school health program is an organized set of policies, procedures, and activities designed to protect and promote the health and well-being of students and staff which has traditionally included health services, healthful school environment, and health education. It should also include, but not be limited to, guidance and counseling, physical education, food service, social work, psychological services, and employee health promotion.

Traditionally, the school health program has consisted of three interdependent components: school health instruction, health services, and a healthful school environment. The three components feed each other, each helping the others to be stronger and more effective. The interdependency of the three components becomes more important as comprehensive school health education (CSHE) evolves.

SCHOOL HEALTH INSTRUCTION

The instructional component is the foundation of the comprehensive school health education program. The 1990 Joint Committee on Health Education Terminology (1991) defined the comprehensive school health instruction component as follows:

> Comprehensive school health instruction refers to the development, delivery, and evaluation of a planned curriculum, preschool through 12, with

goals, objectives, content sequence, and specific classroom lessons which includes, but is not limited to, the following major content areas: community health; consumer health; environmental health; family life; mental and emotional health; injury prevention and safety; nutrition; personal health; prevention and control of disease, and substance use and abuse.

10 Benefits of Comprehensive School Health Education Programs

◆ Less school vandalism

◆ Improved attendance by students and staff

◆ Reduced health care costs

◆ Reduced substitute teaching costs

◆ Better family communication, even on sensitive issues such as sexuality

◆ Stronger self-confidence and self-esteem

◆ Noticeably fewer students using tobacco

◆ Improved cholesterol levels for students and staff

◆ Increased seat-belt use

◆ Improved physical fitness

Source: American Association of School Administrators, *Healthy Kids for the Year 2000: An Action Plan for Schools,* Arlington, VA, 1990. Reprinted by permission.

A number of authors and commentators (for example, Davis et al., 1985, and the National Professional School Health Education Organizations, 1984) have provided rather extensive lists of criteria for, or elements of, comprehensive school health education. Certainly, the concept of CSHE is a departure from the old notions of hygiene class and coverage of health-related topics in isolation. The focus of CSHE is the total person. A number of elements define CSHE.

Element 1

CSHE promotes wellness and motivation for health maintenance and improvement. Although this philosophy implies prevention of disease and disability, it takes a secondary position to the concept of overall wellness.

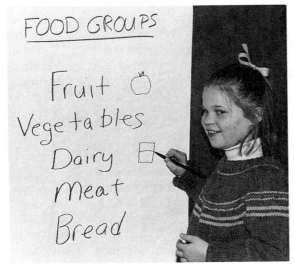

In comprehensive school health education, content areas are addressed with attention to the physical, mental, social, and emotional dimensions.

Element 2

The basis for study is the integration of physical, mental, emotional, and social dimensions of health. Content areas such as substance abuse, consumer health, and environmental health are addressed with reference to each of the health dimensions.

Element 3

Opportunities are provided for pupils to develop and demonstrate health-related knowledge, attitudes, and practices.

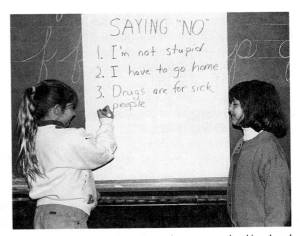

Students should be allowed to demonstrate health-related knowledge, attitudes, and practices.

Element 4

The activities have specific program goals and objectives based upon health-related knowledge, attitudes, and practices, as well as problem-solving skills, intellectual and personal skills, scientific thinking, self-assessment, self-management, and self-discipline.

Element 5

The coursework is in coordination with other subjects. Although a separate course in health instruction is needed, especially at the middle and high school levels, health instruction should be coordinated with most and integrated into some other subject areas. Just as the language arts have promoted "writing across the curriculum," certain parts of health education can be promoted as "health across the curriculum." English teachers can assign compositions and term papers related to health topics. Mathematics courses can utilize health data as examples, problems, and graphing exercises. Likewise, social studies, science and home economics classes can include health-related exercises in a number of creative ways.

Because most of the major health problems facing young people are grounded in a number of factors, a single message delivered by one teacher is not enough to change behavior. Consistent and repeated messages delivered by several teachers, the school staff, peers, and parents can be more effective at altering behavior (Bremberg, 1991; Elder, 1991).

If educators are willing to spend some time together in close communication, the opportunities are endless. As we seek to integrate health education into other disciplines, however, we must be careful not to relinquish the identity and uniqueness of health education as a discipline.

Element 6

The CSHE program offers educational opportunities for the family and community members. This is justified by the fact that the school is a part of the community and that the school is obligated to provide services for members of the community. By providing educational activities for the family and community at large, the school can gain valuable support for CSHE. This often strips away much of the mystery surrounding health education and eliminates a good deal of the opposition from people who do not understand the nature of CSHE.

Element 7

The program is a planned, sequential K-12 (possibly starting at preschool) curriculum, based upon student needs, current and emerging health concepts, and societal issues. The scope of the program, defined as the total range of subject areas or health topics selected to represent the body of knowledge (Pollock and Middleton, 1989), first must be selected. Although they were conceived in the 1960s, the 10 conceptual statements developed by the School Health Education Study (Sliepcevich, 1967) are an excellent place to start in deciding the scope

of the instructional program. They provide a basis for developing goals and objectives leading to instructional strategies and eventually to evaluation. After defining the scope, the ordering of organizing elements, or the sequence, must be dealt with. The ordering of elements through the grade levels is called the vertical sequence. The horizontal sequence is a plan for ordering the elements within the time allotted in a grade or semester. Care must be taken to emphasize the dimensions of health—physical, mental, social, and emotional—in both scope and sequence lest the curriculum degenerate to simply imparting a set of facts.

Element 8

CSHE affords opportunities for family members and concerned community members to provide input into curriculum development and classroom experiences. This can diffuse opposition to health education and give educators insight into community values and attitudes. Historically, most efforts to improve school health education have come from health professionals, with little or no involvement of school educators (Allanson, 1981). Now, we should not overreact and eliminate these health professionals from the curriculum process. Health educators have long been taught the value of involving in the planning process those expected to implement the program (Lewin, 1958). In CSHE, a partnership is struck among health educators, other school personnel, parents, family members, and health professionals to share insights, talents, and concerns for the good of children.

Element 9

CSHE provides leadership and coordination through an effective management system. A number of models can be effective. The most traditional is the *school health council*, set up on the building level. In this model a council made up of teachers, the school nurse, physicians, parents, students, voluntary health agencies, the health department, and other interested parties provides direction to the health education program. The basic functions of the school health council, according to Cornacchia, Olsen, and Nickerson, (1991) are to:

1. Identify health and safety problems of pupils and school personnel;
2. Study these problems;
3. Make recommendations to the school administration for solving the problems.

The council could, however, carry out other functions, such as arranging for speakers and providing necessary materials not supplied by the school district.

In Delaware each school has its own building coordinator for health education, who acts as a liaison with the Department of Public Instruction, interpreting policy decisions and serving on committees that address health education issues. Delaware also has a State School Health Advisory Committee, made up of teachers, district superintendents, representatives from higher education, school nurses, members of the medical profession, and others with expertise in health education or health-related issues. The committee advises the legislature and the Department of Public Instruction on matters relating to health education.

Element 10

CSHE emphasizes resources, and materials appropriate to cultural, ethnic, and geographical traits. Resources include equipment, materials, videos, teachers, and management staff. The materials are directed to a variety of student interests, learning styles, skills, and abilities. Continuing education and staff development are provided.

Element 11

Planned and ongoing inservice programs are provided for teachers and key school personnel, including the principal, nurse, and curriculum specialists. This allows people who are planning and delivering instruction to stay current and continue to improve their skills.

Element 12

CSHE requires continual assessment and evaluation to determine if the objectives are met. Among aspects to be evaluated are student gains in knowledge, attitudes, and behavior; the process of implementing the curriculum; how current the curriculum and materials are; and parent, student, and community perceptions of the program's value.

SCHOOL HEALTH ENVIRONMENT

Even the most carefully planned health instruction program is hindered if it is practiced in an unhealthy environment. Therefore, the school health environment is an important component of CSHE. Unfortunately, schools in the 1990s frequently are beset with hazardous materials and deteriorating construction and are open to community violence. The overall purpose of the environment is to establish a safe climate for children, enabling them to feel good about being in school and enhancing opportunities for learning.

The school environment begins with site selection and design. Most states prescribe the type and amount of land to be used, size of rooms, number of restrooms, drinking fountains, and other construction specifications. Frequently, in planning school buildings, committees are formed to locate a site and draw up specifications within limitations promulgated by the state. Concerned health educators should be included in these committees, as their insight

A 12-Step Action Plan for Developing a Comprehensive Health Education Program

1. **Make the health of students and staff a priority for your schools.**

   When school leaders, including school board members, make the health of students and staff a priority, design policy, and support funding for a program, the chances for the program's success are greatly enhanced.

2. **Make a policy commitment to comprehensive school health education.**

   When developing a sound health policy, school leaders will want to:
   - consider the scope of local health concerns;
   - consider state and federal requirements;
   - review the national health objectives;
   - visit successful programs and bring speakers to talk about school health;
   - be willing to weather controversies related to family, religious, and cultural beliefs and values;
   - be ready to use a reasoned approach in taking stands against local businesses whose products may be damaging to health, even if the taxes help support the school system;
   - prepare a written policy and share it with others, especially school staff and board.

3. **Form a school health education advisory committee or task force.**

   This group can give direction, assist with activities, and provide feedback on health education needs and programs. Keep the committee small with leaders from these and other appropriate groups: parents, students, school board members and administrators, school health education experts, community health professionals, state and county health and education officials, higher education, business and industry, religious organizations.

4. **Assess health, attitudes, behaviors, values, and needs.**

   If staff, parents, and others feel skeptical of a comprehensive approach, you will need to explore the reasons. Take a look at current school courses, and school and community programs and determine if they meet your needs; what attitudes, behaviors, and values are expressed; if they reflect the community's current philosophy about health.

5. **Set goals, objectives, and evaluation criteria.**

   This should be done at both the district and the school levels and communicated to all. Flexibility should be built in and new programs phased in so staff is not overwhelmed. Program goals should address prevention, crisis intervention, and follow-up. Instructional goals and objectives should be age-appropriate and should allow qualitative and quantitative feedback. There also should be goals that relate to school leadership and staffing; staff development; sustained commitment and involvement of the community; and building awareness at the local, state, and national levels. Policies on the overall evaluation of and accountability for comprehensive school health are also a *must*.

6. Decide on curricula.

Before decisions about curriculum can be made, the concept of comprehensive health education must be accepted. Many good curricula are available. Curricula also can be developed locally. Students need candid, age-appropriate information on numerous topics relating to health. Health education and skills development can blend into existing curricula. Whatever curricula are chosen, they should be sensitive to cultural diversity, parental values, and students' needs.

7. Appoint a coordinator.

Choose a strong leader to oversee the program districtwide, preferably a professional health educator. Be sure the coordinator has sufficient time and expertise to make the program work. The coordinator should be knowledgeable about other school health programs and politically astute in working with community groups and coalitions. The coordinator may, among other responsibilities:

◆ coordinate the development of the health curriculum with input from the advisory committee;

◆ train new teachers;

◆ organize and lead parent-information meetings;

◆ write grants;

◆ schedule health screening and follow-up activities;

◆ administer the staff wellness program;

◆ teach portions of the curriculum.

8. Invest in a staff wellness program.

A typical staff wellness program offers periodic physical exams and health screening tests, followed by a meeting with a health educator, school nurse, or other health professional to set goals for better personal health. School-sponsored activities can include smoking cessation groups, stress management workshops, and aerobics groups. The wellness program can build support from employees. Consistent funding and frequent publicity are crucial.

9. Provide staff development to ensure winning teaching methods.

Districts should provide ongoing staff development and training that will enable teachers to incorporate new and different health curricula and instructional strategies that have proven to be effective. Teachers should be comfortable in using action-oriented instruction, enlisting peer leadership and support, involving parents, and engaging students in their own learning.

10. Seek long-term funding and commitment.

To be effective, the program, must be a part of long-term development plans, programming, and budgets. Local commitment is critical and may come from sources outside the district office, including medical and youth-serving agencies, businesses, and service clubs.

11. Foster sustained community involvement.

Success of the school health program is tied closely to community support. Many community members will welcome the opportunity to volunteer time; share expertise; and donate materials, facilities, and money, but you will have to ask. Don't wait for the community to come to you. Build coalitions with organizations to cooperatively plan programs that feature guest speakers and provide school-based services.

12. Ensure evaluation and accountability.

Evaluate regularly, based on the criteria you established in the developmental phase and in light of your objectives. Update and modify the program based upon the results of evaluation.

Adapted from: *Healthy Kids for the Year 2000: An Action Plan for Schools* (American Association of School Administrators, Arlington, VA 1990).

---

into safety and other health concerns may be absent otherwise. The committee's responsibilities might be:

1. To assist in selecting the architect who will design the school (Redican, Olsen, and Baffi, 1993).
2. To review budgetary items, particularly cost-cutting proposals (Jenne and Greene, 1976).
3. To serve in an advisory capacity to the architect, builder, and local board of education (Redican et al., 1993).
4. To the degree members are qualified, to inspect the building during and after construction, keeping alert to obvious safety violations and structural defects (Jenne and Greene, 1976).

Site selection and construction planning should include:

◆ enough space for playgrounds;
◆ adequate space for growth and adaptation;
◆ acceptable water supply and sewage system availability;
◆ access to traffic but away from main traffic arteries;
◆ location away from businesses that generate noise or other forms of pollution and truck traffic;
◆ location away from landfills, dumps, incinerators;
◆ a large indoor space for play;
◆ restrooms and drinking fountains inside classrooms or within sight of classroom door;
◆ sinks with running water inside each classroom;
◆ separate restrooms for teachers.

The playground is an important part of the school environment. It can contribute to children's emotional health or be a virtual minefield of physical hazards. Playgrounds should be fenced and have a large shaded area. Playground equipment should be inspected weekly and repaired immediately. The possibility of student injury and accompanying litigation is great. When children are on the playground, they always should be adequately supervised. The

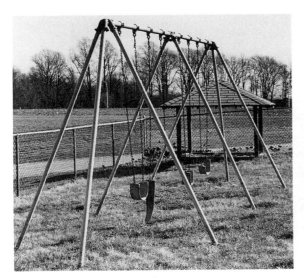

Poorly maintained playground equipment can pose serious safety hazards for children.

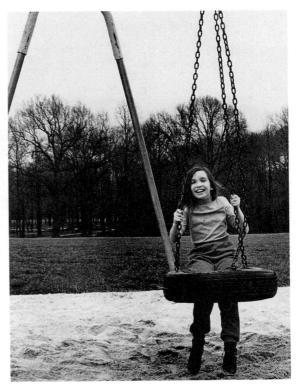

Well planned, well constructed, and properly maintained playgrounds can provide wonderful environments for play and learning.

days when school playgrounds were havens for after-school and summer play are unfortunately in the past. Now we recommend no unsupervised use of a playground after school hours.

Safety procedures should be written and disseminated to each school employee. Appropriate versions of the safety document should be given to parents and children as well. The procedures should include specific instructions on dealing with hazards and emergencies. The buildings and grounds should be inspected regularly for hazards. This is an excellent learning opportunity for pupils.

Teachers, not just the school nurse, should be trained in first aid. A well-stocked first aid kit is imperative.

Traffic safety is a vital element of school operation, as many injuries occur in transit to and from school. It also provides opportunity for teaching and learning. Proper signage and training of crossing guards is a matter of law, and school personnel should be involved. School buses frequently are under school or district jurisdiction. Millions of children ride buses each day, so maintenance, operation, and safety

policies are a grave matter of life and safety. Although much of this is out of the hands of health educators, bus safety education is a practical part of the health instruction. For example, children might be asked to write a safety policy booklet for the bus, incorporating rules they see as important. They might go on a bus inspection with the principal, examining the windows for loose glass; inspecting the seats for safe construction and exposed dangerous surfaces; identifying emergency exits; and examining fire extinguishers, seatbelts (if required), first aid kits, and other features.

School security has become a major issue in modern society. Physical attacks, kidnaping, and weapons have become all too common in America's schools. This situation often makes it

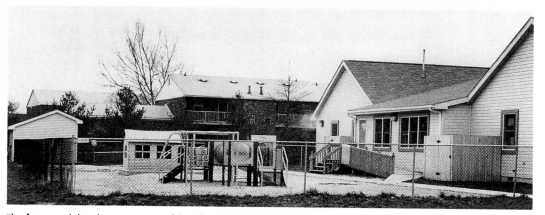

The fence and the close proximity of the playground to the main building at this Head Start center provide security for the children.

difficult for pupils and teachers to concentrate on the teaching and learning for which schools exist. A number of schools have employed police officers to patrol the grounds and halls. Some principals carry two-way radios and clubs to keep order. What are the solutions to this repugnant state of affairs? Although no one solution is satisfactory in every school, a few ideas may be helpful.

A committee should be formed to address school security *before* injuries or threatening incidents occur. The committee should consist of teachers, school board members, parents, police officers, members of the school health council (if any), and parties who command respect in the community, such as ministers. Because of the safety concerns involved, the health educator should be a member of the committee. Each building should be inspected to identify trouble spots. A policy complying with board and state policy, but specific to the school, should be developed. Even though schools should develop individual policies in accordance with their own problems, all policy statements should contain the points that:

◆ any visitors who enter the building will first go to the office;

◆ doors that may present problems will be locked from the inside;

◆ halls and stairwells will be monitored during times of student traffic;

◆ no one will pick up a child from school or a bus without written permission from the parent or guardian.

A great deal has been made of the "drug-free school zone" initiatives. Signs announcing participation adorn many streets leading to schools. We should remember that the drug-delivering product that takes more lives than all the others combined is tobacco. Schools should be totally smoke-free. For those who need assistance, smoking-cessation programs should be provided.

The emotional atmosphere of the school and the classrooms is crucial to learning. All adults who work in the school should strive to make it a warm and friendly place where pupils feel welcome and comfortable. Children should be greeted by name when they approach a teacher, principal, secretary, and other school personnel. It means a great deal to a child to know that the custodian or a teacher down the hall knows his or her name. It means the child is an important part of the school. When a child is not addressed by name, the youngster often infers that he or she is not important enough for people to take the time to learn the child's name.

Teachers should learn the names of their pupils on the first day of school. Likewise, classmates should know each others' names on the first day of school. A number of fun activities promote the learning of names. Individual worth is important to young children, and calling them by name is one way to promote individuality and self-esteem.

Hallways and classrooms should be decorated with pupils' work soon after the beginning of school. Bulletin boards are excellent places to display pupils' work. No pupil should be excluded. Everyone's efforts should be considered worthwhile.

Every child's opinion is important and should be taken seriously. Each child should be encouraged to participate within the bounds of the activity. Although taunting and teasing are almost impossible to avoid, these expressions should be discouraged when they are observed. They only serve to create a negative atmosphere and damage efforts to establish cooperation and equality.

The physical environment of the school and classroom can contribute greatly to the learning process. Therefore, classrooms should be bright, colorful, and lively. Halls and classrooms should be well-lighted. Teachers should make sure that lighting is constant. Desks never should face windows, as children are easily distracted. Teachers should take pains to assure that pupils are not bothered by glare, especially when utilizing video productions.

The classroom should not be drafty. Children are affected more by temperature than adults are. Because they have a higher metabolic rate and often a layer of insulating fat, children are comfortable at temperatures lower than adults usually prefer. The primary consideration should be the children's comfort. This becomes a problem during fall and spring in schools that have no air-conditioning. Often, little learning takes place in classrooms that are too hot.

A classroom with appropriate colors can directly impact feelings of safety and security. It also can produce the desired emotions. For northern exposures, warm colors such as yellow are recommended; for southern exposures, cool colors such as light blue are suggested. Light pastels help to attain proper reflectance. Light colors are recommended for large areas (Redican, Olsen and Baffi, 1993).

Teachers, particularly health educators, should not miss the opportunity to use the school environment as a teaching/learning tool. Occasions frequently arise to discuss sanitation, the role of color and emotions, safety hazards, and a multitude of other environmental factors.

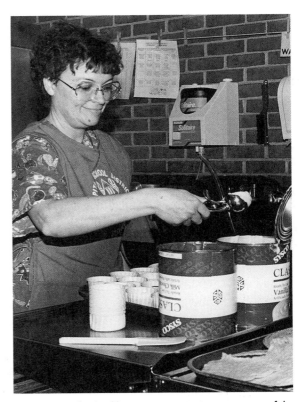

Opportunities for health instruction exist in many areas of the school. The lunch room and kitchen are areas that can be incorporated into health instruction.

SCHOOL HEALTH SERVICES

Schools provide health services daily. These encompass all procedures to promote, appraise, and protect the health of every child in the school. They are provided by physicians, nurses, dentists, teachers, counselors, dieticians, principals, and others. The rationale for school health services is clear and simple: If we receive a healthy child, we are obligated to return the child to the home in at least an equal state of health. Beyond that, we should take every opportunity to improve the child's current health and to enhance his or her chance for future well-being. School health services can reinforce the efforts of parents and the medical community in promoting the health of children.

School health services should be integrated with the health instructional component. Newman (1982) has spoken out quite forcefully against separating health services and health instruction. Asserting that the justification for health services in schools is that they contribute to the schools' educational goals, he suggests that integrating services with instruction provides benefits in three ways:

1. Benefits accrue when health service programs identify problems that interfere with learning.

2. Benefits are seen when health services support the effectiveness of the professional education staff. For example, identifying and proposing solutions to health problems that cause inattention, disruptions to the class, and other disciplinary problems clearly benefit the educational process.

3. Integrating services with instruction benefits the schools' mission when each contributes to pupil's health knowledge and practices. Students assume more responsibility for maintaining their own health.

Schlitt (1992) pointed out that the school's ability to reach children and youth who do not have access to the health care system and who are at highest risk for health problems and potentially life-threatening behaviors is unmatched. The advantages (Klein and Sadowski, 1990) of school health service programs are that they:

◆ are equitable, by offering an entry point into the health care system for all children;

◆ can provide a broad range of comprehensive, preventive services not reimbursed by most health insurance policies;

◆ are confidential;

◆ are user-friendly, because the services are provided in a trusting and familiar environment;

◆ are convenient, making teens more likely to walk in spontaneously.

Appraisal

Appraising aspects of each child's health is an important aspect of school health services. Health care for young people is episodic and crisis-related. Opportunities for preventive health screenings are scarce for many children (Schubiner, 1989), for whom school health appraisals become the only source of early diagnosis. The purposes of appraisal are to:

◆ locate pupils needing medical or dental treatment;

◆ locate pupils who need modified programs;

◆ locate pupils who need thorough medical examinations;

◆ notify parents and school personnel of the child's health status;

◆ help students and teachers make adjustments which promote the learning process;

◆ reduce illness, illness-related disabilities, and their associated costs;

◆ serve as learning experiences for pupils.

Continuous observation

Eisner and Callan (1974) asserted:

The classroom teacher should become the focus of case finding, and the child's behavior and functioning should become the primary indicators of his or her health. If this were done, school physicians could devote their time and attention to those children who have been identified as having problems.

To this end, continuous observation by the classroom teacher can be the most critical part of the appraisal process. The classroom teacher is the one in the school who knows the child best. Not only can the teacher compare the child's appearance and behavior to what is normal for the age group but also to what is normal for that child. Successful appraisal requires some teacher training.

The teacher should be alert for signs of communicable diseases, which include fatigue, flushed face, sleepiness, fever, or rash. The teacher can look for signs of hearing deficiency such as turning the head to one side, cupping the ear, misunderstanding directions, or mispronouncing words frequently. The classroom teacher is often the first person to notice signs of vision problems such as squinting.

Emotional problems may be indicated by a child's behavioral change, such as from being outgoing to being withdrawn. Irritability or hyperactivity also may suggest emotional problems.

Occasionally the family does not notice speech difficulties such as failure to pronounce certain consonants or stuttering. The teacher should not ignore these signs.

Signs of social problems such as child abuse and neglect, drug use, or alcoholism in the family often manifest themselves in children's behavior, appearance, stories they make up, pictures or relationships with other children. In most states, adults, including teachers, are legally mandated to report signs of abuse or neglect.

Procedurally, the elementary school teacher should make an effort to observe each child at some part of the day, paying attention to verbal and nonverbal behavior. Because children of low-income and disadvantaged families have a greater incidence of health problems, these children should get extra attention. Keeping notes on each child to identify patterns is a good practice. At no time should the teacher attempt to diagnose a health problem or to render medical care beyond basic first-aid or emergency care. Any concerns should be referred to the appropriate professional, usually the school nurse or counselor.

Screening

Screening is a preliminary low-cost appraisal technique, the purpose of which is to identify health problems that point to referral and diagnosis by trained specialists. Simply put, it identifies students who deviate from the average on one or more of a series of tests. Screening often is done by teachers, nurses, and trained volunteers.

Health screening can take several forms. Various tests can be conducted separately or, more commonly, as a battery of tests administered in a single session. When a battery of tests is used, it is referred to as *multiphasic screening*. Regardless of the format, screening presents an opportunity for health instruction after administering the tests. When appropriate, teachers should discuss the nature of the test, what it was measuring and evaluating, and possible steps to mitigate any deficiencies found.

Some examples of screening are those for vision, hearing, scoliosis, headlice, overweight, and underweight. Screening also may include blood tests for certain illnesses in high-risk groups. The Boehringer Mannheim Reflotron is a device for yielding measures of cholesterol in about 3 minutes at low cost.

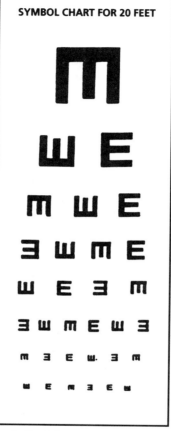

Snellen letter chart

Snellen E chart

Copyrighted by the National Society to Prevent Blindness. Reprinted by permission.

much higher than that of other forms of appraisal. Nevertheless, it provides the opportunity to establish a family doctor-patient relationship where none exists. For this reason, and because the family doctor is more qualified than anyone else to evaluate any change in the child's health status, the physician should conduct these examinations.

Most school districts have their own form for the exam and the health history the physician fills out during the examination. The forms are kept in school records, or the results are entered into the district computer system.

Regular medical examinations have a number of purposes:

1. They may identify problems that have not been identified through other appraisal techniques.

2. They enhance the physician-patient relationship.

3. They present the opportunity for the child and parent or guardian to get the answers to important health questions.

4. Particularly for adolescents, they usually provide reassurance that they are normal.

Medical examination

Comprehensive medical examinations are the best means of appraising a child's overall level of health. Most school districts and states require medical examinations. The number and regularity vary according to state and district policy. At a minimum, at least four regular physical examinations should be required during the K-12 school span.

The examination usually is done by the family physician, health department physician, or a physician or nurse-practitioner employed by the school district. Obviously this makes the cost

Dental examination and services

Dental decay is the most common health defect in school-age children. For this reason, a dentist or dental hygienist should conduct an examination of every child. This also presents an opportunity for young dentists to acquaint themselves with children and their families, so they may be willing to conduct examinations in school at a reduced fee. In some areas, public health dentists perform dental screenings.

The dental examination provides an excellent opportunity for education about diet, flossing, brushing, and fluoride applications. Some school districts provide free fluoride applications to children who live in areas where drinking water is not fluoridated. Information should be sent home to parents, reinforcing this educational program.

Psychological examination and testing

Various procedures are available to test certain aspects of personality, social acceptance, self-concept, intelligence, aptitude, and achievement. These should be administered by psychologists, psychometrists, and specially trained mental health counselors. Only those with specific training should interpret the results. Results can be used to diagnose problems, prescribe therapy, place students in learning groups, and refer students for treatment. The results of these examinations should remain confidential.

Emergency Care

Accidents are the leading cause of death in children. School grounds and buildings frequently are sites of injuries. Children also incur injuries coming to and going from school. The school has a fourfold responsibility in emergency care and accident prevention:

1. We must prevent accidents by foreseeing hazards and correcting them.
2. We must provide a good safety education portion of the health instruction program, including warnings about hazards that are not readily correctable. We also must establish safe habits in children, and a philosophy that accidents are preventable and we all have a responsibility to prevent them.
3. The school must have a written plan for handling emergencies, including access to names,

addresses, and telephone numbers of parents and guardians, as well as a person to contact when parents or guardians are not available. It should include the name of the family doctor, the hospital of preference, and any special medical problems the child may have, such as allergies and chronic disorders.
4. The school should have several employees, in addition to the school nurse, who are trained in first-aid treatment, to lessen the consequences of injuries. First-aid kits, cots or beds, and a quiet place for recovery should be a part of every emergency plan.

The plan should include provisions for transporting children to hospitals if necessary. A policy should be in place for releasing the child to the care of an adult. Under no circumstances should a child be released to another adult without the written permission of the parent or guardian.

School personnel should not administer medication without securing written permission from the parent unless it is deemed a life-threatening situation. Even over-the-counter remedies should be withheld unless written permission is given.

If the child is sent home, calling to check on the child's condition is always a good idea. This reemphasizes the school's commitment to the child's welfare. A report of each incident should be on file in the school office.

Health Guidance

The aim of health guidance is to help pupils discover, understand, and resolve health matters through their own efforts. With guidance, pupils can uncover and use their own natural endowments to acquire the highest level of wellness possible. Teachers, especially at the elementary school level, work closely with children and have a unique opportunity to offer guidance.

Guidance can take many forms, including problem solving and helping children and parents see cause-and-effect relationships between behavior and outcomes. It also can serve as motivation to act.

Counseling is a significant part of guidance. Trained counselors can interpret a problem to students and parents and help them work out solutions so they can achieve high-level wellness through their own actions. Counseling usually takes the form of one-on-one discussions with pupils or their parents, although it can involve both parents and children. Counseling and follow-through can have tremendous input in promoting health.

Regardless of the exact format of the guidance, the teacher, nurse, or counselor should assure that the session receives total attention. Nothing can destroy a guidance session quicker than interruptions.

Communicable Disease Control

On most days in most schools, children come to school ill or become ill after arriving. At these times, decisions must be made to protect other pupils and school personnel. Alert teachers frequently identify sick children during routine observation.

Policies regarding infectious disease and exclusion of students should be well-known to all personnel. Administrators have to be familiar with state laws and school district rules. By consulting pupil records, the nurse can contact parents, guardians, or other adult named on the record to take the child home or to a physician. Someone should follow up by calling about the child later in the day or the next day. The follow-up is important because it emphasizes the school's concern for the child and may provide information about a disease to which other children have been exposed. Policy should dictate the conditions under which a note from a physician is necessary for the child to return to school. Certainly, the teacher should observe the child carefully for a few days for signs of relapse.

Parents should be encouraged to keep the child home if he or she is ill. Unfortunately, many children are allowed to come to school when they are sick because parents feel obligated to be on the job and cannot arrange child care.

The health educator can utilize cases of illness to educate parents about symptoms, means of transmission, prevention, and control of infectious diseases. Flyers sent home with children can be an excellent source of information for parents.

Health Records

A cumulative health record for each child should be stored at the school site or in the computer system so it is accessible to school personnel. This can provide indispensable information regarding reports of teacher observations, screening, medical, dental, and psychometric exams, nurse's reports, and immunization records. It can be a valuable service to the child or parent when emergencies arise or when referral is necessary.

Health records should not contain any subjective statements or value judgments. The only diagnoses to be contained in the record are those by qualified professionals.

Health records should be maintained separate from academic and disciplinary records. Federal law requires that all written records from physicians to schools receiving federal funds be open to parental inspection. Parents may review, challenge the accuracy of, or seek correction of a health record. Health records cannot be released to a third party without the permission of a parent or guardian. Policy should indicate which individuals have access to health records, keeping in mind the children's right to confidentiality.

Health of the Physically Handicapped

Schools are required by law (Palfrey, Mervis, and Butler, 1978; *Irving Independent School District*

v. *Tatro*, 1984) to provide educational opportunities to all children no matter how severe their handicaps. Even though this requirement may present challenges to the school, it does afford the opportunity for communication regarding children with severe special health care needs.

One innovative program addressing these challenges is Project School Care in Massachusetts (Palfrey et al., 1992). Project School Care provides consultation to school systems as they integrate children assisted by medical technology into educational settings. This program emphasizes the importance of early notification of appropriate school personnel about the child who is dependent upon technology (e.g., respirator, tracheostomy, colostomy, urethral catheter, oxygen assistance). A team is created for each child to plan and create a safe environment that enhances the educational experiences of the child with special health care needs. The team usually consists of the child's parents, health care providers, special education or regular education staff (including health educators), and community providers. A health coordinator is responsible for health assessment, training, and monitoring. A Health Care Plan is designed for each child, documenting the child's needs and health condition, technical aspects of the child's health care including nutrition requirements, medication needs, and provision of oxygen or other respiratory supplements. Specific emergency procedures for that child are included in the Health Care Plan.

Prior to the child's enrollment, school personnel are trained regarding the Health Care Plan and the child's special needs. The child's health status is monitored frequently, and the Health Care Plan is reviewed after a major health event, such as hospital admission. Project School Care has enabled children with severe medical conditions to attend school, learn, and become an integral part of their classes.

Health of School Personnel

Even though illness hampers teachers' effectiveness and puts children at risk, the issue of health of school personnel is often ignored. Teachers are role models. When they smoke or are obese, they are giving tacit approval for their pupils to follow suit. When they exercise regularly, maintain ideal weight, and demonstrate other health practices, their pupils also take note.

Frequently, health education programs for school personnel can do wonders in changing adult behaviors. The health educator can easily plan sensible weight reduction programs, smoking cessation programs, and regular exercise opportunities. We should not forget the importance of healthy teachers, principal, and staff.

School-Based Clinics

One in 12 children in the United States does not have a regular source of health care. For African-American children, the rate is one in five. Nearly a fourth of inner-city children rely on "clinic care" through hospital outpatient services, emergency rooms, walk-in care centers, and public health centers (Bloom, 1990). Fortunately, the decade of the 1980s saw growth in the number of school-based clinics or wellness centers. Many of the services discussed here are provided in clinics. In addition, physicians and other health care providers often rotate among a district's clinics. At many clinics a counselor or mental health professional is available at all times. Clinic personnel have access to health records. Services can be conprehensive and self-contained, including testing, diagnosis, counseling, and treatment. In a well-organized school-based clinic, the opportunities for services and instruction are endless. The clinic should not take the place of classroom instruction but can provide a useful supplement.

As early as 1968, the school-based health clinic was implemented in Cambridge, Massachusetts (Nader, 1978). The Cambridge school-based primary care program for children was designed to operate under the auspices of the city's Department of Health and Hospitals and to be the immediate responsibility of the director of the Department of Pediatrics at the Cambridge Hospital. By 1976 five school-based health centers were well-established, providing primary pediatric care as well as accessibility to comprehensive health care.

The program is designed so a single, integrated health service follows the child from birth through adolescence. The stage of the program directed to school-aged children identifies any child who is having trouble adjusting to the classroom. Through nurse practitioner-teacher conferences, children with emotional problems and learning difficulties can be identified and referred for assistance. The nurse practitioner functions as the coordinator of remedial programs between the school consultant and the family and child. Children have access to all levels of care through a coordinated referral system.

As evidence of the educational benefits of the program, the percentage of children entering school from 1965 to 1975 who were immunized for measles rose from 55 to 99. In the fall of 1975, 98% of children entering school had completed the DPT and polio series. Elevated blood levels of lead were found in 7% of the centers' preschool population in 1973. After introducing a lead detection program, the incidence of elevated blood levels of lead was less than 0.5 percent. As a result of nutritional evaluation and obtaining WIC Supplemental Food Program funds (a federal program), iron deficiency anemia in 1- and 2-year-old children dropped from 16% to 4%. In the 2- to 3-year-old age group, the reduction was from 22% to 7%.

In Delaware, since 1986 the state legislature has funded four school-based wellness centers, allocating $100,000 to each yearly. Even in fiscally tight years, the level of funding has been maintained because of the general support the centers have received. New start-up funds will be made available for additional school-based health projects.

In Florida, school districts are given a menu of school health models that can be adopted. Among the choices are health service teams and comprehensive health centers.

For the past decade three publicly funded health provider organizations have been providing services in nine school-based clinics in the Albuquerque, New Mexico, public schools (Pacheco et al., 1991). The three providers—the Albuquerque Family Health Centers, the New Mexico Health and Environment Department, and the Family Medicine Division of the University of New Mexico School of Medicine—had no affiliation with each other for several years, and, thus, there was no coordination between their school-based efforts. The clinics cared for a variety of student health needs such as sports physical examinations, respiratory infections, injuries, depression, and issues regarding sexuality. The school-based clinics represent the major, if not sole, source of health care for many families, mostly indigent.

During the summer of 1987, Albuquerque's school-based clinics came under broad attack from individuals, organizations, and church leaders in the community. After vigorous investigation, the school board voted unanimously to maintain the presence of the clinics in the schools with more uniformity and accountability to the public school administration. The board required regular audits of clinic charts and an assessment of how often contraception was being discussed with students. Uniform parent permission forms, clinic guidelines, and protocols for dealing with special circumstances were developed. The three providers began to meet regularly with the central administration of the public schools. They strengthened their focus on classroom-based health education and streamlined charting and follow-up procedures. They placed more emphasis on notification and involvement of parents in care decisions. In short, the controversy strengthened the Albuquerque school-based clinics and helped them provide the services children need.

More than 50 school-based clinics have been established across the South, many in urban areas with high concentrations of low-income, high-risk families. Reports from clinic administrators reveal that utilization of the centers is extremely high (Schlitt, 1992).

The Congress of the United States, through the Office of Technology Assessment (1991) attested to the usefulness of having health services available on school campuses by stating, "The most promising recent innovation to address the health and related needs of adolescents is the school linked health or youth services center."

SUMMARY

The school health program consists of three interrelated components: school health instruction, healthy school environment, and school health services. The value of each is increased immeasurably when they work in conjunction with and support of one another. If this is done and certain other elements are present in planning and administering the instructional program, the school can boast of quality comprehensive school health education.

REFERENCES

Allanson, J. F. Comprehensive school health education: Maltese chicken or Phoenix? *Journal of School Health, 51* (October 1981): 556-559.

Bloom, B. Health insurance and medical care: Health of our nation's children, United States, 1988. *Advance Data from Vital and Health Statistics* (no. 188). Hyattsville, MD: National Center for Health Statistics, 1990.

Bremberg, S. Does school health education affect the health of students? In D. Nutbeam et al., editors, *Youth Health Promotion: From Theory to Practice in School and Community*. London: Forbes Publications Ltd., 1991.

Commission on the Reorganization of Education *Cardinal Principles of Secondary Education* (Department of Interior, Bureau of Education, Bulletin No. 35, 1918). Washington, DC: U. S. Government Printing Office, 1928.

Cornacchia, H. J., L. K. Olsen, and C. J. Nickerson. *Health in Elementary Schools*. St. Louis: Mosby Year Book, 1991.

Davis, R. L., H. L. Gonser, M. A. Kirkpatrick, S. W. Lavery, and S. L. Owen. Comprehensive school health education: A practical definition. *Journal of School Health, 55* (October 1985): 335-339.

Eisner, V., and L. B. Callan. *Dimensions of School Health*. Springfield, IL: Charles C Thomas, Publisher, 1974.

Elder, J. P. From experimentation to dissemination: Strategies for maximizing the impact and speed of school health education. In D. Nutbeam et al., editors, *Youth Health Promotion: From Theory to Practice in School and Community*. London: Forbes Publications, Ltd., 1991.

Irving Independent School District v. Tatro. 104 S Ct 3371, 1984.

Jenne, F. H. and W. H. Greene. *Turner's School Health and Health Education* (7th ed.). St. Louis: C. V. Mosby, 1976.

1990 Joint Committee on Health Education Terminology. Report of the 1990 Joint Committee on Health Education. *Journal of School Health, 61* (August 1991): 251-254.

Klein, J. D. and L. S. Sadowski. Personal health services as a component of comprehensive health programs. *Journal of School Health, 60* (April 1990): 164-169.

Lewin, K. *Readings in Social Psychology*. New York: Henry Holt and Company, 1958.

Nader, P. R. *Options for School Health: Meeting Community Needs*. Germantown, MD: Aspen. 1978.

National Professional School Health Education Organizations. Comprehensive school health education. *Journal of School Health, 54* (September 1984): 312-315.

Newman, I. M. Integrating health services and health education: Seeking a balance. *Journal of School Health, 52* (October 1982): 498-501.

Office of Technology Assessment. *Adolescent Health: Volume I. Summary and Policy Options* (S/N 052-003-01234-1). Washington, DC: Government Printing Office, 1991.

Pacheco, M., W. Powell, C. Cole, N. Kalishman, R. Benon, and A. Kaufman. School-based clinics: The politics of change. *Journal of School Health, 61* (February 1991): 92-94.

Palfrey, J. S., R. C. Mervis, and J. A. Butler. New directions and evaluation of handicapped children. *New England Journal of Medicine, 298* (April 13, 1978): 819-824.

Palfrey, J. S., M. Haynie, S. Porter, T. Bierle, P. Cooperman, and J. Lowcock. Project School Care: Integrating children assisted by medical technology into educational settings. *Journal of School Health, 62* (February 1992): 50-54.

Pollock, M. B. and K. Middleton. *Elementary School Health Instruction* (2d ed.). St. Louis: Times Mirror/Mosby, 1989.

Redican K., L. Olsen, and C. Baffi. *Organization of School Health Programs* (2d ed.). Madison, WI: Brown & Benchmark, 1993.

Schlitt, J. J. Bringing health to school: Policy implications for southern states. *Journal of School Health, 62* (February 1992).

Schubiner, H. Preventive health screenings in adolescent patients. *Primary Care, 16* (January 1989): 211-230.

Sliepcevich, E. M. Health education: A conceptual approach to curriculum design. *School Health Education Study.* St. Paul, MN: 3M Education Press, 1967.

Seffrin, J. R. The comprehensive school health curriculum: Closing the gap between state-of-the-art and state-of-the-practice. *Journal of School Health, 60* (April 1990): 151-156.

6

SETTINGS FOR HEALTH EDUCATION/PROMOTION

When discussing the settings in which health education or health promotion occurs, we are referring to those that follow a planned process with specific objectives for establishing behavior, increasing knowledge, or changing attitudes, in some combination. Obviously, information can be obtained passively through radio and television. It is also exchanged in a variety of settings such as the playground, the home, or the school bus. Although these settings may qualify as places where true health education *can* take place, they were not established for that purpose, and they seldom provide settings for true health instruction or health promotion. More often they are merely sites of incidental education, usually of little lasting quality.

The president of the Association for the Advancement of Health Education accentuated the need to champion health education in a variety of settings (O'Rourke, 1990):

In order to achieve our mission . . . we should continue to expand our efforts to meet the needs of health educators and promote health education in diverse settings. These include not only the K–12 Schools, but also College/University, Agency/Public/ Community, Clinical/Medical Care/Patient, and Business.

Plainly, the school is the setting where children are exposed to health education most frequently. The school as a health education setting was discussed in Chapter 5. In this chapter, settings for health education and promotion other than the school classroom are explored.

COMMUNITY HEALTH AGENCIES

The United States has hundreds of community health agencies. Some are voluntary, such as the Epilepsy Foundation of America and the American Cancer Society. Some are created by government and funded by taxes, such as state health departments. The latter group of community health agencies is referred to as official or *public health agencies*. Community health agencies perform a variety of functions, such as maintenance of vital records, infectious disease control, research, and provision of direct services to clients. The most important function of community health agencies, however, is education. The Joint Committee on Health Education Terminology (1991) defined community health education as:

> The application of a variety of methods that result in the education and mobilization of community members in actions for resolving health issues and problems which affect the community. These methods include, but are not limited to, group process, mass media, communication, community organization, organization development, strategic planning, skills training, legislation, policy making, and advocacy.

Within the scope of community health education are activities that promote individual behavior conducive to health.

In official health agencies questions often arise concerning the extent of centralization of health education. Should health education in a local health department be centered in one office or unit, or should it be dispersed throughout the department? Certainly, variations are abundant. Centralized health education units sometimes are organized as a separate bureau or office. Health education activities also are frequently decentralized and dispersed throughout the organization. Sometimes health education is placed within a division of vital statistics, of maternal and child health, or of communicable disease control (Pickett and Hanlon, 1990). The key to success of the arrangement is in the department's commitment to health education and the quality of the staff.

Frequently, community health agencies are called upon to reinforce the reasons for and benefits of regulations or environmental controls through health education. For instance, a campaign of public education might be launched about the risks of drunk driving or environmental tobacco smoke before introducing legislation strengthening drunk driving laws or restricting smoking in public places. The combination of education and organizational supports is called *health promotion*. When taxes on tobacco products are raised, states have found it useful to utilize health promotion to clarify the economic reasons for the taxation, the health effects of smoking, and the promise of use of the increased revenue for programs acceptable to the majority of people, such as tobacco education in schools.

Educational Role

Most voluntary health agencies spend a great deal of time and resources in education. For instance, the Epilepsy Foundation of America, through its state and local affiliates, conducts School Alert programs to educate teachers and pupils about epilepsy and to change perceptions and attitudes about the disorder. The American Cancer Society offers its smoking cessation program, called Fresh Start, to businesses and schools. Fresh Start is educational as well as effective at changing behavior. The American Red Cross offers courses to develop individual skills in child care and babysitting, cardiopulmonary resuscitation and first aid, and water safety.

Community health agencies frequently carry out what can be called patient education. In many cases, people who have had the same condition teach others about it. An example is the Reach to Recovery Program of the American Cancer Society, for women who have had a mastectomy. Laypersons can be trained to apply their empathy, understanding, compassion, and enthusiasm in helping another person learn to live with a damaging medical condition.

A critical part of community health education is making people aware of services, programs, and even the agency itself. Frequently, people complain about a lack of services when those services are available at little or no charge in their own communities. This is not the fault of the client or "victim" but, rather, a symptom of the problem of getting the message out that services are available.

Public Relations

Public relations is a vital issue with community health agencies. To be successful, they must make the community aware not only of their services but also of their competence. Public service announcements on television and radio, billboards, flyers, pamphlets, and slogans frequently are used to alert people to the presence of agencies and their programs. In addition to these means, community health agencies must provide quality services including education in accessible locations with warm surroundings and courteous staff.

A major difference between community health education and school health education is that the former has no captive audience. No one is compelled to participate in community education. As Swinehart (1968) observed:

> Information presented through the channels commonly used by public health and voluntary associations is fairly easy for most potential audiences to avoid, since these audiences are not "captive." Even if they are exposed to the communication, there is no guarantee that this will lead to learning and action.

This once again emphasizes the need for good public relations and for sensitizing the community to the presence of services. On the other hand, because participation is voluntary, participants usually are highly motivated to learn and to apply what they learn in their daily lives.

Community health education often suffers from a problem similar to that of school health education when funding is concerned. To the extent health education is considered a secondary service, it will receive inadequate funding, facilities, and equipment. This is probably more of a problem in public health situations than in voluntary health organizations.

Even with all its problems, community health education remains viable, because, among other reasons, it zeros in on readily identifiable community problems and needs. In many cases, elaborate needs assessment is unnecessary. For instance, AIDS education is a need in every community. At other times, a problem specific to a given population, such as water quality or potential dangers of poisoning from lead-based paints, are identified from hospital records or environmental testing. These situations call for alerting the population and immediate educational intervention.

Program Planning

In planning community health education programs, the ultimate goal is to elicit voluntary positive health practices. The role of the health educator is not to coerce or force individuals to adopt lifestyles or habits to which they object. Individuals should freely embrace changes in behavior with full knowledge of the consequences of possible alternatives. Our primary objectives are to develop knowledge about health issues and establish attitudes, values, and beliefs that are positive toward health. A secondary objective may be to fortify the social support of friends and relatives regarding healthy behavior. By establishing this foundation of knowledge, attitudes, and social supports, we hope to reach the paramount goal of a healthy lifestyle.

To have a strong foundation, planning in community health education should be based on sound theory. In addition, it should be rooted in the discovered needs of the target population. It should utilize methods the fields of education, social and behavioral sciences, and communications have established. Planners should involve consumers of services in planning, as consumers often have firsthand knowledge of problems and their causes as well as barriers to change. Chapter 11 explains needs assessment, planning, and implementation of health education programs.

Green (1990) summed up the administrative needs of community health education by stating:

> The educational component of community health programs should have (1) the education plan written not separately or independently but within the context of the larger health program plan, (2) the

responsibility for coordination of the educational component fixed on a designated person, (3) the responsibility for each educational intervention assigned to specific people, and (4) a budget for personnel, materials, and other costs.

WORKSITE HEALTH EDUCATION/PROMOTION

Business and industry is becoming one of the most attractive settings for health education and health promotion. A worksite health promotion program (WHPP) is a combination of educational, organizational, and environmental activities with the purpose of developing and supporting behavior conducive to the employee's health.

For a long time, industry took little interest in the welfare of its employees. Slowly, with changing social values and enlightenment, business leaders began to understand that healthy employees are good for business. Although this may sound callous, businesses exist for the purpose of making money. If they fail, they no longer exist. Therefore, if a business is to provide services for employees, those services must enhance the potential for profit. Indeed, a financial incentive does exist.

Well-designed and well-managed health promotion programs can reduce employee absenteeism (Blair et al., 1984; Cox, Shepard, and Cory, 1981; Chenoweth, 1987), decrease hospital admissions and shorten lengths of stays (Bly, Jones and Richardson, 1986), reduce hospital days and claims of all types (Shepherd et al., 1982), and therefore lower the cost of health insurance and workers' compensation claims (Chenoweth, 1987).

Both workers and employers benefit from reduction in health care costs (Minter, 1986; Bowne et al., 1984). Overall productivity is maximized because more individuals are working closer to their full potential. Productivity also is enhanced as absenteeism and employee turnover are reduced (Berry, 1981). Effective WHPPs also have been demonstrated to increase recruitment capabilities for attracting high-quality individuals (Warner, 1987).

In addition to the financial benefits, WHPPs can produce significant betterment of feelings of general well-being and self-concept (Blair et al., 1984). Improvement in job-related attitudes also are linked to WHPPs (Spilman et al., 1986).

The genesis of the worksite health promotion program was the old industrial medicine and

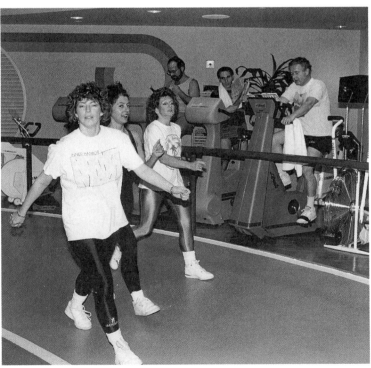

The worksite health promotion program can provide opportunities for activities during or after working hours. The health educator must be capable of "selling" the benefits of the program to both management and labor. Photo courtesy of Johnson & Johnson.

hygiene program. These programs were concerned with first-aid and medical care; environmental hazards, such as toxic components and noise; and safety programs that stressed accident prevention (Breckon, Harvey, and Lancaster, 1985). Legal requirements regarding the protection of workers from injury and illness played a part in the evolution of this movement. Gradually the movement expanded to the level of a wellness orientation and then to include the health of workers' families.

Today's WHPPs offer health education in the form of parenting classes, nutrition and weight control education, stress management, fitness, retirement planning, smoking cessation, cancer risk awareness, and cardiovascular health maintenance. Many programs include health fairs, regular aerobics groups, jogging trails, health screening (e.g., mammograms, chest x-rays, cholesterol level, hypertension), physical examinations, health risk appraisals, support groups, and lending libraries. Employee assistance programs frequently identify employees not necessarily seeking help and refer them for counseling or treatment at agencies outside the worksite. A national survey of worksites with 50 or more employees found that two-thirds had one or more health promotion programs, facilities, or services (Fielding and Piserchia, 1989).

Program Director Skills

The skills the practitioner must bring to the worksite program vary. Managerial skills in planning, implementing, and evaluating programs are critical. The health educator must be able to function in an atmosphere of organizational and policy change.

The health educator must be able to "sell" the program to management and then to workers. Once the program is in place, he or she must keep the workers involved in the program.

Many participants drop out for a number of reasons, including lack of interest, lack of time, inconvenience, and lack of creativity on the part of program directors (Bensley, 1991). McKenzie, Lubke, and Romas (1992) identify this process of keeping participants involved as motivation. Perhaps a more useful way of approaching this aspect of the WHPP is the same as community health education planning takes—namely, assessing the needs of workers and their families, helping them set attainable goals, planning programs and activities to meet those goals, and evaluating the process and the short- and long-term results.

The ability to continue program participation requires organization, administrative support, motivation and reinforcement, and programming that meets the needs of participants (Bensley, 1991). Initiating and continuing participation may require a variety of methods. Bensley (1991) suggests a number of ideas that can keep participants active in health promotion activities:

1. Designing realistic and obtainable goals and objectives, including those that can be attained in a short time.
2. Adhering to motivation theory by stimulating curiosity, incorporating programming directed toward positive external and internal locus of control, identifying health problems, and providing opportunities for socialization.
3. Providing positive reinforcement of individual achievements.
4. Requiring a fee for a program, thereby encouraging personal investment in health promotion.
5. Providing strong leadership and a healthy role model.
6. Providing constant communication between program director and participants, including recognition of individual success.
7. Providing individual and group education.
8. Involving spouses and family.
9. Providing incentives.

These suggestions can help keep participants in the program regardless of setting.

Incentives can incite action in some individuals who otherwise might fail to act. Positive incentives, such as lower insurance premiums for maintaining weight, can increase the perceived value of an activity. Negative incentives, such as a surcharge applied to health insurance for smoking (Penner, 1989), may reduce the value of the harmful activity, increasing the likelihood that it will be discontinued. Incentives should be tailored to individual characteristics including gender, socioeconomic status (Chenoweth, 1987), age (McAvoy, 1979), and psychological differences (Rosenbaum and Argon, 1979).

Incentives come in many packages. One group of incentives consists of those to which McKenzie, Luebke, and Romas (1992) refer as **material reinforcers**. These reinforcers include items such as coupons, merchandise at local stores, token prizes such as T-shirts and caps, lottery prizes in which everyone attending can win a prize, and membership at a fitness club. A popular and effective material reinforcer for many people is to favorably change benefit packages or for the employer to pick up all or part of the health insurance premium to reward healthy practices (Toufexis, 1985). **Social reinforcers** (Feldman, 1983) may be effective with some individuals. This group of incentives includes public recognition, various forms of praise and encouragement, a sense of belonging and acceptance, personal challenge, and competition.

Traditionally, WHPPs have been initiated and sponsored by management. Labor unions recently have shown more interest in a variety of programs (Snow et al., 1986). Feldman (1989) recommended utilizing unions to reach high-risk workers, provide social support for workers, and promote communication among them. In situations in which management has been less than enthusiastic, advocacy by the union may actually spur management to support WHPPs. Joint union and management support undoubtedly have an impact on worker participation.

Recruiting unions or employee organizations to support programs endorsed by management generates a great deal of employee favor and enthusiasm. This kind of support can result in funding materials and allotting of adequate facilities.

The program director must be capable of demonstrating the program's benefits. This requires keen evaluation skills and the ability to interpret data in terms of the company's primary goal—generating income. Businesses that adopt WHPPs do so with the belief that benefits such as favorable publicity, easier recruitment and retention, higher productivity, less absenteeism, and lower health insurance premiums will result. Even though this belief may provide initial commitment and resources, a competent health educator continually justifies the program in ways that impress management.

Because only one health educator may be on staff, that person must be able to implement the program's specific components. The health education administrator may have to change hats and become the health promotion implementer. A solid grounding in adult learning theory is a must. Although some professionals see themselves as specialists, in many settings we also must be generalists, able to field questions and conduct programs in nutrition, stress management, exercise, and a multitude of other content areas.

Criticisms

Worksite health promotion has not been without critics and doubters. Union officials sometimes have expressed concern that WHPPs could shift resources from prevention of occupational hazards in the workplace and negatively affect working conditions. Others have feared that employers might use health promotion to cover poor working conditions. Still others perceive health promotion as a management ploy to elicit more productivity from workers rather than a genuine effort to react to health problems and prevent others. Of course, this is partially true, as management frequently is reluctant to invest in health promotion unless it is convinced that productivity will increase. This does not necessarily mean that increased productivity and income are the sole motives. Even if increased profits is a motive of management, however, the values of the program to individual workers still present a win-win situation.

Occupational health promotion has been disparaged on the basis of its not reaching the people who need it most. To some extent this criticism has merit. Many programs concentrate on managerial, clerical, executive, and professional personnel while not reaching the blue-collar level. One remedy is to involve blue-collar workers in developing and planning the program. Another is to assure release time for workers to participate and make scheduling of services flexible.

One major problem with many WHPPs is a lack of long-term employee and employer commitment. This carries a threat of the "plug being pulled" at any time. Because the program's goals and objectives are not linked directly to the company's production goals, its relevance is being tested constantly and its existence threatened (Greenberg, 1989). This can lead to a stressful work situation for the health educator and staff.

Even though WHPPs have many potential problems, health educators often have found that working in an occupational health program has an advantage that school settings lack: Workers who participate are almost always volunteers and, therefore, are highly motivated. Working with such highly motivated participants is a pleasure and usually produces quick results. These results and the usually responsive attitudes of the worker can make a WHPP a satisfying place to work.

SCHOOLSITE HEALTH PROMOTION PROGRAMS

Our public school systems and private schools employ millions of teachers, nonprofessional staff, and administrators. Schools have a number of reasons for implementing health promotion programs for faculty and staff. One of the most obvious is that students often see faculty as role models. Faculty and staff involvement in health promotion activities frequently leads to student participation. Beyond that, health promotion programs can lead to reduction of direct costs of health insurance and indirect costs of absenteeism, disability, turnover, lower productivity, and faculty and staff recruitment/replacement (LaRosa and Haines, 1986).

A good deal of evidence supports schoolsite health promotion programs (SHPPs) as beneficial to participants. Teachers who have participated in SHPPs report better attitudes about their personal health (Health Insurance Association of America, 1985; Falck and Kilcoyne, 1984), perceptions of increased general well-being (Passwater, Tritsch, and Slater, 1980; Blair et al., 1984; Pine, 1985), less absenteeism and higher morale (Health Insurance Association of America, 1985; Passwater et al., 1980; Falck and Kilcoyne, 1984), and an improvement in quality of their instruction (Health Insurance Association of America, 1985; Passwater et al., 1980).

Two models have been applied to SHPPs. The first, the *clinical model*, uses thorough screening or health-risk appraisals to identify employees at high-risk, who become targets of specialized interventions. The second model, the *community intervention* or *public health model*, attempts to produce mass health changes in all school employees. The public health model seeks to modify the school environment by developing strategies for the cafeteria, school clinic, and instructional programs. This model also attempts to implement policies, such as prohibiting smoking, which encourage healthier behaviors. The public health model may be preferred for some SHPPs because it is likely to attract more participants, is less threatening than screening programs, is easier to evaluate, and offers something for everyone (Blair, Tritsch, and Kutsch, 1987). Regardless of the planning and implementation model, a team composed of faculty, staff, administration, nursing, food service, and maintenance should work together to implement the SHPP. SHPPs have the potential to expand to include the student body, the community, and businesses.

The future of SHPPs may lie in cooperative efforts with the community as a whole and with other worksites. With community involvement, members of boards of health, church groups, local political figures, senior citizens centers, and a host of voluntary health agencies could be absorbed into the process. These groups also could help provide public relations and funding. Large corporate funding could result from a SHPP sporting a company's insignia or mascot. Eventually, a company without facilities for a WHPP may contract with the school program to provide programs for its employees (Richardson and Bensley, 1991).

Community involvement is vital to maintaining the force of the program. When community members and agencies participate in a school program, they benefit from the program and the school benefits from the support they bring.

Topics and content pose another important issue relating to SHPPs in the future. Future programs may include activities to develop skills in parenting, strengthening the family, personal empowerment, promotion of psychological hardiness, self-esteem and self-efficacy. Future programs should be more comprehensive and target a wider range of issues pertaining to healthy behaviors and the school and community environment as a whole.

COLLEGE AND UNIVERSITY WELLNESS PROGRAMS

Colleges and universities have rushed to support the health promotion concept on their campuses

by establishing wellness centers. Frequently, these centers are funded initially by grants and participant fees. After the grants expire, the institutions usually pick up the cost. The philosophy behind colleges' embarking on health promotion is that the institution exists to support the growth and development of the individual student intellectually, socially, and physically. To help the student develop habits that promote wellness optimizes his or her growth and development.

The first formally established wellness program on a university campus was developed at the University of Wisconsin, Stevens Point, in 1972, by the university's Student Life Division. Many schools since then have adopted the wellness center model. Dr. Leafgren, Assistant Chancellor for Student Life at Stevens Point (Clark, 1986), suggested 11 strategies for coordinating and enhancing wellness:

1. Establish administrative leadership (including personal involvement in the process) and support.

2. Inventory existing programs to identify those presently providing wellness services and minimize overlap and duplication.

3. Identify staff members who are interested in modeling a wellness lifestyle and encourage their participation in a wellness committee.

4. Identify students already interested and committed to a wellness lifestyle and encourage their participation in the planning process.

5. Bring all existing personnel resources (faculty and nonstudent affairs administrators) together for brainstorming and goal setting early in the planning process.

6. Involve all student affairs units in a partnership for wellness program implementation.

7. Ask each academic department to inventory its programs and services and identify those that may be related to wellness, if only tangentially.

8. Inform students and faculty about the program and available opportunities. Utilize a regular publication, assessment tools, and so on.

9. Establish priorities for wellness goals and activities.

10. Provide adequate training for professional staff and students involved in implementing the program.

11. Evaluate wellness programs for comprehensiveness and effectiveness in assisting students in their development as persons.

A typical college wellness program attempts to assess the participant's behavior and health status in the initial meeting. This may be done by taking a health history, administering a lifestyle assessment instrument, or conducting a health risk appraisal. Some programs do health screening. Usually a wellness counselor then assists the student in setting goals and prescribes a program tailored to meet the individual's goals. A peer facilitator can be helpful in supporting the student-client in staying with the program.

A thorough health promotion approach to campus life extends to all areas of the institution, including food service, the student health center, counseling services, and academic departments. Each area should have a specific role in promoting students' health.

Colleges and universities present a wonderful opportunity for promoting the health of faculty members and administrators. These individuals often are working under a great deal of stress, have little time for good meals, and may neglect their exercise needs. These campus wellness programs meet the same needs as employee WHPPs. Most university employees believe WHPPs can enhance the quality of worklife (Sarvela et al., 1991). Planners of programs for employees in higher education should conduct screening and implement disease prevention programs to address critical issues employees have. Participation in health programs may be heightened by making the work schedule flexible, making

programs available during employee free time, offering programs at low cost, and introducing incentives such as release time or reduction in cost of health care (Sarvela et al., 1991).

Many innovative programs, such as those at Dundalk Community College in Maryland and at Memphis State University have opened their wellness programs to the public. This enables increased revenue through fees and cost-efficient use of facilities. More important, it provides for a sense of ownership of the school by people who otherwise would have little or no contact with the institution. They become ambassadors for the school.

Whether the program serves only students, employees, the community, or all three groups, adequate assessment of participants is necessary, and the proper medical supervision should be provided if indicated. Only properly trained personnel should be employed in the program. This not only gives the program credibility but also reduces legal liability.

MEDICAL/CLINICAL SETTINGS

Preventive medicine has become part of the scene in American hospitals, physicians' offices, and health maintenance organizations (HMOs). This came about through the prodding of powerful organizations such as the American Hospital Association, the Health Insurance Association of America, and the federal government.

Medical care settings, such as clinics, hospitals, physicians' offices, nursing homes, and health maintenance organizations, can be effective sites for health education/promotion activities, especially if the health educator is perceived as part of the health care team. Health care settings can induce extra motivation in patients because of the perceived level of expertise and because many patients are diagnosed as having a health problem. Most patients understand that education is a means to enhance their prognosis and to help them understand treatment alternatives so they are able to participate in decisions about their care.

Role of the Health Educator

Health education specialists usually are employed as directors or managers of the health promotion program. They serve primarily as administrators. Health practitioners—physicians, nurses, dieticians, pharmacists—provide a unique set of resources to the health educator. In an ideal health care setting professional practitioners do serve as resources to the health educator. In reality they often are the front line of the health education team. The provider is more likely to have the actual patient contact, whereas the health educator plans, implements, and evaluates the program. The program's effectiveness can be compromised, however, if the health care provider carries out health education without the proper preparation. Standards are being developed for patient education training for nurses and other professionals.

The process of health education can be compromised if the patient or the health care delivery team perceives the health educator in an inferior light, a sort of "second-class citizen." Support of management and the staff, including physicians and nurses, is crucial to the success of the education process.

When the health education/promotion program is considered a fringe part of the total operation, this becomes threatening to health educators. Not only are they forced to justify their program from a philosophical point of view, but they also must demonstrate the cost benefit. Unfortunately, this view of health education can lead to a situation in which physicians and nurses have to assume the role of health educator even though they may have no competencies in that area.

Patient Education

Patient education can take place in a variety of settings, including a physician's office, hospital corridor, formalized classroom, or by telephone. It is, of course, most effective as a planned process. The American Hospital Association's *A Patient's Bill of Rights* emphasizes both informing and educating the patient. This education includes treatment options; rights to decline treatment, to have a surrogate make decisions for you if incapacitated, to have advance directive; and perhaps most important, the patient's responsibility for his or her own health.

Patient education traditionally has been mostly the province of nurses and, secondarily, physicians. Ample legal justification exists in the Nurse Practice Acts of each state for the role of nurses in patient education. Legal requirements also exist for continuing education for nurses to

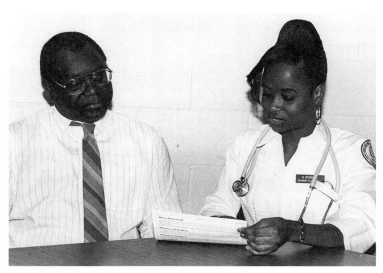

Nurses occupy a vital role in patient education.

A PATIENT'S BILL OF RIGHTS

INTRODUCTION

Effective Health Care requires collaboration between patients and physicians and other health care professionals. Open and honest communication, respect for personal and professional values, and sensitivity to differences are integral to optimal patient care. As the setting for the provision of health services, hospitals must provide a foundation for understanding and respecting the rights and responsibilities of patients, their families, physicians, and other caregivers. Hospitals must ensure a health care ethic that respects the role of patients in decision-making about treatment choices and other aspects of their care. Hospitals must be sensitive to cultural, racial, linguistic, religious, age, gender, and other differences as well as the needs of persons with disabilities.

The American Hospital Association presents *A Patient's Bill of Rights* with the expectation that it will contribute to more effective patient care and be supported by the hospital on behalf of the institution, its medical staff, employees, and patients. The American Hospital Association encourages health care institutions to tailor this bill of rights to their patient community by translating and/or simplifying the language of this bill of rights as may be necessary to ensure that patients and their families understand their rights and responsibilities.

BILL OF RIGHTS*

1. The patient has the right to considerate and respectful care.

2. The patient has the right to and is encouraged to obtain from physicians and other direct caregivers relevant, current, and understandable information concerning diagnosis, treatment, and prognosis.

    Except in emergencies when the patient lacks decision-making capacity and the need for treatment is urgent, the patient is entitled to the opportunity to discuss and request information related to the specific procedures and/or treatments, the risks involved, the possible length of recuperation, and the medically reasonable alternatives and their accompanying risks and benefits.

    Patients have the right to know the identity of physicians, nurses and others involved in their care, as well as when those involved are students, residents, or other trainees. The patient also has the right to know the immediate and long-term financial implications of treatment choices, insofar as they are known.

3. The patient has the right to make decisions about the plan of care prior to and during the course of treatment and to refuse a recommended treatment or plan of care to the extent permitted by law and hospital policy and to be informed of the medical consequences of this action. In case of such refusal, the patient is entitled to other appropriate care and services that the hospital provides or transfer to another hospital. The hospital should notify patients of any policy that might affect patient choice within the institution.

4. The patient has the right to have an advance directive (such as a living will, health care proxy, or durable power of attorney for health care) concerning treatment or designating a surrogate decision maker with the expectation that the hospital will honor the intent of that directive to the extent permitted by law and hospital policy.

    Health care institutions must advise patients of their rights under state law and hospital policy to make informed medical choices, ask if the patient has an advance directive, and include that information in patient records. The patient has the right to timely information about hospital policy that may limit its ability to implement fully a legally valid advance directive.

5. The patient has the right to every consideration of privacy. Case discussion, consultation, examination, and treatment should be conducted so as to protect each patient's privacy.

6. The patient has the right to expect that all communications and records pertaining to his/her care will be treated as confidential by the hospital, except in cases such as suspected abuse and public health hazards when reporting is permitted or required by law. The patient has the right to expect that the hospital will emphasize the confidentiality of this information when it releases it to any other parties entitled to review information in these records.

7. The patient has the right to review the records pertaining to his/her medical care and to have the information explained or interpreted as necessary, except when restricted by law.

8. The patient has the right to expect that, within its capacity and policies, a hospital will make reasonable response to the request of a patient for appropriate and medically indicated care and services. The hospital must provide evaluation, service, and/or referral as indicated by the urgency of the case. When medically appropriate and legally permissible, or when a patient has so requested, a patient may be transferred to another facility. The institution to which the patient is to be transferred must first have accepted the patient for transfer. The patient must also have the benefit of complete information and explanation concerning the need for, risks, benefits, and alternatives to such a transfer.

9. The patient has the right to ask and be informed of the existence of business relationships among the hospital, educational institutions, other health care providers, or payers that may influence the patient's treatment and care.

10. The patient has the right to consent to or decline to participate in proposed research studies or human experimentation affecting care and treatment or requiring direct patient involvement, and to have those studies fully explained prior to consent. A patient who declines to participate in research or experimentation is entitled to the most effective care that the hospital can otherwise provide.

11. The patient has the right to expect reasonable continuity of care when appropriate and to be informed by physicians and other caregivers of available and realistic patient care options when hospital care is no longer appropriate.

12. The patient has the right to be informed of hospital policies and practices that relate to the patient care, treatment, and responsibilities. The patient has the right to be informed of available resources for resolving disputes, grievances, and conflicts, such as ethics committees, patient representatives, or other mechanisms available in the institution. The patient has the right to be informed of the hospital's charges for services and available payment methods.

The collaborative nature of health care requires that patients, or their families/surrogates, participate in their care. The effectiveness of care and patient satisfaction with the course of treatment depend, in part, on the patient fulfilling certain responsibilities. Patients are responsible for providing information about past illnesses, hospitalizations, medications, and other matters related to health status. To participate effectively in decision making, patients must be encouraged to take responsibility for requesting additional information or clarification about their health status or treatment when they do not fully understand information and instructions. Patients are also responsible for ensuring that the health care institution has a copy of their written advance directive if they have one. Patients are responsible for informing their physicians and other caregivers if they anticipate problems in following prescribed treatment.

Patients should also be aware of the hospital's obligation to be reasonably efficient and equitable in providing care to other patients and the community. The hospital's rules and regulations are designed to help the hospital meet this obligation. Patients and their families are responsible for making reasonable accommodations to the needs of the hospital, other patients, medical staff, and hospital employees. Patients are responsible for providing necessary information for insurance claims and for working with the hospital to make payment arrangements, when necessary.

A person's health depends on much more than health care services. Patients are responsible for recognizing the impact of their lifestyle on their personal health.

CONCLUSION

Hospitals have many functions to perform, including the enhancement of health status, health promotion, and the prevention and treatment of injury and disease; the immediate and ongoing care and rehabilitation of patients; the education of health professionals, patients, and the community; and research. All these activities must be conducted with an overriding concern for the values and dignity of patients.

*These rights can be exercised on the patient's behalf by a designated surrogate or proxy decision-maker if the patient lacks decision-making capacity, is legally incompetent, or is a minor.

upgrade their teaching skills. A multidisciplinary teaching staff, including dieticians, social workers, and others, greatly enriches an educational program but demands that careful attention be paid to cooperation, coordination, and continuing communication between staff members (Rorden, 1987).

In this environment the formally trained health education professional serves as a resource person, staff trainer, and usually administrator. The health educator may be called upon to develop the patient education program within the facility. This consists of assessing needs, planning and organizing, marketing, implementing the program, and evaluating it. It may include development of a training program for staff.

Helping patients learn how to care for themselves always has been part of the nurse's role. Recent changes in medical and social attitudes toward health have created more opportunities for patient education. These changes include:

1. *Acknowledgment of the patient's right to participate in decisions about health care and in actually caring for himself or herself.* Exercising this right requires knowledge, acceptance of responsibility for one's own health, and demonstrating that responsibility by acting in a manner conducive to well-being. For most patients, learning is necessary to do these things.

2. *The escalating public interest in wellness.* Individuals frequently turn to health care

professionals for information that will enable them to maintain general well-being.

3. *Increasing costs and rapid technological advances.* Patients now are discharged sooner, often with perplexing care regimens. In addition, people are living longer, require more medical attention, and must comply with complicated treatment and preventive schemes.

Patient education helps prepare patients to deal with these changes in medical care. It takes many forms, including prepared teaching and spontaneous teaching. *Prepared teaching* allows for needs assessment, planning, delivery, and evaluation. An example of prepared teaching is instructing newly diagnosed diabetics about diet, insulin, and exercise requirements. *Spontaneous teaching* happens often without time for preparation, such as a patient or family member asking a nurse for information regarding a case or advice about the case.

The purposes of patient education are to promote health, to prevent illness, and to cope with illness (Narrow, 1979). Examples of promoting health are teaching the young mother the importance of sensory stimulation for her infant and teaching a group of parents the importance of each stage of growth and development. Examples of teaching to prevent illness are genetic counseling about inherited traits parents may carry and helping people reduce stress. Examples of teaching to cope with illness include helping a person cope with residual paralysis caused by an accident and instructing a patient about the importance of following a treatment regimen.

Patient education can serve many functions in a health care setting. Perhaps the most important is helping individuals gain an intellectual understanding of their conditions and encouraging them to bring their feelings into the open. This can assist patients in exploring their own resources for coping and reopening their social spheres.

HMOs and Hospitals

Health maintenance organizations came into nationwide prominence in the 1970s following passage of federal legislation that allowed funding for feasibility studies, start-up, and development of HMOs. One of the criteria for being an HMO is providing health education. Many HMOs took this criterion seriously and, recognizing the cost reduction made possible by effective health education, carried out regular and consistent programs. Many health educators have been employed and have worked effectively in HMOs. Other HMOs did only the minimum to meet the criterion, such as having a physician make a presentation related to a disease once a month. Some designated a nurse as the health educator. During the 1970s and 1980s, it was not unusual to see an announced position for a health educator at an HMO that required no formal education in the field but required the applicant to be a nurse.

In addition to patient education, hospitals have become ideal places for worksite health education programs. Employee programs are more important in health care settings than in other settings because many employees are in direct contact with patients (Breckon et al., 1985).

Nursing Homes

Although nursing homes constitute ideal settings to target health promotion programs (Taylor-Nicholson et al., 1990), this potential has been neglected until recently. Encouraging nursing home residents to practice healthy behaviors in the nursing home as well as at home increases the life span and quality of life.

Breslow and Enstrom (1980) identified behaviors that can significantly improve the health of elderly people. They include abstaining from smoking, using alcohol in moderation or not at all, getting 7 to 8 hours of sleep a night, eating breakfast, cutting down on between-meal snacks, exercising regularly, and maintaining an acceptable weight. These are obvious targets for a nursing home health promotion program.

A number of studies have reported that enhanced physical and mental health status is consistent with an increase in sense of control (Langer and Rodin, 1976; Avorn and Langer, 1982). The feeling that health is influenced by one's own behavior affords a sense of control over one's own welfare. This feeling of control has been demonstrated to affect physiologic processes (Rodin, 1986; Krantz et al., 1981) and it influences people to take better care of themselves, seek health-related information, and comply more frequently with medical instructions (Rodin, 1986). It is indeed past the time when we should be introducing health promotion programs in nursing homes.

SUMMARY

Although we typically think of health education and promotion as taking place in a school-based setting where teachers plan activities and classes for students, the opportunities go far beyond the typical classroom. It would be hard to imagine a setting that would not be appropriate for health promotion activities. The settings discussed in this chapter have relatively short histories of successful programming.

To date, many workers have never been exposed to health promotion in the worksite. Many teachers and school staff have yet to experience the benefits of health promotion. Some health care facilities have only begun to tap the enormous potential of patient education. The reasons are numerous, but many employers obviously have not learned of the financial benefits and esprit de corps generated by worksite health promotion. Many employees and their families have not experienced the improved morale and health advantages gained from well-planned and competently executed health promotion programs. Similarly, some health care providers have not taken to heart the potential of patient and community education for reducing the rising cost of health care.

The potential of the health educator in these settings is only beginning to be tapped. Health educators, however, must "sell" their skills and programs in many cases. We should be on the alert for settings in which to develop programs. Settings such as churches, summer camps, and many military installations are just some of the possible targets for health promotion and education.

REFERENCES

Avorn, J., and E. J. Langer. Induced disability in nursing home patients: A controlled study. *Journal of the American Geriatric Society*, 30 (June 1982): 397–400.

Bensley, L. B., Jr. Schoolsite health promotion: Ways of sustaining interest. *Journal of Health Education*, 22 (March/April 1991): 86–89.

Berry, C. A. *Good Health for Employees and Reduced Health Care Costs for Industry*. Washington, DC: Health Insurance Association of America, 1981.

Blair, S. N., T. C. Collingwood, R. Reynolds, M. Smith, R. D. Hagen, and C. L. Sterling. Health promotion for educators: Impact on health behaviors, satisfaction, and general well-being. *American Journal of Public Health*, 74 (February 1984): 147–149.

Blair, S. N., L. Tritsch, and S. Kutsch. Worksite health promotion for school faculty and staff. *Journal of School Health*, 57 (December 1987): 469–473.

Bly, L., R. C. Jones, and J. E. Richardson. Impact of worksite health promotion on health care costs and utilization: Evaluation of Johnson & Johnson's Live for Life Program. *Journal of the American Medical Association*, 256 (December 19, 1986): 3235–3240.

Bowne, D. W., M. L. Russell, J. L. Morgan, S. A. Optenberg, and A. E. Clarke. Reduced disability and health care costs in an industrial fitness program. *Journal of Occupational Medicine*, 26 (November 1984): 809–816.

Breckon, D. J., J. R. Harvey, and R. B. Lancaster. *Community Health Education: Settings, Roles, and Skills*. Rockville, MD: Aspen Systems, 1985.

Breslow, L. and J. E. Enstrom. Persistence of health habits and their relationship to mortality. *Preventive Medicine*, 9 (July 1980): 469–483.

Chenoweth, D. H. *Planning Health Promotion at the Worksite*. Indianapolis: Benchmark Press, 1987.

Clark, C. C. *Wellness Nursing: Concepts, Theory, Research, and Practice*. New York: Springer Publishing, 1986.

Cox, M., R. J. Shepard, and P. Corey. Influence of an employee fitness program upon fitness, productivity, and absenteeism. *Ergonomics*, 24 (October 1981): 795–806.

Falck, V. T., and M. E. Kilcoyne, Jr. A health promotion program for school personnel. *Journal of School Health*, 54 (August 1984): 239–242.

Feldman, R. H. L. Strategies for improving compliance with health promotion programs in industry. *Health Education*, 14 (July/August 1983): 21–25.

Feldman, R. H. L. Worksite health promotion, labor unions, and social support. *Health Education*, 20 (October/November 1989): 55–56.

Fielding, J., and P. V. Piserchia. Frequency of worksite health promotion activities. *American Journal of Public Health*, 79 (January 1989): 16–20.

Green, L. W. *Community Health* (6th ed.). St. Louis: Times Mirror/Mosby College Publishing, 1990.

Greenberg, J. S. *Health Education: Learner-Centered Instructional Strategies*. Dubuque, IA: Wm. C. Brown Publishers, 1989.

Health Insurance Association of America. *Wellness at the Worksite.* Washington, DC: Health Insurance Association of America, 1985.

Joint Committee on Health Education Terminology. Report of the 1990 Joint Committee on Health Education Terminology. *Journal of Health Education, 22* (March/April 1991): 97–108.

Krantz, D. S., D. C. Glass, R. Contrada, and N. E. Miller. *The Five Year Outlook in Science and Technology, National Science Foundation.* Washington, DC: Government Printing Office, 1981.

Langer, E., and J. Rodin. The effects of choice and enhanced personality responsibility. *Journal of Personality and Social Psychology, 34* (August 1976): 191–198.

LaRosa, J. H., and C. M. Haines. *It's Your Business: A Guide to Heart and Lung Health at the Workplace* (NIH Publication No. 86-2210). Washington, DC: National Institutes of Health, 1986.

McAvoy, L. H. The leisure preferences, problems, and needs of the elderly. *Journal of Leisure Research, 11* (First Quarter 1979): 40–47.

McKenzie, J. F., J. K. Luebke, and J. A. Romas. Incentives: Getting and keeping workers involved in health promotions programs. *Journal of Health Education, 23* (March 1992): 70–73.

Minter, S. G. Occupational health professionals control health care costs. *Occupational Hazards, 6* (April 1986): 63–66.

Narrow, B. W. *Patient Teaching in Nursing Practice: A Patient and Family-Centered Approach.* New York: John Wiley & Sons, 1979.

O'Rourke, T. Challenges, opportunities and future directions: Constancy and change. *Health Education, 21* (May/June 1990): 4–5.

Passwater, D., L. Tritsch, and S. Slater. *Seaside Health Education Conference: Effects of Three 5-Day Teacher Inservice Conferences.* Salem: Oregon Department of Education, 1980.

Penner, M. Economic incentives to reduce employee smoking: A health insurance surcharge for tobacco using state of Kansas employees. *American Journal of Health Promotion, 4* (September/October 1989): 5–11.

Pickett, G., and J. J. Hanlon. *Public Health: Administration and Practice* (9th ed.). St. Louis: Times Mirror/Mosby College Publishing, 1990.

Pine, P. *Promoting Health Education in Schools: Problems and Solutions.* Arlington, VA: American Association of School Administrators, 1985.

Richardson, G. E., and L. B. Bensley, Jr. The future of schoolsite health promotion programs. *Journal of Health Education, 22* (March/April 1991): 90–93.

Rodin, J. Aging and health: Effects of the sense of control. *Science, 233* (September 19, 1986): 1271–1276.

Rorden, J. W. *Nurses as Health Teachers: A Practical Guide.* Philadelphia: W. B. Saunders Company, 1987.

Rosenbaum, M., and S. Argon. Locus of control and success in self-initiated attempts to stop smoking. *Journal of Clinical Psychology, 35* (October 1979): 870–872.

Sarvela, P. D., D. R. Holcomb, J. K. Huetteman, S. M. Bajracharya, and J. A. Odulana. A university employee health promotion program needs assessment. *Journal of Health Education, 22* (March/April 1991): 116–120.

Shepherd, R., P. Corey, P. Renzland, and M. Cox. The influence of employee fitness and lifestyle modification program upon medical costs. *Canadian Journal of Public Health, 73* (July-August 1982): 259–263.

Snow, B. R., D. LeGrande, J. Berek, J. McMahon, R. Wilford, and J. M. Sullivan. Behavioral medicine in industry: A labor perspective. In M. F. Cataldo and T. J. Coates, editors, *Health and Industry: A Behavioral Medicine Perspective.* New York: John Wiley & Sons, 1986.

Spilman, M. A., A. Goetz, J. Schultz, R. Bellingham, and D. Johnson. Effects of a corporate health promotion program. *Journal of Occupational Medicine, 28* (April 1986): 285–289.

Swinehart, J. W. Voluntary exposure to health communications. *American Journal of Public Health, 58* (July 1968): 1265–1275.

Taylor-Nicholson, M. E., D. Brannon, B. Mahoney, and J. Bucher. Assessing the need for health promotion programs in nursing homes. *Health Education, 21* (May/June 1990): 23–28.

Toufexis, A. Giving goodies to the good. *Time, 126* (November 18, 1985): 98.

Warner, K. Selling health promotion to corporate America: Uses and abuses of the economic argument. *Health Education Quarterly, 14* (Spring 1987): 39–55.

7

HEALTH EDUCATION AND HEALTH PROMOTION: PROGRAMS THAT WORK

Health education and health promotion programs have a good chance to be successful in changing behaviors of target groups and in reducing risk factors. The Association for the Advancement of Health Education (1990) has identified five elements known to be related to successful health promotion programs:

1. They are carefully planned.
2. They focus on modifiable risk factors known to be associated with health problems.
3. They use multiple health promotion activities, including health education.
4. The recipients are contributors throughout planning and delivery of the program.
5. Those responsible for delivering the program are qualified and competent.

Unfortunately, health educators must continually justify their existence and the continuation of their programs to administrators and boards of education that, although informed for years or even decades, fail to appreciate the importance of health education in the curriculum. The number of school systems that provide systematic, comprehensive health education is depressingly small. A vicious circle exists in that decision makers must rely on health educators to provide valid and reliable information regarding the impact of health education programs, but often no individual is found in the system who is knowledgeable enough to provide this information.

Those involved in the profession, whether at the national or the neighborhood level, must communicate the need for comprehensive health education programs to those who would influence the system or who are a part of the system. We must not ignore our responsibility to regularly inform members of boards of education, principals and other decision makers, and community leaders of the impact of comprehensive health education.

A number of meta-evaluations have synthesized the findings of several hundred studies conducted to determine the effectiveness of diverse school health education endeavors.* According to Kolbe (1985), the most important generalization supported by this process is that school-based health education programs consistently improve targeted health knowledge, attitudes, and skills, and inconsistently improve targeted behaviors. The probability that any given school-based health education intervention will improve targeted behaviors and the magnitude of the improvement depend on a number of factors. Those factors are the specificity of the intervention in addressing the targeted behavior, sufficient time provided for the intervention, the appraised quality of the intervention, parental or peer support existing or generated for the behavior, the extent to which the intervention was implemented as intended, and reinforcement of the intervention over time.

Kolbe further concluded that ample information suggests that well-planned school health education programs:

— improve student understandings about the scientific and philosophical principles of individual and societal health;

— improve the competencies students need to make decisions about personal behaviors that influence their health;

— improve the skills students need to engage in behaviors conducive to health;

— increase student behaviors that are conducive to health;

— improve the skills students need to maintain and improve the health of the families for which they will become responsible and the communities in which they will reside.

These conclusions provide abundant justification for school-based health education.

A few examples of programs that have been

successful can help explain the benefits of effective programs and how they can be developed. The following examples demonstrate that school health education and health promotion in other settings can change lives and improve health behavior. Administrators and boards of education should be made aware of them.

SCHOOL-BASED HEALTH PROMOTION/EDUCATION PROGRAMS
School Health Education Evaluation (SHEE)

The School Health Education Evaluation is the largest study of health education conducted in the United States (Gunn, Iverson, and Katz, 1985), a 3-year evaluation of the effectiveness of four school health curricula in 20 states. More than 30,000 children in grades 4 through 7 in 1071 classrooms were involved. The four curricula were:

1. Project Prevention.
2. School Health Curriculum Project (SHCP), otherwise known as Growing Healthy.
3. The Health Education Curriculum Guide.
4. 3Rs and High Blood Pressure.

The principal domains measured were (a) overall knowledge, (b) attitudes, (c) practices, and (d) specific knowledge (Connell, Turner, and Mason, 1985).

The SHEE effort found a significant association between time spent in the classroom and learning results, and that teacher inservice training and resource materials influenced the success of the programs on the four domains being measured. In general, with 30 or more hours of classroom instruction, positive effects were found for general health knowledge, general health practices, and general health attitudes (Bedworth & Bedworth, 1992) and, after 50 hours of exposure to comprehensive health education (AAHE,

---

* A meta-evaluation is a secondary analysis of one or more empirical summative evaluations having the power to draw generalizations from the primary evaluations.

1990), statistically significant improvements in knowledge, attitudes, and practices. The advisory panel to SHEE stated:

> The study shows, in general, that health education works; that it works better when there is more of it; and that it works best when it is implemented with broad-scale administrative and pedagogic support for teacher training, integrated materials, and continuity across grades. It works best where there is attention to the building of foundations of basic health knowledge, rather than starting with categorical health problems later in the academic career of pupils. (Green et al., 1985)

As previously stated, the SHEE panel examined four different school health curricula. We shall now consider each of the four.

Project Prevention

The Project Prevention program, implemented in grades K-9 and 11 in Oregon, Washington, and Idaho, was developed by a committee composed of administrators, teachers, students, and community agency personnel to address perceived problems in health instruction in the Chenowith School District, The Dalles, Oregon (*Project Prevention Final Evaluation Report*, 1979). No uniform health curriculum was being taught, and instructional methods and materials were unsatisfactory.

With the aid of a Title IV-C grant, the committee developed a curriculum sensitive to current issues, including alcohol and other drug abuse, cigarette smoking, teenage sexual behavior, and general physical well-being. The curriculum subsequently was expanded to include other issues. The main focus of the program was to develop decision-making and communication skills. Specific goals were established relating to self-concept development, family and society functioning, understanding human growth and development, application of decision-making skills, and awareness of local, national, and worldwide health problems.

The Project Prevention philosophy contends that the primary purpose of health education is to assist people in establishing lifestyles that discourage disease and enhance health. The goal is to provide students with the knowledge, attitudes, and skills that encourage good health. The K-6 curriculum consists of activities that could be conducted throughout the school year. A nine-week unit is provided for each of grades 7 and 8. For grades 9 through 11, a one-semester or 18-week unit is provided. As specific program goals, students will:

— develop a positive self-concept and openness to change;
— know and apply basic first-aid and safety skills;
— understand human growth and development from conception through death;
— know and apply decision-making and communication skills in everyday life as well as in stressful situations;
— function effectively as a family member and as a member of society;
— be made aware of career opportunities in health-related occupations;
— know and be able to evaluate available health resources and services;
— identify and relate more positively to exceptional people;
— know factors and select actions that contribute to good community health;
— understand current local, national, and global health problems, in addition to some of the ways these problems might be solved. (Owen et al., 1985)

Perhaps the success of Project Prevention is attributable to utilization of a curriculum advisory committee composed of concerned and qualified people from a variety of disciplines. The committee developed the curriculum, drawing from the expertise of individual members, concern for students in the system, and realization of local problems.

School Health Curriculum Project (SHCP) Growing Healthy

The SHCP, now known as Growing Healthy, began in the mid-1960s as the Berkeley Project, an effort to combat smoking, alcohol, and other drug use by teenagers. The SHCP was considered an ideal candidate for evaluation because it contains a comprehensive program for grades 4 through 7 and is more widely disseminated than other curricula, having been sponsored and promoted by the Public Health Service since 1967 (Gunn et al., 1985).

Before implementing the program, teachers, school nurses, and support persons attended an intensive training program of 40 to 60 hours. The training involved previewing materials and participation in a complete set of program activities that they would use later in the classroom. The intent of the training was to prepare a core group of people who could train other teachers in their individual districts.

One of the basic premises of SHCP was that children will resist social pressures to smoke, drink, and engage in other forms of substance abuse if they understand how their bodies work and the consequences of poor health (Owen et al., 1985). Consisting of four general areas centering on four systems of the human body, its goal was to impart to pupils a deep appreciation and understanding of the relation of health to care of the body. Each SHCP grade unit targeted a different body system. The program consisted of introduction and motivation activities, followed by five phases.

Phase I: "Awareness" of the general body systems being studied

Phase II: "Appreciation" of the specific body system being studied

Phase III: "Structure and Normal Functioning" of the body system

Phase IV: learning about "Diseases and Disorders" that affect the system being studied

Phase V: "Prevention" of diseases and disorders through good health habits.

The project concluded with presentation of activities the students created, such as skits, papers, demonstrations, and songs, to demonstrate how well they had learned the five phases. One of the findings of the SHEE was a 40% positive difference in smoking behavior of 7th grade students compared to those not in the program (AAHE, 1990).

Health Education Curriculum Guide (HECG)

The HECG came about from the recognition that community health agencies' school health education services in the Canton, Ohio, area were fragmented, that the schools had little control over the content of the presentations, and that instructional time was insufficient to support requests from all agencies. It was thought that classroom teachers had greater and more appropriate skills in delivering education and that the community health agencies had a more proper role as resource and information providers. In 1973, the United Way Health Foundation of Stark County funded a project to develop a comprehensive K-6 school health education curriculum.

A curriculum development committee, consisting of teachers, administrators, a curriculum specialist, parents, a health educator, college health personnel, and community health professionals, developed the curriculum. HECG consisted of three major elements (Bedworth and Bedworth, 1992):

1. The development of a curriculum implemented by teachers but using the expertise of health professionals in community agencies.

2. The formation of an advisory committee made up of school administrators and community representatives to provide guidance and leadership.

3. Coordination, implementation, and evaluation carried out under the leadership of a certified health educator.

The curriculum was based on the School Health Education Study (1967) curriculum design, which is a conceptual approach. The six general concepts selected for HECG were: nutrition; family living; drugs, alcohol, and tobacco; growth and development; environmental, community, and mental health; and safety. The basic goals of the HECG project were (a) to encourage positive health attitudes and behaviors in students; and (b) to help students better understand the health problems and issues they will confront and make decisions about as they become older (Brooks, Kirkpatrick, and Howard, 1981).

The health education curriculum emphasizes the following three components: (Owen et al., 1985)

1. Students must be actively involved in learning.
2. Students must be skilled in decision making.
3. Health knowledge, attitudes, and skills must integrate concepts associated with physical, mental, social, spiritual, and emotional well-being.

The HECG was designed to be flexible enough to allow it to be adapted to the needs of the individual school district. Some possible implementation strategies include:

1. A total health education program utilizing HECG health goals and objectives.
2. Selection of activities or lesson plans supplementing a health text.
3. Integration of activities or lesson plans into other subject areas such as language arts, reading science, home economics, and social studies.

No formal inservice training was built into the HECG. When requested by school district officials, however, a training session designed to introduce teachers to the content of health conceptual areas and to demonstrate hands-on approaches to teaching and learning was arranged.

3Rs and High Blood Pressure

Recognizing that high blood pressure was a major problem in Georgia in the early 1970s, educators decided that a successful approach to the problem might be an effective health education program. The Georgia affiliate of the American Heart Association was the guiding hand in developing the curriculum. The curriculum was based on the hypothesis that 6th-grade students could be taught practical information about high blood pressure and then facilitate the health education of their families and friends to help effect blood pressure control within their community (Owen, 1980).

During development of the program, four preadolescent "readiness" characteristics were considered (Owen et al., 1985):

1. Developing self-concept.
2. Learning to cooperate.
3. Learning self-regulation.
4. Learning about risk-taking and its consequences.

The program was initiated in the 6th grade, based on readiness characteristics of preadolescents, including self-concept development, ability to cooperate, ability to regulate their own basic needs, and ability to learn about risk taking. The program goals were:

— motivate teachers to act as role models, thus reinforcing positive health choices;

— provide information about high blood pressure;

— teach students how to determine high blood pressure;

— enhance communication skills applicable to peers, parents, and siblings.

Learner-centered activities including skill practice sessions were used to achieve these goals.

Ten class sessions, including five devoted to studying the circulatory system, high blood pressure, and risk factors of high blood pressure, comprised the program. Two more sessions dealt with how to use a stethoscope properly and how to measure blood pressure. Three sessions provided practice time. The emphasis was on lifestyle decisions. Participants were encouraged to continue a home practicum involving parents and other family members, encouraging dialogue between parents and children.

The eight objectives of the 3Rs and High Blood Pressure curriculum were for students to (Owen et al., 1985):

— define the term *high blood pressure*;
— describe the basic physiological factors that affect blood pressure;
— explain the seven steps to blood pressure control;
— state the risk factors that affect the blood pressure;
— name the complications that occur from uncontrolled blood pressure;
— identify an elevated adult blood pressure on a given list;
— list the parts of the blood pressure cuff and stethoscope, stating each part's specific function;
— compare systolic and diastolic blood pressure.

Summary of SHEE Findings

Much of the information reported here focuses on four broadly defined student test constructs:

1. Overall Knowledge.
2. Attitude.
3. Practice.
4. Program-Specific Knowledge.

Findings presented here are reported by Connell et al., (1985) unless otherwise noted.

Both the Overall Knowledge and the Program-Specific Knowledge scores increased between the pretest and the posttest. While scores increased in both groups, there were larger gains in those who participated in one of the health education programs (experimental group) than from those who did not participate (control group). Differences for knowledge measures were greater than those for attitudes and practices. Program-specific knowledge gains were 40% greater than for general knowledge.

Students in the health education programs reported healthier attitudes for three of the four subscores. The greatest differences were for attitude toward maintaining a healthy body. All self-reported health skills and practice subscores were greater in health education classes than in the control group, and the largest differences were in decision-making skills. According to their self-reporting, almost three times as many control group students began smoking in the first half of the 7th grade than did students in the health programs. In a midyear report, less than 8% of the 7th grade health education students reported smoking, whereas more than 12% of those in the 7th grade comparison classes were smoking.

All of the findings reported above were statistically significant. Moreover, they were obtained after a relatively short exposure to health education. A substudy of the SHEE indicated that the relatively small gains in attitude and behavior would approach the size of the gains in knowledge after a second year of health education. A coordinated, comprehensive health education program, the results suggest, would have lasting impact on participants' health attitudes and practices. Because this is the objective of health education, practitioners would be wise to make reference to the SHEE in justifying a comprehensive health education policy.

Each of the four SHEE programs described here can be considered successful, as each produced its most conspicuous positive outcomes in the areas targeted as most important by the program developers and teachers. The Growing Healthy project demonstrated the largest student inventory effects across overall domains and content areas as implemented in the "average" classroom. One of the important specific findings relating to the Growing Healthy project was a 40% difference in smoking behavior in 7th grade students in the program compared to 7th grade comparison students (Association for the Advancement of Health Education, 1990). Project Prevention produced its greatest effects in improved decision-making skills. The largest effects for 7th grade SCHP programs were in the areas of smoking incidence and knowledge of growth and development, human sexuality, and substance use and abuse.

The 3Rs and High Blood Pressure provided some insights into the effects of various degrees of implementation of the program. Implementation levels were higher for 3Rs and High Blood Pressure than for the three more comprehensive programs. Program-specific knowledge effects also were greater than those of the other programs. When the program was implemented on a 10-15 hour basis, however, the effects on the general set of attitudes and practices were limited. Yet, when the instructional time exceeded 20 hours, significant improvement in general attitudes and behaviors was recorded. In addition, the extent of parental participation was related to promotion of general health attitudes and behavior. These results strongly suggest that the amount of time devoted to health education influences attitudes and behaviors.

Even though the HECG showed effectiveness in both the areas of general knowledge and program-specific knowledge, program-specific knowledge gain was higher. This is remarkable in that the HECG-tailored knowledge measure was the least specific to program content of the four programs because no HECG-specific tests were contained in the original pool of items.

In addition to the results reported in the SHEE, Brooks et al., (1981) reported positive changes in perceived susceptibility to health problems, perceived seriousness of health problems, perceived preventability of health problems, and self-reported behavior in students in grades 4, 5, and 6 who were exposed to the HECG. Meanwhile, mean changes in beliefs in the control students in most cases did not differ significantly from zero. In every group comparison the mean change in the health beliefs or self-reported behavior of the experimental (HECG-exposed) students was significantly greater than the mean change of the control students. The authors concluded that the HECG was able to change beliefs along several dimensions, including perceived susceptibility, perceived seriousness, and perceived preventability, thereby increasing the likelihood of appropriate health behavior.

COMMUNITY HEALTH PROMOTION

Although we frequently think of health education and health promotion as occurring exclusively in a school setting, many other settings are appropriate. We now examine a few examples of health promotion and health education programs developed by various community members and professionals for application in community locations or community and school situations.

Health on Wheels

The Richmond (Virginia) City Health Department developed a program to deal with the unacceptably high infant mortality rate in that city. The Health on Wheels program has the goal of getting women into care as early in pregnancy as possible. The mobile unit parks at a neighborhood site, and outreach workers spread out in the neighborhood, sharing information, counseling, and going door-to-door to find women in the first trimester of pregnancy. It also visits schools, colleges and universities, street fairs, and athletic events. The Richmond program also has a Teens Only Clinic, a comprehensive prevention clinic operated in a church. The Parent-Child Task Force, a coalition of public and private agencies, works to heighten awareness of health issues concerning children and engage the community in developing strategies to address these concerns. The Richmond City Health Department also administers the

Women, Infants, and Children (WIC) program, providing food and health services and nutrition education. Nonwhite infant mortality dropped from 41% in 1965 to 23.9% in 1986 and to 20.1% in 1987 (Anderson, 1989).

Minnesota Heart Health Program

The Minnesota Heart Health Program utilizes multiple methods, including promoting personal and social skills and parent interviews. It is a 4½ hour program designed for 7th grade students. In one implementation in West Fargo and Fargo, North Dakota, the group of currently smoking students exposed to the program increased smoking amounts by 4% compared to a similar group of students who were not in the program, which increased smoking amounts by 13%. The experimental group had a rate of onset of smoking of 4% whereas the control group had a rate of onset of 12% (Association for the Advancement of Health Education, 1992).

Project Graduation

A community in Maine responded to the high rate of teenage traffic fatalities during the high school graduation season by developing Project Graduation, an alcohol-free program. The program involves the schools and the community at large. Teen alcohol-related automobile fatalities during the graduation season dropped to zero. The plan was so successful that it led to the inception of Project Graduation programs throughout the United States.

The Children Can't Fly

In a 1969 study of child mortality attributable to falls from heights, the New York City Department of Health reported that falls from heights represented 12% of all accidental deaths of children under age 15. The South Bronx initially was targeted for the pilot program because of a reported high rate of infant deaths from falls from windows and high rates of recidivism, or multiple falls in the same household. The program had three principal components:

1. A system of voluntary reporting by police precincts and hospital emergency rooms, followed by home visits by public health nurses.

2. Outreach workers' identifying hazards on a door-to-door basis, counseling parents and providing free window guards where indicated. Community education by public and private agencies and community groups in the form of prevention literature and instruction followed. A media campaign involving radio, television, news stories, and editorials provided prevention education and raised awareness.

3. The distribution of easy-to-install window guards free of charge to families with preschool children living in tenements in high-risk areas.

The program was expanded in 1974 and 1975 to include all five boroughs of New York City. The program also was expanded to include additional visits by public health nurses to provide supportive counseling and referral services to the victim and family.

The Children Can't Fly campaign is credited with a large part of the Bronx' 50% decline in falls reported, from 108 in 1973 to 54 in 1975. Further, during the critical summer months when windows are open more frequently, the percentage declines between 1973 and 1975 during those months were 68% in June, 72.8% in July, 81.5% in August, and 50% in September. Deaths of children as a result of falls from heights citywide, as determined from death certificates, declined from 57 in 1973, to 45 in 1974, and to 37 in 1975 (Spiegel and Lindaman, 1977).

The Battle Creek Schools Healthy Lifestyles Program

In the early 1980s, as the state of Michigan slid into a deep recession and budgets of school districts and state, county, and local health department shrank, school districts in the Greater Battle Creek, Michigan, Area faced a reduction in health services provided by the Calhoun County Health Department. Among these services were provision of school nurses. The role of the school nurse was changed from that of a primary health provider to that of a facilitator, educator, and director. School superintendents of the four school districts submitted to the W. K. Kellogg Foundation a proposal for funding school nurses. After consulting with the foundation, it was decided to include four private school systems in the Battle Creek area, although public schools were to be the primary locus of the health promotion and education initiatives of the project. It also was decided to concentrate on four "risk factors": physical fitness, nutrition, substance abuse, and stress management.

The Educator's Task Force, composed of community health providers, staff of the Kellogg Foundation, and community leaders, was formed to coordinate the project. The project developers also made a conscious effort to include other interested parties in governing and operating the project. They included the Calhoun County Health Department, Kellogg Community College, area hospitals, area nutritionists, Battle Creek Y-Center, parents, school personnel, psychological consultants, United Way, Washington Heights Ministries, and Battle Creek Police. The Healthy Lifestyles Task Force, consisting of representatives of community groups, was formed. Administrators and teachers were surveyed to determine the current scope and sequence of health education/promotion programs and activities they wanted in their schools.

Project initiatives designated teachers and staffs as role models, in the belief that students watch what you do as much or more than listen to what you say. Adult wellness activities were conducted in each school building. To promote physical fitness, all schools in the Greater Battle Creek Area outlined walking courses inside and outside the buildings. Staff members were encouraged to participate in a 6-week shape-up competition augmented with points for weight loss, aerobic activities, smoking cessation, and other healthy lifestyle components. The shape-up program included a health risk appraisal, physical fitness test, and cholesterol tests. More than 300 staff members attended a 4-day summer retreat, receiving information and current health education and health promotion initiatives and developing leadership and enthusiasm.

Traction for Action, a jogging program, was implemented. Walking programs also were started. Students in grades 3, 6, 9, and 12 were tested for physical fitness. Their parents received a report of the results and suggestions for improvement.

A nutritious school lunch program brought significant changes in school lunches. Objectives of the program were to provide students with nutritious food and teach students to become responsible for their own diets.

A student assistance program was initiated. It helped students with issues such as substance abuse, peer pressure, parent interaction, suicide, and teen pregnancy. Teachers were trained in identifying troubled students, and the students were referred to the appropriate community agencies.

The Healthy Lifestyles Program has enjoyed a great deal of parental support. In fact, the school districts have realized more parent support for the overall school program, including school millage campaigns and increases. The project also had increased support from parents for controversial programs, including human sexuality and AIDS prevention. Evaluation of student fitness change and health knowledge is being done and is not yet complete. Faculty absenteeism has been reduced from 623 days in 1985 to 477.5 in 1988, representing a savings of $8,001 in salaries for substitute teachers (Williams and Kubik, 1990).

Heart Beat Campaign

The Ottawa-Carleton (Canada) Heart Beat Campaign was created in 1987. The program seeks to increase public awareness about heart disease, to encourage people to live more heart-healthy lives, and to stimulate and support community activities that promote heart-healthy living. The project is a joint effort of the Ottawa-Carleton Health Department and other health organizations, businesses, and community agencies. Volunteers, a key to the program's success, have helped spread heart health messages throughout the community.

A popular component of the program is the Heart Beat Check. Health department staff, assisted by trained volunteers, tests participants' blood pressure, blood cholesterol levels, height, and weight. It also provides brief counseling sessions and self-help information. High-risk individuals are referred to their physician for follow-up.

The program also offers lifestyle programs designed to support people who are striving to adopt healthy behaviors. Heartstyles, a series of group sessions facilitated by public health nurses, focuses on building skills in personal behavior change, a heart-healthy diet, and stress management. Initial results of Heartstyles showed significant improvement in participants' physical and behavioral measurements.

One of the keys to the success of both Heart Beat Check and Heartstyles is the collaboration with more than 50 local businesses to implement on-site assessment and behavior modification programs. Volunteers and professionals travel the region, setting up portable lifestyle assessment units.

Because of its success, the Heart Beat Campaign is expanding into restaurants and supermarkets. In a study conducted in November 1990, 45% of Ottawa-Carleton residents reported they were exercising regularly, maintaining a healthy weight, and were non-smokers (Heart Beat Campaign, 1992).

Rural Community Health Promotion Programs

In a poor, predominantly black South Carolina county, a program supported by schools, churches, and community was developed to reduce the high rate of teen pregnancy. It was a culturally sensitive, scientifically accurate curriculum emphasizing self-esteem and decision making. The intervention group had an estimated 54% decrease in pregnancy rate, compared to an estimated 29% decrease in the comparison group (Association for the Advancement of Health Education, 1990).

At a small, rural, black-majority senior citizens meal site in Florida, a health promotion demonstration project was undertaken with 22 participants. The program included a weight reduction component with individuals who were 20% above their ideal weight, regular group exercise program, blood pressure referral and reduction program, and community organization. Weight, systolic blood pressure, and diastolic blood pressure all were reduced significantly. In addition, the program generated increases in self-perception related to overall health, physical health, coordination, care of self, strength, hearing, vision, motion, posture, and energy (Sutherland, Cowart, and Heck, 1989).

Health promotion activities addressing community development processes and the cardiovascular risk factors of nutrition, exercise, and blood pressure control were undertaken in six north Florida black churches. A Health Advisory Council was established by recruiting members from church and community leadership in the black population. The council enlisted churches to participate in the project. Leaders from each of the participating churches took part in an 8-week series of church-based health promotion workshops. The workshops consisted of basic cardiovascular knowledge and peer teaching materials and methodologies; health and social service community agencies; necessary program planning and implementation skills to enhance effectiveness of the church committee; and project assessment and reporting procedures. Each church committee planned its initial health promotion programs.

Members of the church communities completed a health assessment instrument consisting of demographic data, family histories for cardiovascular disease and cancer, nutrition practices, and number of months since last visit to a physician. Programs consisted of direct health instruction available to all church community members; Quarterly Health Sundays, focusing upon a physical, mental, spiritual, or emotional aspect of health; integration of health activities into regular church organizations; blood pressure screening; and community awareness activities (Sutherland et al., 1992).

group. The former also exhibited significant behavioral changes. The mortality rate of the group involved in the program was 57% better than that of the control group (Association for the Advancement of Health Education, 1990).

Kent General Hospital in Dover, Delaware, provides an example of community education within a health care setting by offering an annual health fair to residents of central Delaware. Physicians, nurses, dieticians, and other professionals, assisted by volunteers, present informal education at booths set up at the hospital. One of the most important functions is explaining risk factors of chronic diseases and lifestyle changes that can reduce the risks. Literature about nutrition is passed out, and healthy foods are given away. A play with a theme such as the importance of self-concept is presented several times during the day. Physicians explain some of the technology available to them for diagnosis, treatment, and surgery. The hospital's wellness program, Lifestyles Fitness Center, is open to the public, where physical therapists do screening for posture and flexibility.

CLINICAL SETTINGS

As discussed in Chapter 6, health education and promotion frequently take place in medical care settings. An example is the successful long-term health education program for low-income minority hypertensive patients developed and tested in a 5-year study. The primary program focus was weight reduction. Four hundred patients were exposed randomly to various educational experiences including counseling which explained and reinforced doctors' orders, a series of group sessions, and health education sessions centering on hypertension management and compliance. The control group received the usual treatment. In the 5-year analysis, the experimental group was significantly better at controlling blood pressure than the control

WORKSITE HEALTH PROMOTION

Health promotion at places of employment has expanded rapidly in recent years. The following examples illustrate the reasons for adopting worksite health promotion programs.

Campbell Soup Company

The Campbell Soup Company offers a comprehensive health/fitness program to employees. In 1968, the medical department of the company began offering a cardiovascular disease prevention program. The program included medical screening, diet and weight-reduction counseling, serum-lipid modification, smoking cessation, and exercise. Campbell's Institute for Health and Fitness publishes a newsletter that carries information on health promotion topics such as nutrition and fitness. Inhouse diagnostic and treatment services are offered along with behavior modification programs (Patton et al., 1986).

Johnson & Johnson—Live for Life

Johnson & Johnson, one of the nation's largest companies, implemented the Live for Life program, the goal of which was to provide the means for Johnson & Johnson employees "to become the healthiest in the world" and to control the increasing illness and accident costs of the corporation (Wilbur, 1983). LFL is a comprehensive endeavor aimed at aiding individuals to develop and maintain healthy lifestyles. The lifestyle seminar addresses many areas of health promotion and education, including nutrition, stress management, blood pressure control, and

elimination of smoking. Employee participation is voluntary and free of charge.

In one study, 2,000 employees were exposed to the comprehensive LFL Program, and an additional 1,700 were exposed to only a small part of the program. The results of a 2-year evaluation showed that participants in the comprehensive Live for Life Program recorded daily increases in energy use in vigorous physical activity of 104% compared to 33% in the comparison group. Higher levels of physical activity are associated with reduction in coronary risk. In a 5-year study, medical costs of nonparticipants were 200% more than the LFL participants, hospital admissions were more than double that of the participants, and the number of hospital stays also were more than double. Johnson & Johnson concluded that the program reduced medical costs by 40% and absenteeism by 18% (Association for the Advancement of Health Education, 1990).

In another study (Bly, Jones, and Richardson, et al., 1986), the LFL program cut employee

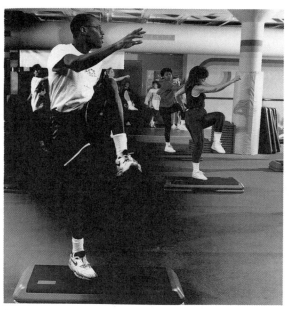
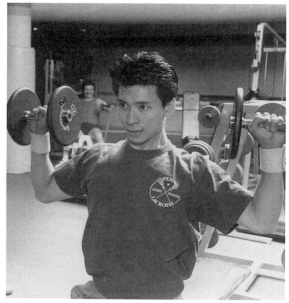

The Johnson & Johnson program of employee health promotion addresses employee wellness in a number of active ways, including safe low impact aerobic classes and strength development. Photos courtesy of Johnson & Johnson.

hospital-cost increases nearly in half at participating facilities, compared to facilities without the program.

IBM Corporation: A Plan for Life

A Plan for Life is a comprehensive health education program employing a full medical staff of 50 physicians and 150 nurses at several sites around the country. The primary objectives of the program are to encourage employees to take personal responsibility for their health, to offer health education programs, and to encourage employees to become members of health maintenance organizations.

Voluntary health screening, medical examinations, and health education programs are offered. Health education topics include weight control, exercise, nutrition, smoking cessation, prevention of back problems, first-aid and CPR, and stress management. Outside agencies as well as staff members conduct education programs. In 10 years, more than 190,000 employees had health examinations, and 41% of them were found to have unsuspected medical problems (Patton et al., 1986).

Blue Cross and Blue Shield of Indiana (BCBSI) Health Promotion Program

Blue Cross and Blue Shield of Indiana initiated a comprehensive health risk identification and reduction program for employees in 1978. The program was designed to reduce behavioral risk factors associated with the leading causes of death. Disease prevention was the primary thrust of the program.

The BCBSI program consisted of four phases:

1. *Employee health risk education.* This first phase, which lasted 2 months, involved mass health awareness/information strategies. Health risk appraisal questionnaires were sent to all employees following the education campaign.

2. *Brief physical exams and counseling.* All employees who returned health risk appraisals were given short physical examinations that measured blood pressure, height, weight, blood cholesterol, carbon monoxide, blood sugar, and hemoglobin. Individual counseling then was conducted to review the preliminary results. Based on disease risk, employees were encouraged to enroll in a worksite health promotion class or to work on their own at reducing their risk factors.

3. *Health promotion classes.* These classes, with topics such as smoking cessation, nutrition education, and weight reduction, promoted positive health behavior change. They were conducted on company time and offered free of charge to the employees.

4. *Maintenance of the new behavior.* This final phase included periodic telephone contact with individuals who had participated in the health promotion classes to check on their progress, to encourage continuation of healthful behavior, and to urge the involvement of significant others in maintaining of new behaviors (Sciacca et al., 1990).

The BCBSI program is particularly interesting because of its philosophy of enrolling only those who have demonstrated risks. Although many worksite health promotion programs implement more universal primary prevention, this one, sponsored by a health insurance company, implements primary prevention only to the extent of identified risk factors.

SCHOOL SITE HEALTH PROMOTION

A number of school districts have discovered the benefits of health promotion to their employees. These benefits range from those affecting health to those affecting the financial strength of the district.

A Texas program for teachers included health education in nutrition, exercise, and stress management. The experimental group increased physical activity and levels of fitness, lowered weight and blood pressure, and reported greater well-being than the comparison group. In an ensuing study, the experimental group reported 1.25 fewer days absent per teacher. Translated into dollars, at $47 per day per substitute, the districts realized a savings of nearly $150,000 from the 2,546 participants in the program (Association for the Advancement of Health Education, 1990).

SUMMARY

Effective and productive health promotion/ education programs are abundant. The examples set forth in this chapter are only a selected few. Sample school-based health promotion/ education successful programs are Project Prevention, Growing Healthy, HECG, and the 3Rs and High Blood Pressure, all part of the School Health Education Evaluation (SHEE). Community health promotion is exemplified by Health on Wheels, the Minnesota Heart Health Program, Project Graduation, The Children Can't Fly, the Battle Creek Schools Healthy Lifestyles Program, and the Heart Beat Campaign, along with some exemplary rural community programs. Health education and promotion, too, often take place in medical care settings. Worksite programs have been carried out by the Campbell Soup Company, Johnson & Johnson, and Blue Cross/Blue Shield, among others. A number of school districts also conduct health education programs for their employees.

Most of the programs described here have been studied for effectiveness and have been shown to meet their objectives. All of them have had positive impact on the lives of those they serve.

REFERENCES

Anderson, S. The role of health education in reducing infant mortality in Richmond, Virginia. *Health Education, 20* (October/November 1989): 35-43.

Association for the Advancement of Health Education. *Health Education Works!* Reston, Virginia: AAHE, 1990. (video)

Bedworth, A. E. and D. A. Bedworth. *The Profession and Practice of Health Education.* Dubuque, IA: Wm. C. Brown Publishers, 1992.

Bly, J. L., R. C. Jones, and J. E. Richardson. Impact of worksite health promotion on health care costs and utilization. *Journal of the American Medical Association, 256* (December 19, 1986); 3235-3240.

Brooks, C. H., M. Kirkpatrick, and D. J. Howard. Evaluation of an activity-centered health curriculum using the Health Belief Model. *Journal of School Health, 51* (October 1981): 565-569.

Connell, D. B., R. R. Turner, and E. F. Mason. Summary of findings of the School Health Education Evaluation: Health promotion effectiveness, implementation, and costs. *Journal of School Health, 55* (October, 1985): 316-321.

Green, L. W., T. D. Cook, M. E. Doster, S. W. Fors, R. Hambleton, A. Smith, and H. J. Walberg. Thoughts from the School Health Education Advisory Panel. *Journal of School Health, 55* (October, 1985): 300.

Gunn, W. J., D. C. Iverson, and M. Katz. Design of the School Health Education Evaluation. *Journal of School Health, 55* (October, 1985). 301-304.

Heart Beat Campaign. *Health Promotion, 30* (Spring 1992): 30-31.

Kolbe, L. J. Why school health education? An empirical point of view. *Health Education, 16* (April/May 1985): 116-120.

Owen, S. When the student is ready, the teacher will come. *Journal of the South Carolina Medical Association*, September 1980, pp. 25-28.

Owen, S. L., M. A. Kirkpatrick, S. W. Lavery, H. L. Gonser, S. R. Nelson, R. L. Davis, E. F. Mason, and D. B. Connell. Selecting and recruiting health programs for the School Health Education Evaluation. *Journal of School Health, 55* (October 1985): 305-308.

Patton, R. W., J. M. Corry, L. R. Gettman, and J. S. Graf. *Implementing Health/Fitness Programs.* Champaign, IL: Human Kinetics Publishers, 1986.

Project Prevention Final Evaluation Report. Portland, OR: Northwest Regional Education Laboratory, July 1979.

School Health Education Study. *Health Education: A Conceptual Approach to Curriculum Design.* St. Paul, MN: 3M Education Press, 1967.

Sciacca, J., R. Seehafer, R. Reed, and C. Berry. Evaluating worksite health promotion programs. *Health Education, 21* (May/June 1990): 17-22.

Spiegel, C. N. and F. C. Lindaman. Children Can't Fly: A program to prevent childhood morbidity and mortality from window falls. *American Journal of Public Health, 67* (December 1977): 1143-1147.

Sutherland, M., M. Cowart, and C. Heck. A rural senior citizens health promotion demonstration project. *Health Education, 20* (October/November 1989): 40-43.

Sutherland, M., M. Barber, G. Harris, and M. Cowart. Health promotion in southern rural Black churches: A program model. *Journal of Health Education, 23* (March 1992): 109-111.

Wilbur, C. S. The Johnson & Johnson program. *Preventive Medicine, 12* (September 1983): 672-681.

Williams, P., and J. Kubik. The Battle Creek (Michigan) Schools Healthy Lifestyles Program. *Journal of School Health, 60* (April 1990): 142-146.

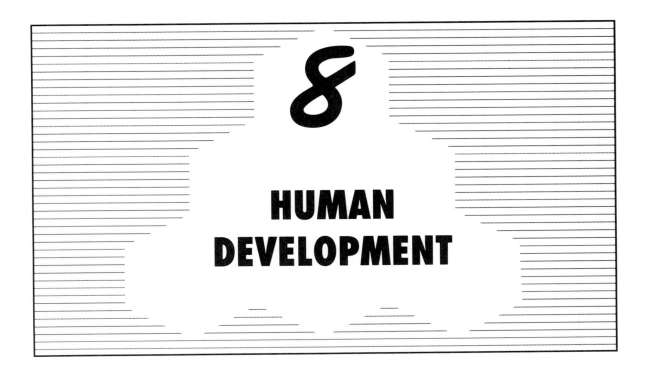

HUMAN DEVELOPMENT

Much of human behavior is based upon the individual's current level of development. Three well-known models explain the development of humans from birth through old age. These models are explained and summarized here not only to acquaint the prospective health educator with their content but also to make their content relevant to the profession. When curricula are developed, they have a basis in the development, the "readiness," of the person to whom they are addressed. The daily activity of the classroom should be carried out with the developmental stages of the student in mind.

Community health educators also frequently deal with challenges of adults and children relating to developmental tasks. These professionals should be cognizant of that reality when initiating programs and activities.

Although a number of similarities are evident in the models of Erikson, Havighurst, and Coleman, they are presented individually to better note their unique messages for health educators and for teachers in general. Students of

health education should endeavor to isolate the differences in the models.

ERIKSON'S MODEL OF HUMAN DEVELOPMENT

Erik Erikson (1963) explained the development of humans as an eight-stage process involving a dichotomy at each stage. These stages also are referred to as *developmental phases*. As the individual matures, he or she is faced with a basic task. Meeting the task prepares the person for success in meeting the task at the next stage. The stages are summarized by Carroll and Miller (1991) in Table 8.1.

Teachers spend a good deal of their professional lives assisting in the development of the positive side of the dichotomies, at least through adolescence. Many educators deal with adults through college instruction, community organizations, and other settings. Recognition of individual's efforts to meet the developmental tasks and assisting him or her to do so can be a

Table 8.1.   Erikson's Eight Stages of Human Development

Developmental Phase	Basic Task	Characteristics of Psychosocial Crises
Infancy (first year)	Basic trust vs. mistrust	Confidence originates in mother's consistent actions and care of infant's needs; mistrust develops from a sense of abandonment and deprivation.
Early childhood (1–3 years)	Autonomy vs. shame and doubt	Expressions of independence, coupled with parental protection, surface; failure to achieve autonomy results in self-consciousness, feelings of inadequacy, and self-doubt.
Preschool (3–5 years)	Initiative vs. guilt	Pleasure derived from attack and conquest, self-observation, and identification with same-sex parent in work roles; denial and inhibition give rise to guilt.
Elementary school (6–11 years)	Industry vs. inferiority	Desires for production, use of tools, doing things with others; nonaccomplishment results in a sense of inadequacy and mediocrity and in conformity.
Adolescence (12–19 years)	Identity vs. role confusion	Concern with other persons' views of oneself and with the search for continuity, values, and commitment to ideals; failure to achieve identity gives rise to role confusion and doubts about one's sexual and occupational identity.
Young adulthood (20+ years)	Intimacy vs. isolation	Willingness to enter affiliations, to make self-committments and close friendships, and to express heterosexuality; avoidance of intimacy related to fears of losing self and to developing sense of isolation and self-absorption.
Middle adulthood	Generativity vs. stagnation	Capacities of teaching, guiding, producing, and creating evolve; without generativity, a feeling of personal impoverishment and nonaccomplishment develops, along with psychological nonmovement.
Late adulthood	Ego integrity vs. despair	Embraces the order and meaning of one's life cycle, with its joys and sorrows; defends dignity of the life cycle; the sting of death is diminished; without enough time to start life anew, feelings of disgust and fear of death predominate.

Source: C. Carroll and D. Miller, *Health: The Science of Human Adaptation* (5th ed.) (Dubuque, IA: Wm. C. Brown Communications, 1991). All rights reserved. Reprinted by permission.

crucial role in education as well as other areas of society.

Erikson's Eight Stages

Basic Trust vs. Mistrust

According to Erikson, trust coincides with confidence. The infant relies on sameness and continity of the provider, primarily the mother. The baby is dependent on the quality of the relationship with his or her mother. Mothers create a sense of trust in their children by combining sensitive care of the baby's individual needs with a firm sense of trustworthiness. This treatment exists within the framework of the culture and lifestyle.

Autonomy vs. Shame and Doubt

As the surroundings encourage the child to "stand on your own feet," he or she must be protected against arbitrary experiences of shame and doubt. The caregiver also must provide well-guided experiences of free choice and avoid the development of precocious conscience and obsessiveness. It is a tightrope of responsibility that requires sensitivity and awareness. Too much shaming can lead to a secret need to get away with things or even defiant shamelessness. According to Erikson, this stage is decisive for the ratios of love and hate, cooperation and willfulness, freedom of self-expression and its suppression.

Initiative vs. Guilt

Initiative adds to autonomy the quality of undertaking, planning, and attacking a task for the sake of being active and on the move. Loco-motor skills have developed to the extent that the child can transport himself or herself without aid and can perform many complex movements. These skills elicit tremendous enjoyment in the freedom of movement and the mental power it brings. The danger of this stage is a sense of guilt regarding the goals contemplated and the acts initiated. Although the child is capable of manipulation, indeed overmanipulation, he or she can gradually develop a sense of moral responsibility. The child can gain insight into institutions, their functions and roles, which permit limited and reasonable participation.

The child finds blissful accomplishment in handling and using tools, toys, and other implements. He or she may even take some pride in caring for younger children. The child is eager to do things cooperatively. He or she is willing to learn and benefit from teachers and to emulate models. The child is ready to learn and capable of doing so quickly.

Industry vs. Inferiority

The child rapidly learns to win recognition by producing things. He or she learns the pleasure of completing a task. During this stage the child is willing to learn from older children. The school becomes a culture unto itself, with its boundaries, goals, and limits, its achievements and disappointments.

If the child feels insecure or inadequate with his or her skills or tools, or of his or her status in the group, the loss of identification with them and with a section of his or her tool world may become evident. This may lead to isolation and less industry. The child may consider himself or herself doomed to mediocrity and inadequacy.

Erikson (1968) described this stage as a most decisive one socially. Much of the child's success comes from outside himself or herself; industry involves doing things with others and in their company. At this fourth stage the development of many children is disrupted if family life has failed to prepare them for school life or when school life fails to sustain the promises of early age.

Identity vs. Role Confusion

The fifth stage of development, adolescence, marks the ending of childhood and the beginning of youth. Physiologically, the body is undergoing a tremendous reformation. Adult roles and tasks lie ahead, visible on the horizon. Adolescents are concerned primarily with what they appear to be in others' eyes compared with what they feel they are. They also are concerned with issues relating to connecting the roles and skills developed earlier with occupational paradigms. They seek to merge the future with the recent past.

Adolescents also become concerned with ideals and idols. They search for someone in whom to place their faith and may become too strongly identified with their heroes. Erikson (1968) attributed this to the inability to settle on an occupational identity. Frequently, the well-meaning people in their lives, teachers and parents, are placed in the roles of antagonists. As Erikson (1963) stated:

> The integration taking place in the form of ego identity is . . . more than the sum of childhood identifications. It is the accrued experience of the ego's ability to integrate all identifications with vicissitudes of libido, with the aptitudes developed out of endowment, and with opportunities offered by social roles.

Ego identity is the confidence that the sameness and continuity of one's past and one's meaning for others are the same. This confidence forms the basis of the promise of a "career."

Role confusion, which Erikson blames to a large extent on "strong previous doubt as to one's sexual identity," may produce deliquency, antisocial behavior, and what is sometimes called "psychotic episodes." Simply put, it is a lack of occupational identity.

One result of role confusion is "falling in love," which may be asexual or have little sexual substance. Adolescent love is an attempt to arrive at a definition of one's identity by projecting one's own scattered ego on another and observing it reflected and gradually clarified. This is the young love that usually is more conversational than physical.

Adolescents also become quite cliquish. They exclude others on the basis of seemingly irrelevant issues such as dress and tastes in music and cars. They also may make exclusions based upon more concrete concerns such as race, cultural background, and neighborhood. This clannish behavior may be a defense against identity confusion.

The adolescent intellect is at a stage between childhood and adulthood. It has arrived at a confusing place between the morality learned as a child and the ethics developed by the adult. Perhaps no stage in human development is as crucial to the social and occupational success of the person as adolescence.

Intimacy vs. Isolation

After searching for identity, the young adult is ready and impatient to merge his or her identity with that of others. The individual is ready for intimacy. In Erikson's parlance, intimacy is the capacity to commit oneself to real and serious affiliations with others and to develop the ethical strength to abide by those commitments, even though they may depend upon significant sacrifices and compromises. Avoiding close friendships, possible sexual unions, inspirational experiences by those who are respected, and other close affiliations may lead to a deep sense of isolation and self-absorption. Avoiding sexual unions as a possible inducement to isolation should not be construed as encouraging sexual promiscuity. Sexual alliances do not necessarily involve physical sexual activity. Unfortunately, young people who are not sure of their identity may avoid interpersonal intimacy, preferring promiscuous acts without true intimacy and self-abandonment. As adulthood progresses, intimacy and the questions surrounding it become subject to the ethical sense, which is the stamp of mature adulthood.

Generativity vs. Stagnation

Generativity is the concern for the next generation, the desire for developing and passing on to the next generation a fair and better world. It is evidenced in the need to guide and instruct.

Mature parents and grandparents, after years of comfortable intimacy, demonstrate the creative and productive urge to advise and counsel their children and grandchildren as well as others who are their junior. Unfortunately, young parents often do not have the ability to develop this stage, leaving their children with insufficient guidance. Societal institutions, such as the family, work, and church, codify the ethics of generative succession, safeguarding and reinforcing the continuation of generativity.

Ego Integrity vs. Despair

Ego integrity means acceptance of the life cycle as singular and inevitable. It allows acceptance of the end of the life cycle so death loses its pain. Whereas ego integrity is comfort with the life cycle, despair is the fear of death. For a person who has not established ego integrity, time is short; he or she cannot accept the inevitability of the life cycle and its necessary end. It is easy to see how lack of career success influences despair as well. The person looks back on life as incomplete and realizes there is not enough time to do the things that would make life complete. Failure to achieve intimacy and generativity frequently lead to despair in late adulthood.

Erikson's Development Stages and Health Education

An integral part of any successful health education program is enhancement of the individual's development. This is as true in the community program for the senior citizen as it is in the middle school class. The relevant issues are the "hows."

Curriculum development always should emphasize development of the person. Whether directly or indirectly, curricula have done so for years with varying degrees of success. They even have dealt with development of the preschool child and infant. A good example of this is the fairly recent phenomenon called *family life education*. These programs consistently broach issues relating to parenting and child development. Many home economics classes also venture into the arena of parenting with sensitivity and expertise.

Community organizations frequently deal with infant and preschool development. Many hospitals and organizations such as the American Red Cross offer courses on the basic skills of parenting. These courses touch on the infant's basic needs and the skills necessary to meet those needs. Daycare center licensure should be based in part on knowledge of child development, because daycare workers daily affect the health, values, and physical and emotional development of children.

Many learning experiences relating to parenting fail to give adequate attention to the father's role in childrearing. Erikson writes a good deal about the mother's role, especially in infancy when trust is established, but much less about the father's role in the child's development. Curricula should be developed so the importance of both parents is understood. The idea of the mother rearing the children and the father providing the income is, for most families, obsolete.

Two issues stand out in the stages Erikson identified: self-concept and values. *Self-concept* is emphasized in infancy as not only trust of the caregiver but of self. Avoiding shame and doubt is an obvious self-concept issue of early childhood. Circumventing feelings of inferiority during the elementary school stage also is clearly tied to self-esteem. The joy of handling tools, toys, and other devices is an overt indication of self-esteem. Because successfully completing a task greatly encourages the development of esteem, the teacher must assign tasks in which the child is likely to find success. As the child masters tasks, the complexity of work and play can increase gradually.

Adolescents are concerned primarily with others' perception of them; their self-esteem is determined largely by others. Sensitive parents and teachers should be aware of this. The emotional issues attached to adolescents, including adolescent love and rejection by peer cliques, are issues that only sensitive adults can deal with successfully.

Textbooks and workbooks devoted to developing self-concept recently have targeted the health education market. Health educators would do their students a great service by investigating this literature. A great many activities directed toward generating positive self-concept have been developed and tested and are readily available.

Values and morals are emphasized throughout Erikson's stages. Even in infancy, trustworthiness becomes a value upon which to base others. The balance between autonomy and shame often can be expressed in terms of values. During the preschool years, moral responsibility can be developed gradually. The school, a microcosm of society, becomes a culture unto itself, with its rules, limits, achievements, and various forms of feedback. Erikson described the adolescent mind as a stage between childhood and adulthood and between the *morality* learned by the child and the *ethics* developed by the adult. Erikson claimed that one mark of adulthood is when intimacy becomes subject to ethics. Although values are not the same as morality and ethics, Erikson's reference to morality and ethics carries an implied reference to values.

In this text we have discussed values as they involve health-related behavior. At no stage in a child's development is the question of values to be ignored. Although his description of the stages of development do not specifically address many health issues and behavior related to them, Erikson has indirectly given a framework for the development of values in children that can affect their health-related behavior throughout life.

Good teachers know how to assist the individual's development. They know how to alternate play and work. They know how to alternate games and study and how to integrate them. They also should know how to utilize the prevailing technology to develop and sustain industry. In the 1990s, high technology computers dominate, but many schools do not have enough funds to provide them. This has severe implications for maintaining industry and developing subsequent tasks.

Good teachers know how to utilize others' skills and experience. Generativity can be a powerful tool. One way is to invite adults with specific expertise to share and instruct in class. This represents a virtually untapped resource in health education.

Erikson provides valuable insights to all of education. The wisdom he offers to health educators is more than valuable; it is indispensable.

HAVIGHURST'S DEVELOPMENTAL TASKS

Robert Havighurst (1952, 1972) presented the development of humans in six age periods similar to Erikson's. Havighurst, however, provided specific developmental tasks that dominate each stage. He stated that development was tied strongly to learning and, to understand development, one must understand learning. We learn our way through life.

Havighurst (1972) defined a developmental task as:

> A task which arises at or about a certain period in the life of the individual, successful achievement of which leads to his happiness and to success with later tasks, while failure leads to unhappiness in the individual, disapproval by the society, and difficulty with later tasks.

Developmental tasks arise from three sources:

1. *Physical maturation,* as evidenced by learning to walk, and to behave in ways acceptable to the other sex during adolescence.
2. *Cultural pressure of society,* as evidenced by the need to read, and to participate as a citizen in a socially acceptable manner.
3. *Personal values and aspirations* of the individual.

Havighurst's developmental tasks are summarized in Table 8.2.

Havighurst's Developmental Tasks and Education

Havighurst confirms strong links between development and learning, stating that individuals learn their way through life. Therefore, rather than amplifying on Table 8.2 and then establishing links between education and health education and the developmental tasks, the two objectives are addressed simultaneously here.

Formal education is in reality a means generated by society to help its members achieve certain developmental tasks. Tasks such as establishing autonomy and learning a masculine or feminine role are *recurring;* they must be achieved in various degrees throughout the life cycle. Early success in recurring tasks is an indication of success in later phases, making the critical period that point at which the task first appears. The school is not alone in its role of assisting the development of these tasks. It aids and is aided by other institutions of society such as the family, church, and community organizations.

Havighurst alludes to a number of issues that have strong implications for health education and education in general. A number of references are made to sexuality, family life education, including education for parenting, development of values, social development and health, and general health. These references can be utilized to make a convincing argument for comprehensive health education.

Sexuality and the development of attitudes about sex form a central core of human developmental tasks. As Havighurst (1972) said with reference to the infant and early childhood task of learning sex differences and sexual modesty: "Attitudes and feelings he develops about sex in these early years probably have an abiding effect upon his sexuality throughout his life." We learn early in life what it means to behave like a boy or a girl. Planning for this socializing process begins even before birth as parents select the color scheme for the nursery, and it continues with clothing and toy selections for the crib. Certainly, it is important that this happens. It is

---

Table 8.2.   Havighurst's Developmental Tasks

Age Period	Developmental Task	Nature of the Task
Infancy and Early Childhood (through fifth year)	Learning to walk	
	Learning to take solid food	To be weaned from breast or bottle
	Learning to talk	To learn to make meaningful sounds; to communicate with others through use of these sounds
	Learning to control elimination of body wastes	To learn to urinate and defecate at socially acceptable times and places
	Learning sex differences and sexual modesty	
	Forming concepts and learning to describe social and physical reality	To learn that certain images and sounds are associated with people; to learn that particular perceptions can be grouped together and called by one name
	Getting ready to read	To learn that signs stand for words; to discriminate among a variety of signs; to acquire a vocabulary of at least several thousand words
	Learning to distinguish right and wrong and beginning to develop a conscience	To learn concepts of good and bad; to give content to those concepts
Middle Childhood (6–12 years)	Learning physical skills necessary for ordinary games	To learn the physical skills necessary for games and physical activities highly valued in childhood
	Building wholesome attitudes toward oneself as a growing organism	To develop habits of body care, of cleanliness and safety, a sense of normality and adequacy, the ability to enjoy using the body, and a wholesome attitude toward sex
	Learning to get along with agemates	To learn the give-and-take of social life among peers; to learn to make friends and to get along with enemies; to develop a "social personality"
	Learning an appropriate masculine or feminine social role	To learn to be a boy or a girl — to act the role that is expected and rewarded
	Developing fundamental skills in reading, writing, and calculating	To learn to read, write, and calculate well enough to get along in American society
	Developing concepts necessary for everyday living	To acquire a store of concepts sufficient for thinking effectively about ordinary occupational, civic, and social matters
	Developing conscience, morality, and a scale of values	To develop inner moral control, respect for rules, and the beginning of a rational scale of values
	Achieving personal independence	To become an autonomous person, able to make plans and to act in the present and immediate future independently of one's parents and other adults
	Developing attitudes toward social groups and institutions	To develop social attitudes that are basically democratic
Adolescence (12–18 years)	Achieving new and more mature relations with agemates of both sexes	To learn to look upon girls as women and boys as men; to become an adult among adults; to learn to work with others for a common purpose, disregarding personal feelings; to learn to lead without dominating
	Achieving a masculine or feminine social role	To accept and learn a socially approved adult masculine or feminine social role
	Accepting one's physique and using the body effectively	To become proud, or at least tolerant, of one's body; to use and protect one's body effectively and with personal satisfaction
	Achieving emotional independence from parents and other adults	To become free from childish dependence on parents; to develop affection for parents without dependence upon them; to develop respect for older adults without dependence upon them

— Continued

Table 8.2.   Havighurst's Developmental Tasks — *Continued*

Age Period	Developmental Task	Nature of the Task
	Preparing for marriage and family life	To develop a positive attitude toward family life and having children; to get the knowledge necessary for home management and child rearing
	Preparing for an economic career	To organize one's plans and energies so as to begin an orderly career; to feel able to make a living
	Acquiring a set of values and an ethical system as a guide to behavior — developing an ideology	To develop a rational body of ideas, images, and ideals upon which to base future decisions and behavior
	Desiring and achieving socially responsible behavior	To develop a social ideology; to participate as a responsible adult in the life of the community, region, and nation; to take account of the values of society in one's personal behavior
Early Adulthood (18–30 years)	Selecting a mate	
	Learning to live with a marriage partner	To learn to express and control one's feelings — anger, joy, disgust, love — so one can live intimately and happily with a mate
	Starting a family	To have a first child
	Rearing children	To learn to meet the physical and emotional needs of young children
	Managing a home	To manage and share the physical and financial responsibilities of a home
	Getting started in an occupation	
	Taking on civic responsibility	To assume responsibility for the welfare of a group outside of the family — a neighborhood or community group or church or lodge or political organization
	Finding a congenial social group	To form new friendships
Middle Age (30–60 years)	Assisting teenage children to become responsible and happy adults	To cooperate with adolescent children, to become emotionally independent from parents, and to become emotionally mature
	Achieving adult social and civic responsibility	
	Reaching and maintaining satisfactory performance in one's occupational career	To achieve flexible work role that is interesting and productive and financially satisfactory
	Developing adult leisure-time activities	
	Relating oneself to one's mate as a person	
	To accept and adjust to the physiological changes of middle age	
	Adjusting to aging parents	To meet the responsibility for the needs of aging parents; to promote the happiness of the middle-aged generation
Later Maturity (60+ years)	Adjusting to decreasing physical strength and health	
	Adjustment to retirement and reduced income	
	Adjusting to death of mate	
	Establishing an explicit affiliation with one's age group	To accept one's status as a member of the elders of a society; to become a constructive participant in one's age group
	Adopting and adapting social roles in a flexible way	
	Establishing satisfactory physical living arrangements	To find the kind of living quarters that are most comfortable and convenient

Adapted from R. J. Havighurst. *Developmental Tasks and Education* (3d edition) (New York: David McKay Company, 1972).

just as important that young parents recognize that it happens and are able to focus their interactions with their infants in positive ways.

The developmental tasks of middle childhood grow out of three outward pushes: the child being thrust out of the home and into the peer group; the child being thrust into the world of games requiring neuromuscular skills; and the mental thrust into the world of adult concepts, logic, symbolism, and communication. Attitudes about many of life's intricacies are formed out of these pushes. Attitudes, particularly toward sex, are affected by these changes and are established early in life. By middle childhood, the youngster should have developed a wholesome attitude about sex. The culture of the home and community often affects the development of attitudes about sex. The teacher should understand the peer culture of the school and community and, in multicultural situations, pay attention to cultural interactions and differences.

Adolescence is the most critical time in developing and establishing of sexual identity and attitudes. Havighurst referred to learning to look upon girls as women and boys as men and accepting socially approved masculine and feminine roles. Although traditional education regarding sexuality has found it easy to identify the components of these masculine and feminine roles, our changing society blurs the lines and can easily cause confusion in young people.

The debate rages over how to address sexual orientation and androgyny. Virtually all adolescents sometimes feel they are not "normal." This feeling is intensified if they are uncomfortable in "traditional" sex roles. Only a few generations ago, women were expected to remain in the home and men were expected to earn the living. Women were once looked upon as "loose" or immoral if they wore pants. Men were almost forbidden from wearing earrings by common social mores. All of these standards have been weakened or thoroughly destroyed. For most teens, the school is a social laboratory for adolescent experimentation. It takes a sensitive educator to assist students who are dealing with reconciling their own feelings and standards with those of the community.

The role of *family life education* is strengthened by Havighurst's developmental tasks. Family life education is a multiphasic curriculum component, including aspects of managing the finances of a family, sexuality and sex education within a family, decision-making skills, coping skills, parenting skills, and a plethora of other subjects. The developmental tasks address a great many issues specific to parenting, such as toilet training, role modeling, and providing rewards and punishment leading to development of a conscience. They also confront issues of maturation such as developing autonomy and gradual independence from parents. This is a particularly touchy area for many parents. Effective family life programs assist students in becoming ready for independence and also provide conferences and parent education to help parents deal with their children's need for independence.

A significant part of any family life education program is helping adolescents to develop a positive attitude toward family life. This is especially important when dealing with today's nontraditional families. Each family member has certain responsibilities worked out within the group. Whether traditional or otherwise, each family member must accept his or her responsibilities if the family is to flourish. Understanding the significance of the individual's culture to the family unit and roles within it is also important. Different cultures have different role expectations for family members. This diversity can present problems for the teacher or for students who have not been exposed to different cultures. Havighurst asserted that the best preparation for marriage and family life is through achieving satisfactory relations with people of similar age and of the other gender. This is related to earlier tasks.

Skills in home management also are needed, and can be attained through a complete family life curriculum. The adolescent can profit a great deal from experience with young children.

During the adolescent period, there is need for well-trained, sensitive, expert advice concerning sex and courtship problems. Frequently, the health educator is the person the student goes to for advice. This indicates that perhaps the student does not feel comfortable discussing these subjects with family members. The health educator should maintain confidentiality with the student but also should have formal authorization to take on this role. A well-trained educator can be a helpful resource to students during adolescence.

Although Havighurst addressed the need for effective high school and college courses in marriage and family, the current philosophy is to include family life education in a comprehensive health education program. A well-designed, comprehensive health education program utilizes other disciplines and the expertise of other faculty members. This comprehensive program should be a part of the curriculum at all levels of schooling.

The value of a comprehensive health education program is carried throughout life. The difficult developmental tasks of learning to live with a partner, starting a family, rearing children, and managing the home are part and parcel of family life education and comprehensive health education. Learning to express feelings and to let others do so are necessary to happy family living. Health education has been useful in preparing young people for their first pregnancy and childbirth. Adjusting to the considerable changes in the lives of future parents can be aided by well-planned family life programs.

Acquiring *values* and morals is a critical theme throughout the developmental tasks. The issue of education relating to morals is often controversial because of fears that it may contradict cultural and religious teachings. Nevertheless, when the issue is values, the basic guides that give direction to our lives and behavior, the concensus is that the schools have a responsibility to be involved in their development. There is also agreement that the comprehensive health

education program is a viable modality for identifying and stimulating the acquisition of the values that are inherent in our society and that produce consistency in our behavior.

Many real life situations require the individual to choose between two or more values. Thus, the child has to develop a scale of values. In this way he or she can make sensible, consistent, and steady choices.

Havighurst alluded to learning during the infancy and childhood phase as distinguishing between right and wrong and the concepts of good and bad. The content associated with these concepts form the basis for values. During the middle childhood years, health educators provide the basis to establish those values and concepts. Respect for rules of behavior and for authority are acquired in school. In adolescence, the individual must fine-tune a set of values and develop a system of ethics to guide his or her behavior. Havighurst specified the educational implications to this acquisition as:

1. To help students acquire a worthwhile combination of expressive and instrumental values that will maintain the positive qualities of a highly productive economy and add to aesthetic and ethical values which bring more beauty and love into the lives of people.

2. To help students learn how to apply these values in their personal and civic lives.

Havighurst emphasized the role of *social development* throughout the life span and the importance of language as a central focus during infancy and early childhood: "The human mind literally grows on the basis of the language environment provided for it during the preschool years." A developmental task of middle childhood is to learn to get along with same-age peers. This includes making friends and, perhaps as important, getting along with enemies. This is the age that, having left the protection of the home for the first time, the school child learns the exchanges of social life. The peer group provides increasingly for the social approval the child needs. This means the child has to recognize and deal with peer pressure. Part of the health educator's role is to help pupils consistently apply their own set of values to decisions that frequently are affected by peer pressure. Exercises in dealing with peer pressure involving use of drugs, including alcohol and tobacco, sexual activity, and maintaining friendships, are useful for this purpose.

Kohlberg and Turiel (1971) offered a useful approach to the development of decision making in light of personal values and morals and the pressure from peers and family, incorporating three levels: preconventional, conventional, and autonomous. During the *preconventional* level, we behave in a way that brings pleasure or avoids discomfort. This is exemplified by the infant who cries for food even when the mother cannot readily deliver it. At the *conventional* level, we behave in ways that bring approval from others who are important to us, such as parents, teachers, and peers. Many people never progress past this level. Certainly, children and even adolescents operate at this stage of moral development. During the *autonomous* or *post-conventional* stage, the individual makes decisions based upon his or her own set of values and beliefs, with little consideration of positive or negative feedback from others.

As mentioned previously, the school is a laboratory for social discovery and experimentation. This is especially true during adolescence. Young people typically achieve the goals of cooperation in working toward a common goal and learning to lead without dominating. They become less dependent upon parents and develop the beginnings of the autonomy that will stand them in good stead throughout adulthood. The typical adolescent struggles and falls many times along the road to social maturity and autonomy. This teen needs guidance from home and school even as he or she rebels against what seems like the foundations of each.

The adolescent faces the task of achieving socially responsible behavior. This means developing a social ideology that allows for participation in social institutions, taking into account the values of society and the need to sacrifice for the group.

As the individual matures into early adulthood, the lessons learned in school and community help to develop the ability to mold new friendships and to take on a degree of civic responsibility. Certainly, schools should encourage participation in community activities. Every community has plenty of health and social service organizations that welcome the help of volunteers.

As the adult matures, the opportunity and responsibility to participate in community and social activities increase. Community leadership arises from early opportunity and encouragement in school.

Another major theme running through the developmental tasks is *general health*. During infancy, the tasks include the largely maturational examples of learning to take solid foods and toilet training. In middle childhood, building healthful attitudes about oneself as a growing organism requires learning to care for the body, cleanliness, proper diet, and safety, as well as the previously discussed wholesome attitude about sex. These areas of content have been part of elementary health education for years.

During adolescence, accepting one's physique becomes an important task. This requires some tolerance for one's body and the changes through which it passes and is complicated by the variability of development in teens. Health educators need compassion to explain this variability as a normal part of adolescence. Pupils also must be made comfortable in asking questions.

The information gained and the attitudes developed during the school health education experience are useful throughout life in making decisions regarding general physical health. It also is valuable as one ages and the body no longer responds as it did during youth. Loss of youthful strength, gradually diminishing sex drive, and menopause are examples of issues that can cause anguish to those who are unprepared and uneducated.

Havighurst's developmental tasks provide a blueprint for development of the person. They also provide a framework for planning comprehensive school health education. Careful attention to development of children, especially in the areas of sexuality, family life, values development, social health, and general health, provides the skills and attitudes necessary for the individual's continued successful development throughout life. Attention to the developmental tasks of middle age and later maturity by those in community health education and services contributes to the continued health of the community.

COLEMAN'S DEVELOPMENTAL TASKS

James Coleman (1969) took the work of Erikson (1963) and Havighurst (1952) a step further by developing a six-stage process of developmental tasks interwoven with specific behaviors characteristic to each stage. Coleman's tasks are presented in Table 8.3.

Coleman and Health Education

Coleman's developmental tasks present many interesting connections to health education. We concentrate here on the first three stages, in order to apply the theory to the school setting. Health educators, of course, frequently work outside the school setting with adults, and the remaining stages have meaning for those individuals as well.

Although one might assume from a study of Coleman's work that children come to the school setting with the tasks of the early childhood stage fully developed, this, unfortunately, is not the case. The family of the 1960s, when the tasks were identified, is considerably different from that of the 1990s. With many more single-parent homes, an increase in daycare services, and the dramatic increase in the teenage birth rate, many children do not have the benefit of time spent with mature, loving parents to achieve these tasks. For instance, a startling number of children enter school with little respect for rules and authority. In addition, the question has been raised repeatedly: How can children (especially boys) identify with their own sex and develop sex role models when the same-sex parent is often absent from the home? These and other issues require the classroom teacher to be more sensitive to the development of these and other tasks than may have been necessary in the past.

Preschool programs such as Head Start may see these tasks as a focus of their programs. Certainly, the development of family life education programs beginning in kindergarten is appropriate for developing family group membership, identifying with one's own sex, appropriately giving and receiving affection, and learning social realities.

During the elementary school and middle school years (middle childhood), health educators can play significant roles in attaining successful development of many of the tasks Coleman identified. Erikson, Havighurst, and Colemen all provide justification for a well-planned and sensitive family life education program implemented by competent, well-trained educators, particularly health educators, which can assist greatly in developing masculine and feminine social roles. As emphasized previously, health behavior and decision making are largely a function of attitudes about self and one's health and the values one develops about health and society. Most knowledgeable health educators strive to develop these attitudes and values as defined by the community and the curriculum.

Health educators should support our physical education colleagues in the development of physical skills and neuromuscular coordination. Among other benefits, physical educators assist students in learning how to win and how to give and take in social situations.

Perhaps nowhere in the development of the person is successful attainment of the necessary

---

TABLE 8.3.   Coleman's Developmental Tasks

1.	Early Childhood (Birth–6 years)	Acquiring a sense of trust in self and others. Developing healthy concept of self. Learning to give and receive affection. Identifying with own sex. Achieving skills in motor coordination. Learning to be a member of family group. Beginning to learn physical and social realities. Beginning to distinguish right from wrong and to respect rules and authority. Learning to understand and use language. Learning personal care.
2.	Middle Childhood (6–12 years)	Gaining wider knowledge and understanding of physical and social world. Building wholesome attitudes toward self. Learning appropriate masculine or feminine social role. Developing conscience, morality, a scale of values. Learning to read, write, calculate, other intellectual skills. Learning to win and maintain place among agemates. Learning to give and take and to share responsibility.
3.	Adolescence (12–18 years)	Developing clear sense of identity and self-confidence. Adjusting to body changes. Developing new, more mature relations with agemates. Achieving emotional independence from parents. Selecting and preparing for an occupation. Achieving mature values and social responsibility. Preparing for marriage and family life. Developing concern beyond self.
4.	Early Adulthood (18–35 years)	Seeing meaning in one's life. Getting started in an occupation. Selecting and learning to live with a mate. Starting a family and supplying children's material and psychological needs. Managing a home. Finding a congenial social group. Taking on civic responsibility.
5.	Middle Age (36–60 years)	Achieving full civic and social responsibility. Relating oneself to one's spouse as a person. Establishing adequate financial security for remaining years. Developing adult leisure-time activities, extending interests. Helping teenage children become responsible and happy adults. Adjusting to aging parents. Adjusting to physiological changes of middle age.
6.	Later Life	Adjusting to decreasing physical strength. Adjusting to retirement and reduced income. Adjusting to death of spouse and friends. Meeting social and civic obligations within one's ability. Establishing an explicit affiliation with age group. Maintaining interests, concern beyond self.
	Tasks at All Periods	Developing and using one's capabilities. Accepting oneself and developing basic self-confidence. Accepting reality and building valid attitudes and values. Participating creatively and responsibly in family and other groups. Building rich linkages with one's world.

Source: J. C. Coleman. *Psychology and Effective Behavior* (Chicago: Scott, Foresman, 1969).

---

tasks so important as in the adolescent stage. The body is changing so rapidly that often the child cannot make the necessary mental, emotional, and social adjustments. These adjustments can be supported by sensitive health educators. On a cognitive level, we help young people know what to expect in terms of physical changes. This is only the beginning, though. We must support children as they deal with all of the attendant changes that occur as their bodies mature. A well-ordered curriculum will help achieve this support. Unfortunately, a number of school districts still are dominated by conservatives who believe that discussing issues related to sexuality should be omitted from schools. This

battle will continue to be fought on both national and local levels.

Maturing and looking to the future are tasks implied by Coleman for adolescents. Young people must develop more mature relationships with people of their own age. Relationships require more than play. They require trust, commitment, support, sacrifice, and a number of other qualities that were not necessary as young children. This development is a social task that leads to long-term relationships, and for most people, marriage and family life. Health educators can help adolescents recognize the importance of friendships and commitment to others. Social and emotional development is a duty of many disciplines in the school, including health education.

A crucial component of the health education program is the development of an understanding of the importance of family. Schools have been guilty in the past of presenting only one model of the family. This may have made some students feel excluded. While the structure of the family in America is changing and may have connotations dependent upon economics and culture, certain values—commitment, sharing, nurturing, responsibility, sacrifice of one's personal wants for the good of the group— are common to all families. These values are unarguably necessary to successful family membership, and developing of them is a joint task of the family, community, and school.

SUMMARY

The stages of human development set forth by Erikson, Havighurst, and Coleman provide somewhat similar descriptions of the challenges confronting humans as we grow and mature. Each of the three authorities, in his own way, provides a basis for implementing comprehensive health education. More important, each model provides guidance to the health educator in designing programs and experiences to assist learners in achieving the positive tasks.

Although identifying the differences in the three versions of development would make an interesting study, it perhaps is more important to note the similarities and consistencies. These consistencies are what give strength and credibility to the objectives for which we strive in health education.

REFERENCES

Carroll, C., and D. Miller. Health: *The Science of Human Adaptation* (5th ed.). Dubuque, IA: Wm. C. Brown Publishers, 1991.

Coleman, J. C. *Psychology and Effective Behavior.* Palo Alto, CA: Scott, Foresman, 1969.

Erikson, E. H. *Childhood and Society.* New York: W. W. Norton & Co., 1963.

Erikson, E. H. *Identity: Youth and Crisis.* New York: W. W. Norton & Co., 1968.

Havighurst, R. J. *Developmental Tasks and Education* (2d ed.). New York: David McKay Co., 1952.

Havighurst, R. J. *Developmental Tasks and Education* (3d ed.). New York: David McKay Co., 1972.

Kohlberg, L., and E. Turiel. Moral development and moral education. In G. Lessor, editor, *Psychology and Educational Practice.* Chicago: Scott, Foresman, 1971.

9

PRINCIPLES OF LEARNING AND THEORIES OF HUMAN BEHAVIOR

The goals of health education basically involve either changing human behavior or establishing preferred behavior. Principles of learning and theories of human behavior provide models and frameworks for understanding how people learn and how and why people behave as they do, as well as bases for interventions to effect behavior change.

No single theory dominates research or practice in health education. Health education and its determinants are much too complex to be explained by a lone theory. The health educator is best advised to apply the most appropriate of the various theories to the situation and setting. The principles of learning, the domains of learning, and several theories of human behavior presented in this chapter are easily applied to health education. In addition, several theories of human behavior developed specifically to explain health-related action are explored.

SIGNIFICANT PRINCIPLES AND CONCEPTS OF LEARNING

Health educators, indeed all educators, are devoted to promoting change. Change can occur in three ways: maturation, learning, or a combination of maturation and learning. *Maturation* is a developmental process within which a person manifests traits, the blueprint of which is carried on the genes. *Learning* is change of behavior brought about by experience, insight, perception, or a combination of the three, which causes the individual to approach future situations differently.

Learning is not static. It is a dynamic process beginning with some motivation (desire, urge, drive) and leading the learner to be receptive to outside stimuli. As Knutson (1965) wrote, if the learner trusts and is satisfied with his or her present facts, perceptions,

135

values, and assumptions, he or she will have no need to seek new knowledge, skills, or attitudes. A learning environment and activity must be present. Learning also requires a process of some kind. Finally, the learner must be able to use the new knowledge or skills in future applications.

According to Coleman (1969), the learning process consists of four critical factors: the learner, the task, the procedure, and the learning situation.

1. The *learner* brings all of his or her experience to the situation, including successes and failures. The learner also brings his or her resources, skills, motivations, and tendencies. Moreover, the learner's own personal frame of reference may greatly affect his or her ability to comprehend and apply what is to be learned. A certain level of maturity and adjustment affects factors such as patience, concentration, and objectivity.

2. The *task* itself is defined by its size, complexity, and clarity. The task also is affected by the conditions and procedures applied to the learning experience. Familiarity with the task makes for a more suitable beginning. A small, simple body of knowledge is easier to assimilate, especially if it is built upon existing skills and knowledge.

3. The *procedures,* or learning opportunities, are critical to the learning experience. College level "methods and materials" courses emphasize the selection and implementation of procedures to best suit the learner, based on a multitude of factors such as age and maturity, proficiency in the language, reading level, gender, and other readiness indicators.

4. The *learning situation,* the time and place of the experience, is expedited by using the best and most appropriate resources and facilities available for the individual learner.

Kolb and Fry (1975) advocate a responsive learning environment. According to them, a responsive learning environment includes:

◆ permitting free exploration and opportunity to discover the problem;

◆ giving immediate feedback about the consequences of actions;

◆ permitting full use of the capacity for discovering various kinds of relations;

◆ structuring so the learner is likely to make interconnected discovery about physical, social, and cultural aspects of the world.

Principles of Learning

The following principles are applicable to health education:

1. Learning is continuous; it is not a single event.
2. People learn by doing.
3. Without sufficient readiness, learning is inefficient and possibly harmful.
4. Motivation is necessary for learning.
5. Immediate responses, or reinforcement, enhance effective learning.
6. Transfer does not automatically occur; the learning situation must provide for it by presenting responses in the way they are going to be used.
7. People vary in how they perceive a stimulus, and their responses vary according to their perceptions.
8. Responses vary according to the learning environment.
9. We cannot teach another person, only facilitate his or her learning.
10. The learner learns only what he or she perceives as relevant.
11. Experiences that involve a change in the self tend to be resisted, and experiences that are

perceived as inconsistent with the self can be assimilated only if the organization of the self is relaxed.

The final three principles, attributed to Carl Rogers (1967), are particularly interesting to health educators. Lest we deemphasize the learner's role in his or her own learning, we have to recognize our role as facilitator and accept the learner's role as more important. As a kindly professor always announced to her students on the first day of class: "You have two teachers: you and me. By far, you are the most important." The final principle implies that the most effective learning situations are those that reduce to a minimum the threat to the learner. If the student is relaxed and comfortable, he or she will be more able to learn.

The Domains of Learning

Traditionally, learning has been categorized into three domains: cognitive, affective, and psychomotor (sometimes called action). Briefly, the cognitive domain involves acquiring knowledge and information on an intellectual level. The affective domain involves acquiring and changing emotions, feelings, and attitudes. The psychomotor domain involves acquiring physical skills, and also the aspects of learning in which the individual applies accumulated knowledge and attitudes to behavior or action.

Public health learning often is explained in a hierarchy of learning (see Figure 9.1) with reference to the cognitive and affective domains affecting action. In the hierarchy (Knutson, 1965), the first learning situation utilizes health facts, imposed in regulations and statutes, to require public action. In the second situation, the public is encouraged to act based upon recommendations of authority. The assumption in this situation is that people will act in the best interests of society through recommendations as a result of attitudes and information the public already has acquired. In the third situation, the public acts in a self-directed way because of the

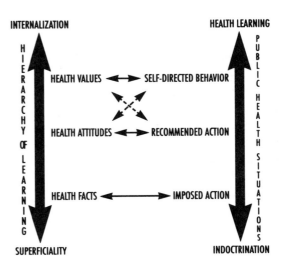

Source: D. A. Bedworth and A. E. Bedworth, *Health Education: Process for Human Effectiveness* (New York: Harper & Row, 1978). Reprinted by permission of HarperCollins Publishers.

FIGURE 9.1. Public Health Learning Situations

goals it chooses based upon its own values. Health education programs act primarily on the second and third situations, which are education-oriented.

Cognitive Domain

Learning within the cognitive domain principally involves the acquisition of knowledge and facts. In recent years, acquisition of knowledge has lost some of its emphasis among health educators, supplanted by more emphasis on attitudes and values. In truth, both domains affect behavior. Rudd and Glanz (1991) wrote, "Knowledge is considered necessary but not sufficient . . . to guide . . . health actions and to stimulate health-enhancing behavior." Certainly, to minimize the significance of cognitive learning would be a mistake.

The cognitive domain traditionally has been depicted in terms of Bloom's (1956) *Taxonomy of Educational Objectives*. The taxonomy is arranged from simple to complex and implies intellectual abilities. The taxonomy and some examples of cognitive abilities of each objective are:

1. **Knowledge**—naming, defining, listing, identifying.
2. **Comprehension**—explaining, describing, interpreting.
3. **Application**—illustrating, predicting, applying.
4. **Analysis**—analyzing, categorizing, classifying, differentiating.
5. **Synthesis**—concluding, proposing, synthesizing.
6. **Evaluating**—contrasting, comparing, evaluating.

Teacher training programs and, therefore, public and private schools have leaned heavily upon Bloom's taxonomy. Although it still forms the basis of much of cognitive teaching-learning strategy, it is challenged by a number of theories. Currently, the most prominent challenger is constructivism (discussed in detail later in this chapter). Regardless of one's view of Bloom's taxonomy, its vast following and its historical significance demand that educators be familiar with it.

Affective Domain

The affective domain consists of emotions, personal interests, values, and attitudes. As mentioned earlier, knowledge is necessary to guide behavior choices, but knowledge is not enough. Knowledge coupled with affective associations can be highly effective in shaping health-related behavior. Attitudes can be described as perceptions that people have about their environment and the things in it. Attitudes can be a reason to act. Attitudes, however, are influenced by the acquisition of health concepts that result from knowledge, comprehension, and application of health knowledge. The development of positive health attitudes is a fundamental factor

in improving health behaviors and, therefore, health status.

Krathwohl, Bloom, and Masia (1964) suggested several processes, from simple to complex, associated with affective learning:

1. **Receiving**—awareness, willingness to receive controlled or selected attention.
2. **Responding**—acquaintance, willingness to respond, satisfaction in response.
3. **Valuing**—acceptance, preference, commitment.
4. **Organization**—conceptualization of a value, organization of a value system.
5. **Characterization** by a value or value complex—generalized set characterization.

Affective development can be influenced in a number of ways. The long-term goal of health education, however, is *voluntary* behavior that is conducive to health. To inflict health attitudes upon learners is unethical. Choices should remain personal and individual and not the result of indoctrination or brainwashing. The development of attitudes and feelings conducive to health should be the result of rational reflection, not authoritarian strategy. This rational reflection, coupled with knowledge, produces attitudes, beliefs, and values.

Psychomotor Domain

The psychomotor domain is concerned with human movement, including motor skills and coordination. It also is interpreted to refer to the development of behavioral patterns. This, of course, is the essence of health education.

Behavioral patterns are made by choice. Thus, certain variables must be prerequisite to making the choice from different alternatives. These variables include knowledge, attitudes, beliefs, and feelings. Therefore, the cognitive and affective domains affect the psychomotor domain. Health education can instill the variables that encourage people to behave in ways which enhance their health. This is its purpose.

WHY THEORY?

Theory and its value to education sometimes are underrated. Failure to appreciate the relationship of theory and real-world practice has damaged academic endeavors and research for years. Two definitions of "theory" help to clarify its nature:

> A set of interrelated constructs (concepts, definitions, and propositions) that present a systematic view of phenomena by specifying relations among variables, with the purpose of explaining and predicting phenomena. (Kerlinger, 1986)

> A systematic explanation for the observed facts and laws that relate to a particular aspect of life. (Babbie, 1989)

Concepts are major components of a theory. When concepts are developed or adopted for use in a particular theory, they are called *constructs* (Kerlinger, 1986). *Variables* are the operational definitions of concepts (Green and Lewis, 1986); they specify how a concept is to be measured.

Theory can be applied in the real world of health education in a number of ways:

1. Theory can *explain* relationships, the whats, hows, whens, and whys.

2. Theory can be used as a *basis for research* and a *basis for formulating hypotheses.*

3. Theory can be used as a *basis for intervention.*

4. Theory can be used to *predict outcomes* of interventions and research procedures.

5. Theory aids in *measuring the impact* of interventions.

Health educators are action-oriented interventionists (Glanz, Lewis, and Rimer, 1991). We use our knowledge, experience, and education in planning activities that influence people to act in positive ways. Designing effective interventions can be done best by understanding theories of behavioral change and stages of human development.

No single theory or even conceptual framework dominates the practice of health education today. A review of 116 theory-based articles published between 1986 and 1988 in two major health education journals revealed fifty-one distinct theoretical formulations (Glanz, 1988). The theories discussed in this chapter have their foundations in different disciplines. Although this text is not designed to delve deeply into psychology, sociology, or similar discipline, it is fashioned to help the aspiring health educator comprehend some of the theories explaining the processes that affect behavior relating to health. If health educators are successful in changing or establishing health behavior, they must be cognizant of the factors affecting behavior. This chapter's explanation and interpretation of several theories of human behavior can be applied to the work of health educators.

MASLOW'S THEORY OF HUMAN MOTIVATION

According to Abraham Maslow (1943), people have at least five sets of goals, usually referred to as *basic needs*, which are common to all: physiological, safety, love, esteem, and self-actualization (see Figure 9.2). These are related to each other, arranged in a hierarchy. Maslow's theory often is identified mistakenly as a "theory of

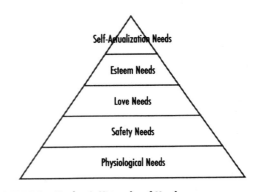

FIGURE 9.2 Maslow's Hierarchy of Needs

human needs." In reality, Maslow has identified human needs in a theory of *human motivation*. Maslow's theory explains how our needs contribute to motivating actions or behavior.

Physiological needs are considered the most basic and influential. The major motivation of the human who is missing everything in life in an extreme fashion is most likely physiological needs. Although an exact and total listing of these needs is not possible, certainly the needs for freedom from hunger, sufficient oxygen, and adequate water have to be included. Arguably, for some individuals, sleep, the freedom to move, sexual activity, and addictive drugs are basic physiological needs. If a person who is in extreme distress to satisfy a basic need, say hunger, no other interests exist except food. Food dominates the person's thoughts, dreams, and emotions. He or she wants only food and will risk all else to obtain food.

Safety needs surface if the physiological needs are relatively well satisfied. The need for safety can surface during a quarrel, the threat of physical battery, or isolation. Behavior then will be oriented toward reducing the danger and increasing safety. For children, being confronted with unexpected changes in the environment or new, unfamiliar situations can provide reason for terror.

Unfortunately, in today's society children frequently are deprived of a safe, orderly, predictable, and organized world. The shield of family and parents often is either nonexistent or inconsistent. All too often children carry with them fears and lack of trust of adults, which can hamper their learning experience and their ability to relate to others.

Love needs comprise the next level in Maslow's hierarchy. Once physiological and safety needs are well met, love, affection, and belongingness needs emerge. The individual acutely feels the absence of friends, or a sweetheart, or children, or a mate. Individuals strive intensely for affectionate relationships with others. The thwarting of these needs frequently is at the core of maladjustment and severe

psychopathology. Love needs necessarily involve both giving *and* receiving love.

Esteem needs, the fourth level of the hierarchy, mean that all people have a need or desire for a stable, firmly based high evaluation of themselves, for self-respect, for self-esteem, and for esteem of others. This esteem should be based upon reality—real capacity, achievement, and respect from others. These needs may be for achievement, adequacy, confidence, and independence. They also take the form of desire for reputation, prestige, recognition, and appreciation.

Self-actualization, the highest level on the hierarchy, is the need or desire to become more and more of what one is, to become everything one is capable of becoming. Upon satisfying the other levels of the hierarchy, Maslow states, the individual attempts to meet his or her needs to self-actualize. It may be a creative urge, a desire to be an ideal mother or father, the desire to be a great athlete, or the need to accumulate great wealth.

The eminent need, or the one that is superior in power, force, or influence, motivates our immediate actions. It monopolizes our consciousness and tends to organize the recruitment of our various skills and talents. The less superior needs are minimized, forgotten, or denied. When a need is fairly well satisfied, however, the next most prominent or higher need emerges to dominate the conscious life and serve as the center of organization of behavior. For instance, a person will not seek safety or love until his or her basic physiological needs (including freedom from hunger and sufficient oxygen) are met. Then the individual will be motivated to satisfy his or her needs for safety and security. Once the needs for safety and security are met, the individual acts upon the now predominant need for love.

Although satisfying these wants and needs is not altogether mutually exclusive, it tends to be. The average member of our society most often is partially satisfied and partially unsatisfied in all of his or her wants. The principle of hierarchy usually is observed in terms of higher percentages of nonsatisfaction as we go up the hierarchy.

Thus, in the example given in the previous paragraph, the individual may not be totally free from hunger to begin acting on his or her needs for safety—only "free" to the point that that individual can begin to act on the need for safety. Of course, the relative degree of satisfaction varies from individual to individual. It also varies among the need levels of the hierarchy. For instance, an individual may have a relatively low level of need for safety to act on needs for love and require a high level of need satisfaction for love before acting on needs for esteem.

Of course, there are exceptions. For instance, Dr. Martin Luther King predicted his death shortly before he was assassinated, yet continued his work, forsaking safety for self-actualization. Mother Teresa has sacrificed safety, and at times physiological needs, to meet her love, esteem, and self-actualization needs. There are examples of martyrs who, throughout history, gave up everything for the sake of ideals.

It is often said that a good teacher motivates students. Perhaps in light of Maslow's work, it is more accurate to say that good teachers recognize children's needs and design ways to meet those needs. From Maslow's work, true motivation seems to come from within.

The accomplished teacher frequently can recognize when children are not having their needs met for adequate food, security, and love. The continuous observation (see Chapter 5) yields evidence of these deficits in many ways. If a child is hungry, he or she will not learn to his or her potential. The teacher then might refer the child for counseling or suggest to the parents that the school breakfast or lunch program may be of help to the student. When a child shows signs of insecurity, it may be a symptom of divorce or separation in the home, or of abuse. The teacher should handle this situation carefully, enlist the aid of counselors, and alert the principal to potential problems. Frequently, the same signs of lack of safety indicate lack of love and affection.

Children want an orderly, predictable world—an indication of the need for safety. For this reason, teachers must exercise consistency and fairness when dealing with pupils. Changes in standards, schedules, or classroom arrangements can be threatening to children.

The central role of parents and family is indisputable in meeting children's needs for safety and love. Arguing, physical assault, separation, divorce, and death may be particularly terrifying to children. Outbursts of rage, threats, rough handling, or physical punishment can elicit panic and terror in the child. Unfortunately, many children are subjected to this sort of treatment regularly. Teachers need to temper their expectations of children undergoing these hardships. They also have a legal responsibility to report cases of suspected abuse or neglect.

Fortunately, in recent years, courses called *family life education* have made their way into the curricula of many school districts. Comprehensive school health education programs also are being implemented. Health educators generally see these steps as positive developments. We should not treat the "family" as simply and exclusively the concept of the traditional nuclear family though. With the changing nature of families, children from single-parent households and other nontraditional families should not be given the impression that their homes are somehow unsatisfactory. This could challenge the child's sense of safety and could inhibit efforts at achieving esteem. Various circumstances, however, should not result in suppressing discussion about positive and negative aspects of different family structures and characteristics.

Teachers often perpetuate artificial gender differences in the classroom. Many teachers unintentionally push boys toward mathematics and sciences and steer girls away from these areas. Sometimes girls are directed toward language skills and the arts and boys are discouraged from these interests. Most teachers recognize on a cognitive level that boys and girls do not have innate abilities or disabilities in these areas because of their gender. They should assess their own behavior and make sure they do not practice this form of subtle discrimination. Certainly, implications for meeting esteem needs and even self-actualizing needs are enormous. On the surface, this does not seem to be an issue for the health educator, but health educators often become unofficial counselors to many students and are asked for advice in career choices and class selection.

Perhaps no level of the hierarchy is more directly applicable to health education than the area of love and affection. Love and affection, as well as their possible expression in sexuality, generally are looked upon with ambivalence and customarily are couched in many restrictions and inhibitions. This is nowhere more true than with adolescents. Their needs for love and affection are taking new turns. The love expressed in the family no longer suffices. Our curricula in the area of interpersonal relationships and sexuality frequently have fallen short of reality and of the responsibility to help young people address their needs for love and affection while dealing with their emerging desires for sexual contact.

The consequences of adolescent sexual activity are documented thoroughly in this text. Nevertheless, simply recognizing the possible negative outcomes have not served to diminish those consequences and certainly do not help young people make decisions that will help them meet their needs for love and affection. This is the reason parents, clergy, students, and other interested people should be involved in developing sensitive, effective curricula in the area of human sexuality. Simply preaching abstinence has proven to be ineffective and certainly does not address the child's needs. The person teaching in this area must be sensitive, well-educated in this specialty, have the trust of students and parents alike, and desire the involvement.

The health educator should address the self-esteem of every pupil. Every child should be made to feel confident, capable, and worthy. People react to the world in terms of the way they perceive it. The most conspicuous feature of the individual's world is the self as he or she sees, perceives, and experiences it. Therefore, the self-concept becomes the frame of reference through which the individual interacts with the world.

According to Rogers (1951), the self-concept is a reflection of an individual's mental health. Because health education is so directed toward action, the health educator should be sure to incorporate activities that develop positive self-esteem in the pupil.

Upon reviewing several studies regarding the self-concept of delinquents, Fitts and Hamner (1969) concluded that delinquents see themselves as undesirable people who do not like, value, or respect themselves. A number of researchers, including Butler (1982), Rosecrans and Brignet (1972), and Braucht et al. (1973), have found relationships between frequent or abusive use of drugs and low self-esteem. The implications of these findings for health educators are huge and obvious.

LEWIN'S FIELD THEORY

Kurt Lewin (1948, 1961) provided an extremely useful tool for diagnosing the forces at work in situations involving group or individual change. The tool, *force-field analysis*, is referred to as field theory. It proposes that the forces existing in group situations are accessible to systematic analysis. It further suggests that the continuing forces within a group situation influence one another.

According to field theory, behavior results from two sets of forces: *change* or *driving forces* and *resisting* or *restraining forces*. Change forces are those that pressure the group or individual to move toward a goal. Resisting forces are those that resist change. The two sets of forces are constantly working against one another (see Figure 9.3).

When the total influence of the change and resisting forces is equal, the individual is immobilized, producing no action. When the resisting forces outweigh the change forces, the individual's behavior is blocked and no action is produced. When change forces are strong and resisting forces are weak, however, the individual behaves so as to attain the goal. In all cases, the

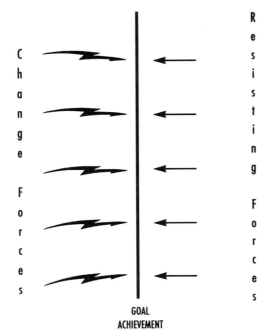

FIGURE 9.3. Lewin's Force Field Concept

total weight or total influence of the combined change and resisting forces is uniform. The relative influence of the change and the resisting forces can and often does increase and diminish.

Health educators can utilize force-field analysis to understand why certain behaviors are motivated or blocked (Ross and Mico, 1980). They also can suggest strategies for change. These strategies involve (a) increasing the influence of driving or change forces, (b) reducing the influence of restraining or resisting forces, or (c) concurrently increasing change forces and decreasing resisting forces. Although this may seem simple, it requires identifying and understanding both change and resisting forces. Educators must understand why behavior is blocked and from where the forces are coming. They then must identify ways to increase change forces and reduce resisting forces. Fortunately, well-prepared health educators are skilled in doing this. One way is to allow individuals to air their own feelings and involve them in planning ways to

solve the problem. Through open exchange, health educators can identify the resisting forces and guide students in reducing them.

A good example is smoking cessation. The change forces may be knowledge of the health risks of smoking on the individual and on his or her family members, the expanding social isolation of smokers, and the inconvenience caused by legislation restricting smoking in public places. The resisting forces may be the pleasure derived from smoking, the feeling of being accepted by some peers, and the fear of withdrawal from the addictive drug nicotine. Once the health educator has identified these factors, he or she can manipulate them to change behavior. For instance, the health educator may persuade family members to encourage smoking cessation. He or she may suggest that the smoker sit in the "no smoking" section of restaurants, if they are so differentiated, to make it even more inconvenient to smoke. He or she may suggest a smoking cessation program for the smoker. All these are efforts to maximize change forces. Resisting forces can be minimized by encouraging peers to assure the individual that they will still like the person when he or she stops smoking. (Indeed, it may make the person a more pleasant companion.) Perhaps a physician can prescribe a nicotine patch to reduce withdrawal sensations.

To reduce resisting forces while increasing driving force pressure is crucial. Changes brought about only by increasing change forces are likely to be temporary because, when pressures are relaxed, people tend to revert to the previous behavior. On the other hand, change rising exclusively from decreased restraining forces has a greater likelihood of being permanent because it reduces or removes resistance to change.

Lewin explained the action-planning procedure in five phases of learning and change called unfreezing-to-refreezing theory:

1. Unfreezing.
2. Problem diagnosis.
3. Goal setting.

4. The new behavior.
5. Refreezing.

Unfreezing means becoming ready to consider change. Examples include the smoker who has decided to try to stop smoking and the overweight person who is thinking seriously about beginning to exercise. Through *problem diagnosis* the person achieves a better understanding of the problem. At this stage the health educator can be vital to success. Helping the smoker to question why he or she smokes and helping the overweight person to conduct a force-field analysis around the goal of reducing caloric intake and increasing activity are illustrative of this phase. Once the person understands the problem, *goal setting* becomes crucial in planning the behavior change. Intensive help from the health educator can be useful at this stage. It may include strategies to integrate new behaviors into one's lifestyle or workshops on skills development, to mention just two methodologies. At this point the individual tries out new alternatives, practices the *new behavior.* For the smoker, this may mean gradually tapering off or quitting "cold turkey." For the overweight person, it may mean walking regularly and eating a salad for lunch. *Refreezing* occurs when the new behavior becomes a routine, ongoing, and stabilized part of the person's behavior.

Of course, success is a major motivating force in maintaining the behavior. The health educator can plan for milestones to mark successes in the individual's lifestyle. Occasionally, the person may backslide to former behavior. The smoker may be tempted to try a cigarette. The health educator must put this temporary lapse into perspective and not allow it to seem to be a failure of the entire process.

Although designing curricula to address each student as an individual is difficult, curricula can be designed in such a way as to identify the phases in the action-planning procedure and provide opportunities for application to individual behavior. This type of flexibility is essential to successful curriculum development.

SKINNER AND BEHAVIORAL MODIFICATION

B. F. Skinner (1938), perhaps the best known behaviorist, formulated a widely accepted hypothesis that the frequency of a behavior is determined by its consequences, or reinforcement. Skinner (1953) demonstrated that the observable behaviors of humans can be changed by manipulation of rewards. Learning, in his view, results from events (reinforcements) that reduce physiological drives that activate behavior. This is a cornerstone in the science of behavior change. Skinner showed that people will behave in ways that get them the rewards they need and will stop the behavior if it is ignored and does not get them the rewards they need. He also showed that people will continue a behavior that avoids punishment, thereby learning the behavior because it reduces the tension set up by the punishment. Hence, behavior frequently is modified by external forces that produce rewards.

An interesting facet of Skinner's work is the absence of mental concepts. According to this theory of behavior, no reasoning or thinking is required to explain behavior.

All too often, behaviors and lifestyles resulting in loss of health, high risk for accidents, and premature death are those that produce immediate rewards for the individual. A few of the abundant examples of these behaviors and rewards are:

◆ the immediate pleasure of sexual intercourse;
◆ the pleasure derived from use of psychoactive drugs;
◆ the peer acceptance derived from smoking cigarettes;
◆ the thrill of traveling down the road at high speed;
◆ the enjoyment of consuming some tasty high-fat foods.

The challenge to health education is to overcome the immediate rewards of these behaviors by replacing them with other rewards. This approach can entail a number of strategies. Rewards can be designed and manipulated so alternative behaviors become the choice. For instance, many teens are choosing abstinence from sexual activity as a way to avoid the risk of acquiring AIDS. The education leading to this decision has successfully provided a long-term reward for behavior change: life. In some teen peer groups, virginity is being touted as a badge of respectability and, therefore, popularity. The immediate reward can be peer acceptance. As this attitude becomes more popular, its rewards become more socially expressed.

In another strategy the *attitude* about engaging in the behavior is changed. For example, many teens smoke cigarettes because it is the "in" thing to do in their peer group. Incentives (rewards) for cessation must be stronger than the rewards gained from smoking. This is difficult when the change must come from within a group. Recognition of the reward gained from the behavior, however, clearly signals to the educator that simply teaching or preaching about health consequences is not enough. Developing self-esteem and the strength to

make independent decisions is the basis for this change. Development of self-esteem is an exercise in positive rewards, usually delivered immediately. The long-term rewards may include leadership status in the group or respect from other students.

Parents should be educated in delivering positive rewards for their children's actions. As parents, we frequently deliver only negative comments and punishments. We often see discipline as causing children to *not* do what we *do not* want them to do. Instead, inducing desired behavior by rewarding that behavior when it occurs is more positive. This approach also can be applied to the development of healthy lifestyles.

Some commercial weight reduction programs have utilized behavior modification successfully by providing appropriate rewards. Educators have not made maximum use of positive stimuli to promote learning and behavior change in children.

SOCIAL LEARNING THEORY

Social learning theory (SLT) was first introduced by Miller and Dollard (1941) and later refined by Bandura (1965), who referred to it as *social cognitive theory*. SLT can be applied to health education and health promotion activities in assorted ways. SLT involves a broad range of conceptualizations, based on the central idea that a person's behaviors are responses to which other people apply reinforcements. These reinforcements splice the response to specific stimuli and thereby increase the likelihood that those responses will occur. Bandura and Walters (1963) concluded that children learn by watching other children and, to learn a new type

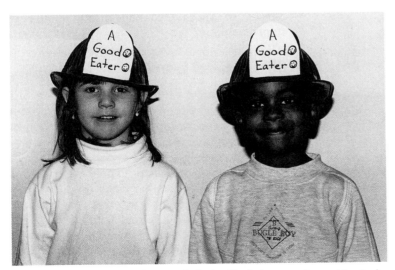

It is an easy matter to provide rewards for healthy behaviors. Recognition in the form of ribbons, articles of clothing, hats, and praise reinforce behavior.

of behavior, do not need to be rewarded directly. They change their behaviors because they desire to emulate role models who are being rewarded for their behaviors.

An underlying assumption of SLT is that behavior is dynamic and depends on the environment and personal constructs that influence each other simultaneously. A continuing interaction occurs among (a) a person, (b) the behavior of that person, and (c) the environment within which the behavior is performed. This interaction is called *reciprocal determinism* (see Figure 9.4). Because the three components are interacting constantly, a change in one may result in a change in the others (Bandura 1978, 1986).

Reciprocal Determinism

The environment encompasses all the physical factors that are not part of the individual and his or her objective notion of those factors. It consists of other people, including those who supply social supports, such as friends and family; the room; the climate; and the playground.

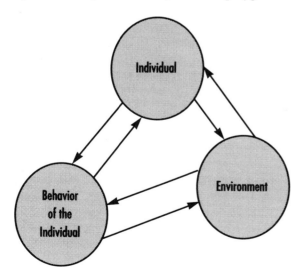

FIGURE 9.4.   Reciprocal Determinism, the Underlying Assumption of Social Learning Theory

The person's perception of the environment is the *situation*. It includes real, distorted, and imagined factors such as time, place, activity, and participants. The environment can affect the individual's behavior or the individual. Likewise, the individual or his or her behavior has the potential to affect the environment. The situation guides and limits the person's thinking and behavior and provides cues about what is acceptable. These cues, or consequences, may be positive or negative.

Another important concept of reciprocal determinism is *behavioral capability*. This concept holds that if a person is to engage in a given behavior, he or she must know what the behavior is and how to perform the behavior.

Expectancies or incentives are the values a person places on a specific outcome. If all other things are equal, a person will choose to perform an activity that maximizes a positive outcome and minimizes a negative outcome (Perry, Baranowski, and Parcel, 1991). Therefore, if trying to eliminate a behavior that brings pleasure or other positive outcome, the health educator must stress the positive outcomes of the change. For instance, to encourage overweight people to reduce weight, the positive aspects of appearance and health should be emphasized.

Observational Learning

The environment is considered critical in SLT because the environment provides models for behavior. *Expectations* arise from observing or experiencing a situation and the consequences of action. According to SLT, expectations may be learned from one's own experience or from observing others in similar situations. The latter is called observational learning or *vicarious experience*. It takes place without any real reward for the learner. Observational learning sometimes can be a shortcut to learning because the learner uncovers rules for behavior without the trial-and-error of personal experience. It is the basis for *modeling*. By simply observing others, we may find that a certain behavior or response is socially acceptable or reinforcing and adopt that behavior ourselves. Conversely, we may find that a behavior is not socially acceptable if our observation recognizes no reward or even notes punishment. This logically leads to our not adopting the behavior.

Observational learning and modeling have been used to explain why inner-city children become involved in illegal activities and become less interested in school. They see neighborhood toughs gaining respect and the trappings of wealth by engaging in behaviors such as selling drugs, promoting prostitution, joining gangs, and gambling. This argument leads to the conclusion that more role models are needed to depict positive social behaviors and illustrate the rewards gained from these behaviors.

According to Bandura (1977a), observational learning, as identified in social learning theory, has four sequential stages:

1. *Attentional processes,* which are influenced by an individual's needs and wants and the degree of attractiveness of the model activity under scrutiny.

2. *Retention processes,* which entail remembering what has been observed so the behavior can be imitated.

3. *Motor reproductive processes,* the physical activity necessary to replicate the situation.

4. *Motivational processes,* or reinforcement, in which the individual experiences reward from or satisfaction in the process. The reward may come from the environment, another person, the self, or vicarious reinforcement. When it occurs, it may become an integral part of the person's behavior pattern.

The motivational processes, or *reinforcement,* incorporates three types of reinforcement: (a) *direct* reinforcement (operant conditioning), (b) *vicarious* reinforcement (observational learning), and (c) *self*-reinforcement (self-control). Reinforcement can be categorized further into external or internal. *External* reinforcement is supplied by an event or act having predictable reinforcement value not necessarily of personal value to the individual. For example, a person may lose weight to keep his or her job. *Internal* reinforcement is a person's own experience or perception that an event has some value to him or her (Perry, et al., 1991). For instance, a person may lose weight to feel better.

Bandura (1977b, 1978) suggested that *self-efficacy* is the most important prerequisite for behavior change. Self-efficacy is confidence a person feels about his or her ability to perform an action. It affects how much effort an individual applies to a task and what levels of performance are attained (Ewart et al., 1983). Among the ways to develop self-efficacy are to use incremental short-term goals, simplify actions that consist of several steps, and use repetition.

SLT and Health Education

The trio of factors that interface with each other in reciprocal determinism—the individual, his or her behavior, and the environment—have implications for health educators. They should recognize that any action that addresses any of the factors singly is likely to affect the others. As an example, think about a young man who considers reducing his heavy alcohol consumption. Drinking has become an integral part of his life. He drinks heavily with many meals, drinks heavily during recreational outings, drinks when he enjoys a televised sports event with friends and at most other social occasions. A dramatic event, such as the death of a friend in an alcohol-related accident, may suddenly occur in the man's life, forcing him to consider his own drinking. Having decided to reduce his consumption of alcohol, the man is faced with all his old drinking buddies in his old locations. These environmental settings exert negative pressure on his decision, forcing him to seek out new friends, places, and activities. His attitude and actions may influence some of his old chums to make a similar decision.

As health educators, we must strive to enhance individuals' capacity to behave in healthy ways. To know the most healthy behavior is not enough. A person also must know how to perform the behavior. The coping skills and decision-making skills, as well as comprehension of the physical action required for the behavior, is part of the responsibility of health education. Closely related to behavioral capacity is self-efficacy. The individual must believe he or she has the capacity to attain the goal. Simple, attainable, short-term objectives often are successful at developing self-efficacy.

Health educators have a remarkable opportunity to present themselves as role models for children. By exhibiting the kind of lifestyles we encourage in our pupils, we provide the model for their behavior. Educators who exhibit negative behavior such as excessive alcohol consumption, smoking, using smokeless tobacco, and driving without buckling seatbelts cannot realistically expect their pupils to behave any differently. On the other hand, teachers who maintain a trim, strong body through regular exercise and proper diet present the kind of image young people can emulate. Expressing satisfaction with healthy lifestyles is critical to the potential of the motivational processes. A key to application of modeling and vicarious reinforcement in health education is pointing out examples of people to emulate and discuss. These examples can be the well-known and the not-so-well-known. Young people can be influenced greatly by a healthy successful senior citizen or middle-aged person.

SLT lends itself to inappropriate applications if the planner of interventions is careless. To be effective, planners should first identify the behavioral outcome and the SLT variables most likely to influence change in the behavior. At that point, the intervention methods can be matched to SLT variables to influence the behavioral outcome. The last step is to translate the theory into practical and effective strategies that help change people's lives.

HEALTH BELIEF MODEL

Over the last three decades, the health belief model (HBM) has been one of the most influential and widely used psychosocial approaches to explaining health-related behavior (Rosenstock, 1991). It is an explanation of preventive health behavior, concentrating on the relation of health behavior to the health and medical services available (Rosenstock, 1974). According to Creswell and Newman (1989), it is "the most extensive work done thus far in an effort to develop a theory and science of health behavior change." Since its development in the 1950s to explain people's widespread failure to participate in programs to prevent or detect disease, it has been revised to include general health motivation, people's responses to illness (Kirscht, 1974), and behavior in response to diagnosed illness, particularly compliance with medical regimens (Becker, 1974). The HBM now provides an excellent means to analyze forces that influence health behavior. It also has applications in program planning and implementation.

Although the model deals with illness behavior and sick-role behavior, this discussion will deal with health behavior only. Health behavior, as defined by Becker (1974), is any activity undertaken by individuals who believe themselves to be healthy, for the purpose of detecting and preventing disease in any asymptomatic stage. From the health educator's standpoint, we can emphasize the portion of behavior that has as its aim the prevention of disease and disability. The model postulates that:

1. Health behavior of all kinds is related to a general health belief that one is susceptible to health problems.

2. Health problems have undesirable consequences.

INDIVIDUAL PERCEPTIONS	MODIFYING FACTORS	LIKELIHOOD OF ACTION

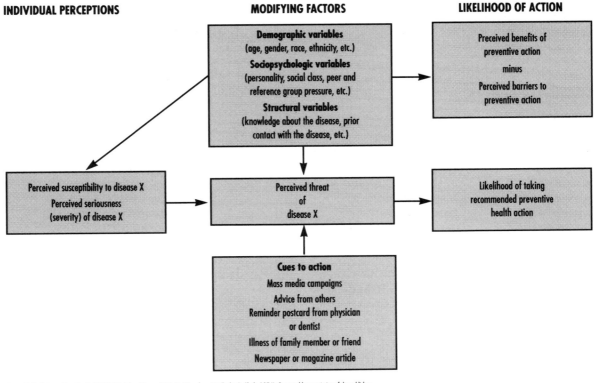

Source: M. H. Becker, editor, *The Health Belief Model and Personal Behavior* (Thorofare, NJ: Charles B. Slack, 1974). Reprinted by permission of the publisher.

FIGURE 9.5.   The Health Belief Model

3. Health problems and their consequences usually are preventable.

4. Barriers or costs have to be overcome if health problems are to be overcome.

The health belief model consists of three distinct phases (see Figure 9.5) that lead up to an action related to health: individual perception, modifying factors, and likelihood of action.

Individual Perceptions

Individual perceptions are of two basic types: the individual's subjective perception of risk of contracting the health condition (*perceived susceptibility*), and *perceived severity* of the condition, such as disability or injury, dying, or other negative consequence. A good example is teenage sexual intercourse and the consequences of contracting a sexually transmissible disease (STD), such as AIDS, or producing a pregnancy. According to the model, the teen will be less likely to engage in sexual activity, especially unprotected sexual activity, if he or she perceives the effects of sexual activity as a threat to himself or herself and that STD's and pregnancy are serious conditions. Further, the sexual activity must be perceived as causing or at least greatly increasing the likelihood of these outcomes. The two perceptions of personal susceptibility and severity of the condition are necessary for modifying behavior or maintaining (in this example) abstinence behavior. Many investigators label the combination of susceptibility and severity as *perceived threat*.

Modifying Factors

If the perceptions or conditions are present, modifying factors now come into play. The ultimate decision to engage in the behavior is influenced quite heavily by modifying factors. Modifying factors can be demographic variables, such as age, gender, and educational level; sociopsychologic variables, such as personality and peer pressure; and structural variables, such as knowledge about the condition or disease.

In the example of the teenager trying to make a conscious decision about sexual intercourse, the religious and moral values of the home may play a serious role in the decision. Peers' actions and attitudes and the individual's perceptions of those actions and attitudes also may affect the decision. If the individual wrongly perceives that all of his or her friends are sexually active, he or she may be encouraged to be sexually active. Another modifying factor is the knowledge gained in health education class about the risk of contracting an STD or the fact that no part of the menstrual cycle is really "safe" as far as pregnancy is concerned. Perhaps a greater modifying factor is the student's self-esteem which allows him or her to have the confidence and independence to make important decisions without fear of being ridiculed. All of these factors and more can combine to influence the behavior.

The model refers to the mass media and other sources. These sources may act as calls to action (or inaction) based on how the individual interprets their messages in the context of perceptions. Media messages discouraging adolescent sexual activity may be consistent with messages from home, school, and church supporting the abstinence position. Many advertisements, music videos, and television programs may be seen as encouraging sexual activity but may be rejected because of their inconsistency with the major predisposing factors related to the situation. Under some common circumstances, however, these messages can be consistent with some predisposing factors and can serve as a key factor in the decision to engage in sexual activity. For example, media messages about the use of condoms as a protection against AIDS may be confusing in the face of abstinence ideology. Before we become too simplistic, let us recognize that modifying factors can and often do provide both positive and negative values for the decision maker.

Likelihood of Action

Individual action is determined by the balance or imbalance between the individual's perceived positive and negative forces affecting his or her health behavior (Creswell and Newman, 1989). In the example, the action of abstinence or at least the use of condoms gains positive feedback from family and friends. It also is consistent with the knowledge that the individual has acquired in the health education class.

Action is related to the appraisal of susceptibility. The individual acts only when he or she acknowledges personal susceptibility to undesirable consequences of the act or failure to act. The person also must desire to lower susceptibility or possess motives to reduce the threat. Action also depends upon the perceived severity of the health problem. Finally, the action is related to the individual's estimation of the *benefits of the action* minus the *barriers to the action*. This estimate can be a daunting task for young people to make without the help and guidance of concerned adults. The individual must estimate the effectiveness of the action and the potential negative aspect of the action. A nonconscious, cost-benefit analysis is thought to occur wherein the individual weighs an action's effectiveness against perceptions that it may be expensive, dangerous, unpleasant, inconvenient, time-consuming, and so forth (Rosenstock, 1991).

In 1977, Bandura introduced the concept of self-efficacy, or efficacy expectation as distinct from outcome expection (Bandura 1977a, 1977b, 1986). This concept has been added to the HBM. Self-efficacy is "the conviction that one can successfully execute the behavior required to produce the outcomes" (Bandura, 1977a). For example, for an obese person to lose weight, he or she must believe that losing weight will benefit his or her health and also that he or she is capable of losing weight.

An individual's perceptions are crucial to beliefs and actions. Beliefs are predicated on the *perceived* seriousness of the health problem or situation, the *perceived* susceptibility of the individual, the *perceived* benefits from taking the action, and the *perceived* barriers to taking action. Actions are predicated on all of .these perceptions plus modifying factors such as demographic, sociopsychologic, and structural variables, as well as confidence that one can implement the action.

Dignan and Carr (1987) stated that the effectiveness of the health belief model is based upon three essential factors:

(1) the readiness of the individual to consider behavioral changes to avoid disease or to minimize health risks; (2) the existence and power of forces in the individual's environment that urge change and make it possible, and (3) the behaviors themselves. Each of these factors is influenced by a complex set of forces that relate to the personality and environment of the individual, as well as past experiences with health services and providers.

An essential element should be added to that cogent statement: the health educator.

Health Education and the Health Belief Model

The health belief model has broad implications for health educators. Virtually every statement made thus far about the model provides opportunity for health educators to influence the behavior of young people. Programs should be based at least in part on how many and which members of the target population feel susceptible and believe the threat could be reduced by some action on their part at an acceptable cost. Programs also should be based upon the extent to which students, patients, or clients feel competent to carry out the prescribed actions over long periods (Rosenstock, 1991).

Perhaps the most obvious role of health educators lies in affecting the students' perceptions. According to Bedworth and Bedworth (1992), before perception can take place, the individual must be exposed to an educational experience that deals with perceptions as its outcome. Even though youngsters frequently understand the seriousness of health situations, they do not perceive themselves as susceptible. Teenagers are notorious for their feelings of invulnerability. This is a difficult perception to overcome, but overcoming it is a prerequisite to healthy lifestyles. It is more than simple knowledge; it is also attitude. Educators should address this point in curriculum development and in everyday instruction. It is not a matter of imposing scare tactics on students; it is a matter of facing reality. A positive way of attaining this goal is to emphasize the benefits of the behavior. When a young person internalizes the benefits of action, logic leads to the perception of personal susceptibility.

We must recognize, however, that experiences and messages that reinforce negative perceptions also are a form of education. The plethora of advertising and media that seem to invite indiscriminate sexual behavior is an example of a message that says, "Do what you want; there is no risk!" One lucky, intoxicated trip home behind the wheel of a car provides an experience that may encourage repetitions of that behavior. Experiences such as this further strengthen the sense of invulnerability.

The health educator is a modifying force in the student's environment. By providing knowledge, the teacher is affecting a structural variable. By providing advice and support for the decision, the health educator is acting as a cue to action. The health educator can organize peer support for the action. Although the results of the Just Say No movement have been questioned, the idea of organizing Just Say No clubs can serve as support for abstinence from drugs in the same way as Students Against Driving Drunk organizations have provided support for abstaining from alcohol and from driving after drinking. In this case, the name of the organization is not what is important. Rather, the quality of the interaction and the group support are the critical elements.

Self-efficacy may be increased in a number of ways. One well-documented method is to set short-term rather than long-term goals (Bandura and Schunk, 1981). The teacher or provider should give reinforcement as the client or student moves toward the goals.

SELF-CONCEPT THEORY

Drawing upon the self-concept as a well-documented aspect in the prediction of human behavior and success, Beatty (1968) has developed a unique theory of self-concept and learning that integrates personality development, motivation, and learning in a solitary construct. Beatty's theory presents the self-concept as a group of self-images perceived through feedback or judgments of others—the perceived self. On the basis of this perceived self, the concept of how to behave to be effective, or adequacy, is developed. Therefore, the self-concept is made up of the *perceived self* and the *adequate self*. The individual's task is to make the perceived self as similar as possible to, or to overlap, the adequate self.

Unfortunately, the two selves do not overlap most of the time. Motivation, according to Beatty, is the work of making the perceived self more like the adequate self. Learning comes from using feedback from others and the environment and acting to determine which behaviors will lead to the adequate self.

Beatty identified four areas of experience and learning that contribute to the overlapping of perceived and adequate selves, reducing the discrepancies between them. These four areas are *worth, coping, expressing,* and *autonomy*.

1. By experiencing love or other forms of inclusion, the individual gains a sense of *self-worth* without an accompanying sense of defensiveness.

2. By learning how to do something that previously could not be done, the individual feels better able to *cope* effectively.

3. By means of affective (pleasant or unpleasant) experiencing of sensations, the individual becomes more *self-expressive* and relatively more free of tension and anxiety.

4. By making *autonomous* choices, the individual develops a greater range of choices for controlling his or her own future.

Experiencing these areas develops maturity.

As individuals strive, often without their own knowledge, to reconcile differences in the perceived and the adequate self, health educators should help with this task. The teacher can have a great deal of influence on development of the perceived self. The perceived self is an accumulation of information provided by others and the environment. Frequently, teachers fail to acknowledge children's positive behaviors. We often spend so much time correcting behavior that we miss opportunities to provide feedback about children's effective and useful behavior. These rewards can take the forms of verbal acknowledgement, notes on papers, awards, "I Caught You Being Good" tickets, and hundreds of others. We also should encourage a positive environment in the classroom, one that encourages students to reassure one another and provides cooperation among students.

A child's idea of the adequate self often is skewed by a few children who, through the force of their personalities, popularity, physical size, athletic ability, or strength, intimidate others. In these cases, what is adequate to the child is not what the society sees as adequate. Children may be challenged to smoke cigarettes to be a part of the group or to escape harassment. They may be discouraged from studying because the peer group does not reward good grades. These are examples of how the adequate self can be built around peer acceptance or even survival rather than success in school or in adulthood. Clarifying these issues is not an easy task, but it is one that every school, teacher, and parent should address.

The classroom teacher can enhance the four areas of organized learning and experience Beatty identified (worth, coping, expressing, and autonomy). Although not every child comes from a loving home environment, the classroom should be accepting and psychologically affectionate. All children should be included in activities whenever possible. Each child should have opportunities to develop a sense of worth by successfully participating in classroom work, field trips, and decision making relevant to the group.

Frequently, children do not wish to try an unfamiliar activity. For example, children often do not want to take swimming lessons because they do not yet know how to swim! Children may refuse to speak in front of the class or to read aloud because they are unfamiliar with the task. Children may ignore a homework assignment simply because they have no experience with using the library. These are examples of opportunities for developing coping skills. The opportunities exist almost constantly in school. Careful attention to challenging students within their capabilities is a talent that good teachers develop and exhibit. The recognition of one's feelings through experiencing sensations, both new and old, helps the individual to become more self-expressive. The affective (feeling) domain often is addressed poorly in health education, yet most decisions about health behavior are based on feelings and attitudes. Expressing feelings and emotions can reduce tension and anxiety. A good many diseases and disorders originate in stress and tension. Therefore, by

addressing the affective experience of sensations, we can enhance the self-concept and the physical self as well.

Our society asks a lot of our adolescents when we require them to make decisions about sexual activity, substance use, and a variety of other issues. This task becomes even more difficult when the young person has little or no experience making autonomous choices. The question arises: How can kids be expected to make sound decisions when they have never made them before? Parents frequently are guilty of making all the choices for children—when to eat, what to eat, when to sleep, what to wear. The children miss opportunities for practice at decision making. For instance, asking a child if he or she would rather have broccoli, green beans, or asparagus gives him or her some autonomy in meal selection and practice at living with his or her own choice.

Schools should provide the opportunity for choices as well. Of course, living with the consequences of the choice is part of making the choice. A health educator may give choices for assignment topics—for example the consequences of teenage pregnancy, how to say no to a sexual advance, or planning for a safe prom date. Once the student has chosen the topic, the choice now might be the format of the assignment. It could be a paper, a skit, a video production, a speech, or other form. Once the choices are made, the student and the teacher must live with them and face their consequences, both positive and negative. This is just one example of a way to give students practice in making autonomous choices. As the student develops more skill and responsibility, he or she can be given more and more autonomy in making choices as practice for real-life decisions.

CONSTRUCTIVISM

Constructivism is the new rallying theme in education. Part of its popularity derives from its origins in a variety of disciplines, most notably philosophy of science, sociology, and psychology. Some professional groups, such as the National Association for the Education of Young Children and the National Council of Teachers of Mathematics have based revisions of their standards on the constructivist assumption that learners do not passively absorb knowledge but, rather, construct it from their experiences. Constructivism is not a new idea. It has roots in classical philosophy of science as well as in the educational theories of Montessori, Piaget, Dewey, and others (Ashton, 1992).

Definitions and Principles

Constructivism deals with questions of knowledge and is, therefore, considered an exercise in epistemology (the study of the nature, origin, methods, and limits of knowledge). It stresses pupil engagement in learning and the importance of understanding the student's current conceptual scheme in order to teach effectively. For this reason, the student's experiential world upon entering the learning situation is crucial to constructivists. Constructivists emphasize dialogue, conversation, argument, and the justification of student and teacher opinion in a social setting (Matthews, 1992). Confrey (1990) wrote:

> Constructivism can be described as essentially a theory about the limits of human knowledge, a belief that all knowledge is necessarily a product of our cognitive acts. We can have no direct or unmediated knowledge of any external or objective reality. We construct our understanding through our experiences, and the character of our experience is influenced profoundly by our cognitive lens.

Confrey's powerful words indicate that, to the constructivist, knowledge does not exist to the individual unless he or she has produced the knowledge through his or her own actions and experiences.

Constructivism comes in at least thirteen different varieties. The common thread running

through all of them is that constructivism is subject-centered, experience-based, and relativistic. Wheatley (1991) expressed this commonality by stating:

> The theory of constructivism rests on two main principles . . . Principle one states that knowledge is not passively received, but is actively built up by the cognizing subject . . . Principle two states that the function of cognition is adaptive and serves the organization of the experiential world, not the discovery of ontological reality . . . Thus we do not find truth but construct viable explanations of our experiences.

Piaget developed his constructivist theory in opposition to another scientific theory, associationism. According to associationism, and its better known outgrowth, behaviorism, knowledge is acquired by *internalizing* certain connections, contingencies, and stimuli from sources external to the individual. Constructivism, by contrast, holds that humans acquire knowledge by building it *from the inside* in interaction with the environment (Kamii, Manning, and Manning, 1991).

Constructivists do not view curriculum as a daily course to be run, consisting of preset means, certain material to cover, and predetermined ends in the form of a discrete set of skills. Instead, they endorse a more interactive and dynamic approach to curriculum. They view curriculum as more of a matrix of ideas to be explored over time. The students enter the matrix at various points, depending upon where they are in their current understanding. The students' experience and context rule their learning.

In the constructivist view, there is no distinction between learning and problem solving, or between comprehension and application. To learn is to actively solve problems; to comprehend is to apply. This, of course, poses some opposition to Bloom's taxonomy and is not surprising, because Bloom relied heavily on the literature on transfer of learning. Constructivists hold that transfer never has been validated fully, and they prefer an alternative, the idea of connectedness. Connectedness, according to Prawat (1992), is the assumption that:

> Knowledge is more accessible, and thus more likely to be transferred to novel situations, when it is a central or integral part of one's cognitive structure.

As a part of one's cognitive structure, it becomes more difficult to separate learning, application, understanding, problem solving, comprehension, or any cognitive function.

Radical constructivism, one of the varieties of constructivism, currently is receiving much attention. One of its chief proponents, von Glasersfeld (1992), contends that just because something works (is viable) does not mean that it therefore is a representation of the "real" world that prevents other things from working. That "real" world remains unknowable no matter how well we manage in the domain of our own experiences. Thus, this branch of constructivism attempts to withdraw from the tradition that knowledge must be a representation of reality, in which reality means a world prior to having been experienced. It holds that we cannot put any meaning to the "real" world's existence in the sense that it exists by itself prior to our noticing, perceiving, and thinking about it. To radical constructivists, "to exist" means to be experienced. Applied to learning, radical constructivism asserts that knowledge is a result of constructive activity and cannot be transferred to a passive learner.

Radical constructivism replaces the idea of truth with viability, which limits knowledge to what a person has experienced. The ability to predict what will happen in the future is based solely on the knowledge that already proved viable under the unique circumstances of the case. This rather extreme view is reflected and perhaps carried a step further by Nadeau and Desautels (1984):

> Science as knowledge is an intellectual construct, and what are referred to as the laws of nature are merely the result of this human activity. Nature as such does not have laws.

Constructivism, its critics argue, short-circuits the process of working intellectually with real objects that others have described and experienced or that, so far, defy description. This seems to violate the premise of science that we comprehend things outside ourselves. Making sense of the things that provide input to our senses, Matthews (1992) claims, is not enough to warrant the science (or, for that matter, health) teacher's disturbing children's deeply ingrained and important beliefs. Finding out the truth might provide such warrant. Starting out with what makes sense to students, as constructivists advocate, following those students through what we know to be false views while encouraging them along to the current scientific view raises serious questions to some educators. Many hold that the reasons science and human behavior make sense cannot be spelled out in terms of sensory inputs only. Although these arguments certainly add fuel to the debate about constructivist education, we recognize some practical implications for the health education classroom.

Implications for Health Education

Constructivist learning is viewed as more concerned with understandings achieved through relevant experience than with accumulated facts received from others. Constructivists see learning as more imbued with meaning, more influenced by social and cultural contexts and, in general, less purely cognitive and less governed by abstract principles than traditional conceptions of learning (Black and Ammon, 1992).

The critical element is the child's own experience. The constructivist teaching role is to build on the child's experience and to draw on subject matter knowledge to help the child make better sense of present life experiences and thus be better able to form decisions about future life behaviors. The teacher must embed the learning experience with real-world activity. In this way the teacher can orient the student in a general direction and set up limitations that prevent the student from constructing a direction that seems unsuitable to the teacher.

Radical constructivists (e.g., von Glasersfeld, 1992), carry this practice a step further by stating that as a teacher, you should not tell students the reality you have constructed is the one that they ought to believe. They even hold that knowledge in textbooks and documents is an illusion and advocate "group learning." This type of learning, practiced in a number of subject areas, allows students to work on problems together, generating reflection and discussion regarding thinking and doing.

Perhaps no discipline has more opportunity to apply the most useful of constructivism's principles than health education. Children come to school with a variety of home and social experiences. They interpret the world in terms of their world. It takes little imagination to find examples of baggage children bring to school that often make everyday cognitive schooling seem irrelevant. Many children's experiences make talk of two-parent homes irrelevant. Some children experience violence and drug abuse as casual ways to deal with stress and disagreements. Indeed, some children's experience makes illicit drugs a legitimate income source. Health education offers great opportunity to utilize these schema to develop ideals of values, attitudes, and behavior.

Brown, Collins, and Duguid (1989) suggested that perhaps educators should begin with activities and situations, then work back to relevant skills and concepts. Certainly, health education scenarios and simulations offer the opportunity for these applications.

The child's own thinking processes are important to the constructivist teacher. Asking a student how he or she got to an answer is a good way to discover information about his or her thinking. It allows for explanation in a way that is clear to the student that a specific answer may not be useful under certain circumstances. For example, a student may be asked to respond to a scenario in which, as a new student in school, he or she is asked by an attractive opposite-sex classmate to trade lunches. The student's response may indicate need for affiliation and opposite-sex companionship. This indication could be verified by asking the student if he or she ever had been in a similar situation or to explain why he or she felt the answer was realistic. Whatever the student answers to a question or problem such as this makes sense to the student at the moment and should be taken seriously. The teacher then may rephrase the question, substituting an offer for drugs or a request for sexual activity. This allows for observation of the student's thought processes and also allows the student to think about similar situations that may require different responses.

Simply answering "correct" to a question usually does not do much for the student's conceptual development if he or she is not interested. Creating situations that present opportunities for the gratification inherent in solving a problem may pique students' motivation to delve further into questions that at first are of little interest to them.

On the other hand, simply telling students they are wrong may crush their motivation. To change their way of acting and thinking, students need to see in their own experience that what they did was not the most successful way of behaving.

Constructivist theory insists that content be accessible, oriented toward student experiences. It also insists that content be powerful and correct in the sense that it meets standards of the discipline. If these criteria are met, the theory holds that application of knowledge contributes to the development of that knowledge and vice versa.

SUMMARY

Principles of education guide the development of curricula. They also direct the planning of classroom activities and student-teacher encounters. Acquisition of knowledge is not a one-dimensional task. Neither is the evolution of feelings and attitudes. Because the cognitive and affective domains both affect behavior, establishing health-related behavior through education cannot be a unidimensional effort.

Theories that allow for the prediction of human behavior and explain its motivation are of great value to health educators. Understanding the reasons for behavior, the aspects of personality that affect decisions, and the multitude of variables that are forced on individuals are basic to changing unhealthy habits and establishing healthy behaviors.

Appreciation of the value of self-concept, especially in children, is important to any teacher. To health educators, however, it it critical, as so many choices are based upon self-esteem.

Identification of factors that influence behavior—change forces and restraining forces—can be pivotal in establishing healthy behavior. When combining this knowledge with the ability to identify motivating factors, health educators are well-armed in their quest to win students' trust and help them adjust their behavior.

Behavior modification and modeling can be effective tools in addressing others' actions. Health educators have the unique opportunity to utilize these vehicles in helping young people improve their lives.

Constructivist theory provides the basis for a truly nontraditional way of conducting health education. Educators often talk of meeting the child where he or she is and bringing that child to a new level. Health educators may apply constructivist theory to help children look at their world and their behaviors in a different light. The result could be incredible!

Theories of learning afford a way to formalize an approach to teaching. If applied faithfully, they provide defense and justification for curriculum and classroom activities. Although learning theories have inconsistencies, the ideal for the health educator is to formalize teaching around a demonstrated, systematic explanation of interrated educational constructs.

REFERENCES

Ashton, P. T. Editorial. *Journal of Teacher Education, 43* (November-December 1992): 322.

Babbie, E. *The Practice of Social Research* (5th ed.). Belmont, CA: Wadsworth Publishing, 1989.

Bandura, A. Influence of models' reinforcement contingencies on the acquisition of initiative responses. *Journal of Personality and Social Psychology, 1* (June 1965): 589–595.

Bandura, A. *Social Learning Theory.* Englewood Cliffs, NJ: Prentice-Hall, 1977a.

Bandura, A. Self-efficacy: Toward a unifying theory of behavioral change. *Psychological Review, 84* (March 1977b): 191–215.

Bandura, A. The self system in reciprocal determinism. *American Psychologist, 33* (April 1978), 344–358.

Bandura, A. *Social Foundations of Thought and Action.* Englewood Cliffs, NJ: Prentice-Hall, 1986.

Bandura, A. and D. H. Schunk. Cultivating competence, self-efficacy, and intrinsic interest through proximal self-motivations. *Journal of Personality and Social Psychology, 41* (September 1981): 586–598.

Bandura, A., and R. H. Walters. *Social Learning and Personality Development.* New York: Holt, Rinehart & Winston, 1963.

Beatty, W. *Emotions: The missing link in education.* Paper presented at Conference on Issues in Human Development: Present and Future, at Institute for Child Study, University of Maryland, April 20, 1968.

Becker, M. H., editor. The health belief model and personal health behavior. *Health Education Monographs* 2 (Winter 1974): 404–419.

Bedworth, A. E. and D. A. Bedworth. *The Profession and Practice of Health Education.* Dubuque, IA: Wm. C. Brown Publishers, 1992.

Black, A., and P. Ammon. A developmental-constructivist approach to teacher education. *Journal of Teacher Education, 43* (November-December 1992): 323–335.

Bloom, B. S. editor. *Taxonomy of Education Objectives, Handbook I: Cognitive Domain.* New York: David McKay Co., 1956.

Braucht, G. N., D. Brakarsh, D, Follingstad, and K. L. Berry. Deviant drug use in adolescence: A review of psychological correlates. *Psychological Bulletin*, 79 (February 1973): 92–106.

Brown, J. S., A. Collins, and P. Duguid. Situated cognition and the culture of learning. *Educational Researcher* August-September 1989: 32–42.

Butler, J. T. Early adolescent alcohol consumption and self-concept, social class and knowledge of alcohol. *Journal of Studies on Alcohol, 43* (May 1982): 603–608.

Coleman, J. C. *Psychology and Effective Behavior.* Palo Alto, CA: Scott, Foresman and Company, 1969.

Confrey, J. What constructivism implies for teaching. In R. B. Davis, C. A. Maher, and N. Noddings, editors. *Constructivist Views on the Teaching and Learning of Mathematics.* Reston, VA: National Council of Teachers of Mathematics, 1990.

Creswell, W. H., Jr. and I. M. Newman. *School Health Practice* (9th ed.). St. Louis: Times Mirror/ Mosby College Publishing, 1989.

Dignan, M., and P. A. Carr. *Program Planning for Health Education and Health Promotion.* Philadelphia: Lea and Febiger, 1987.

Ewart, C. K., C. B. Taylor, L. B. Reese, and R. F. Debusk. Effects of early post-myocardial infarction exercise testing on self-perception and subsequent physical activity. *American Journal of Cardiology, 51* (April 1983): 1076–1080.

Fitts, W. H. and W. T. Hamner. *The Self Concept and Delinquency* (Research Monograph no. 1.) Nashville, TN: Nashville Mental Health Center, July 1969.

Glanz, K. *Can health education research and practice be more successful by using behavioral theory?* Paper presented at American Public Health Association annual meeting. Boston, November 14, 1988.

Glanz, K., F. M. Lewis, and B. K. Rimer, editors. *Health Behavior and Health Education: Theory, Research, and Practice.* San Francisco: Jossey-Bass Publishers, 1991.

Green, L. W. and F. M. Lewis. *Evaluation and Measurement in Health Education.* Mountain View, CA: Mayfield Publishing, 1986.

Kamii, C., M. Manning, and G. Manning, editors. *Early Literacy: A Constructivist Foundation for Whole Language.* Washington, DC: National Education Association of the United States, 1991.

Kerlinger, F. N. *Foundations of Behavioral Research* (3d ed.). New York: Holt, Rinehart & Winston, 1986.

Kirscht, J. P. The health belief model and illness behavior. *Health Education Monographs, 2* (Winter 1974): 387–408.

Knutson, A. L. *The Individual, Society, and Health Behavior.* New York: Russell Sage Foundation, 1965.

Kolb, D. A. and R. Fry. Toward an applied theory of experiential learning. In C. L. Cooper, editor, *Theories of Group Process.* New York: John Wiley and Sons, 1975.

Krathwohl, D. R., B. Bloom, and B. Masia. *Taxonomy of Educational Goals, Handbook II: Affective Domain.* New York: David McKay Co., 1964.

Lewin, K. *Resolving Social Conflicts.* New York: Holt, Rinehart & Winston, 1948.

Lewin, K. Quasi-stationary social equilibria and the problem of permanent change. In W. G. Bennis, K. D. Benne, and R. Chin, editors, *The Planning of Change.* New York: Holt, Rinehart & Winston, 1961.

Maslow, A. H. A theory of human motivation. *Psychological Review, 50* (July 1943): 370–396.

Matthews, M. R. Constructivism and the empiricist legacy. In M. K. Pearsall, editor, *Relevant Research, Volume 2.* Washington, DC: National Science Teacher Association, 1992.

Miller, N. E. and J. Dollard. *Social Learning and Imitation.* New Haven, CT: Yale University Press, 1941.

Nadeau, R., and J. Desautels. *Epistemology and the Teaching of Science.* Ottawa: Science Council of Canada, 1984.

Perry, C. L., T. Baranowski, and G. S. Parcel. How individuals, environments, and health behavior interact: Social learning theory. In K. Glanz, F. M. Lewis and B. K. Rimer, editors, *Health Behavior and Health Education: Theory, Research, and Practice.* San Francisco: Jossey-Bass Publishers, 1991.

Prawat, R. S. Teachers' beliefs about teaching; A constructivist perspective. *American Journal of Education, 100* (May 1992): 354–395.

Rogers, C. R. The interpersonal relationship in the facilitation of learning. In Association for Supervision and Curriculum Development, *Humanizing Education: The Person in the Process.* Washington, DC: National Education Association, 1967.

Rosecrans, C. J., and H. P. Brignet. Comparative personality profiles of young drug abusers and nonusers. *Alabama Journal of Medical Science, 9* (October 1972): 397–402.

Rosenstock, I. M. Historical origins of the health belief model. *Health Education Monographs, 2* (Winter 1974): 328–335.

Rosenstock, I. M. The health belief model: Explaining health behavior through expectancies. In K. Glanz, F. M. Lewis and B. K. Rimer, editors, *Health Behavior and Health Education: Theory, Research, and Practice.* San Francisco: Jossey-Bass Publishers, 1991.

Ross, H. S. and P. R. Mico. *Theory and Practice in Health Education.* Palo Alto, CA: Mayfield Publishing, 1980.

Rudd, J., and K. Glanz. How individuals use information for health action: Consumer information processing. In K. Glanz, F. M. Lewis and B. K. Rimer, *Health Behavior and Health Education: Theory, Research, and Practice.* San Francisco: Jossey-Bass Publishers, 1991.

Skinner, B. F. *The Behavior of Organisms.* East Norwalk, CT: Appleton & Lange, 1938.

Skinner, B. F. *Science and Human Behavior.* New York: Macmillan, 1953.

von Glasersfeld, E. Questions and answers about radical constructivism. In M. K. Pearsall, editor, *Relevant Research, Volume 2.* Washington, DC: National Science Teachers Association, 1992.

Wheatley, G. H. Constructivist perspectives on science and mathematics learning, *Science Education, 75* (January 1991): 9–22.

10

COMPETENCIES AND SKILLS OF THE HEALTH EDUCATOR

For several years professionals have been attempting to identify competencies for the practice of health education. On occasion we have recognized the need to determine the relative importance of the various competencies. Some professionals have perceived the need to differentiate the perceived importance of various requisite competencies by practice settings, such as school, worksite, or voluntary health agency. Although identifying competencies is important at all strata of the profession, nowhere is it more important than at the level of professional preparation. The Role Delineation Project has formed a firm foundation for the identification of competencies. The work of others, however, demonstrates that there are alternative ways of addressing the problem.

More than 20 different institutions in the United States offer degrees in public health such as the Master of Public Health (M.P.H.), Doctor of Public Health (Dr.P.H.), and Doctor of Philosophy (Ph.D.) in Public Health. The approach of these degrees is usually directed toward groups rather than individuals and frequently has a lesser emphasis on education and more emphasis on service delivery. Of the 300 or more institutions that grant degrees in Health Education, many are located in Departments of Health Education or Health, Physical Education, and Recreation, or some similar configuration. They frequently are linked to a College of Education or School of Public Health. These institutions grant a variety of degrees including Bachelor of Science (B.S.), Master of Education (M.Ed.), Doctor of Education (Ed.D.), and Doctor of Philosophy (Ph.D.) in Health Education. These degrees usually are rooted in the process of education (teaching) and frequently are preparatory for school health education.

Unfortunately, "health educators" emerge from other programs with little or no health education preparation *per se*. Some of these individuals are assigned health education duties by virtue of their backgrounds in nursing, medicine, home economics, biology, or psychology. These are essentially laypeople, the most dedicated of whom become effective through on-the-job training, workshops, conferences, and college courses. The least effective situation occurs when lack of funding forces those with no interest in the field to take over the responsibilities of health education.

Although the nature of an individual's education and training is an important issue, regardless of how we come to the profession, a certain level of proficiency in a select set of competencies must be attained if the individual is to be successful in meeting his or her responsibilities. Professional preparation and credentialing must establish standardized qualifications for entry into the profession, and formalized entry routes for employment must be established. As Neutens (1984) stated so clearly, we "must not become a refuge for the unqualified."

Most professionals would agree that some general skills are necessary to health educators. The more obvious of these include:

1. Written and oral communication;
2. Ability to apply theories of learning and behavior;
3. Ability to develop appropriate materials for education;
4. Ability to work with people of various educational backgrounds and social and cultural groups;
5. Ability to access information and resources;
6. Ability to think critically;
7. Ability to understand research and evaluate research findings.

The undergraduate educational experience should help to develop these skills. Too frequently, however, students delay in taking speech and writing courses, causing them to struggle when they are asked to perform tasks related to these skills later in their academic careers. Sometimes students never recover from this loss of time and preparation. The ability to work with people of various social and cultural groups has been enhanced greatly by the recent

trend in education requiring exposure to multicultural experiences.

IDENTIFICATION OF COMPETENCIES

During the decade of the 1970s, the professional organizations identified with health education prepared statements on professional preparation for health educators. These amounted to policy statements. The School Health Division Task Force of the American Association for Health, Physical Education, and Recreation (AAHPER) (1974) published a document determining that the undergraduate preparation should produce health educators who show competency in the following major areas:

1. Health content
2. Allied health fields
3. Professional education
   Curriculum
   Methodology and materials
   Evaluation and measurement
   Organization and administration
   Public relations
4. Personal qualifications
5. Practicum

The American School Health Association (ASHA) (1976) published a slightly different report, listing "skills and knowledge" rather than competencies. The report was prepared by the ASHA Committee on Professional Preparation and College Health Education. The fundamental areas identified were:

1. Content areas in health education
   Direct health content
   Related health content
2. Educational skills
   Learning theory applied to health behavior
   Verbal and nonverbal communication
   Curriculum planning and implementation
   Methodology applied to direct and related health content

Resources applied to direct and related health content

Evaluation techniques

3. Orientation to the profession

Philosophy

Organization/administration

School health program

Community health program

Process skills

4. Demonstration of skills and knowledge

Student teaching

Community health practicum

The Society for Public Health Educators (SOPHE) (1976) published *Guidelines for the Preparation and Practice of Professional Health Educators*. It is competency-driven and identifies the following major areas to be achieved at both the baccalaureate and the master's level:

1. Foundations of health education

2. Administration of health education

3. Program development and management

Planning for change: planning process for health education

Health planning methods

Training theory and skills

Group dynamics theory and skills

Community organization

Information and media

4. Research and evaluation

5. Professional ethics

6. Special applications

Examination of the major areas (competencies) from AAHPER, ASHA, and SOPHE uncovers some significant differences. As Neutens (1984) observed, the underlying assumptions for which the listed competencies and objectives originally were intended were quite different. Whereas the AAHPER and ASHA documents emphasize preparation of the school health educator, the SOPHE document leans toward health education in the community setting.

In 1978, the National Task Force on the Preparation and Practice of Health Educators, made up of representatives from national organizations with health education constituencies published its landmark *Preparation and Practice of Community, Patient, and School Health Educators* (Sliepcevich, 1978). The work was the culmination of the efforts of what has come to be known as the Workshop on Commonalities and Differences. The workshop identified three functions that are instrumental to health educators in all settings:

1. Function I of a Health Educator: Assess health and educational needs and interests of the target population.

2. Function II of a Health Educator: Design, implement, coordinate, and evaluate health education activities that meet the goals of health education.

3. Function III of a Health Educator: Coordinate multidisciplinary resources to enable an educational planning and implementation process to exist.

Implications of the findings of the Workshop on Commonalities and Differences are enormous to the profession of health education. This marked a movement toward the philosophy that, regardless of setting, the competencies necessary to practice health education are the same. Previously, professional preparation programs could operate from a variety of assumptions and goals, based on the belief that health educators working with different populations and in different settings function in different ways and apply different skills. With the Workshop on Commonalities and Differences, the trend had begun to enforce a large measure of conformity on the preparation of health educators. Neutens (1984) seemed to support this position when he declared, "For too long, graduates in health education have been the product of individual program interests rather than the product of a unified set of experiences common to everyone who has the title of health educator."

In 1978, a contract between the National Center for Health Education and the Bureau of Health Professions Division of Associated Health Professions (Department of Health and Human Services) was signed to initially specify the responsibilities, functions, skills, and knowledge of entry-level health educators; to define entry level into health education; and to identify levels of supervision required for entry-level personnel (Henderson, McIntosh, and Schaller, 1981). This endeavor became known as the aforementioned Role Delineation Project. The major assumption that formed the foundation of the project is that responsibilities, functions, requisite skills, and knowledge of health educators are common to all health educators, regardless of setting or constituency. Thus, all the competencies the Role Delineation Project identified apply to school health educators, community health educators, patient educators, and others who identify themselves as health educators.

Several definitions are important to understanding the Role Delineation Project. The following are taken from the Glossary of Terms (Bureau of Health Education, 1980) of the Role Delineation Project:

> *Health Educator:* An individual prepared to assist individuals, acting separately or collectively, to make informed decisions regarding matters affecting their personal health and that of others.
>
> *Role:* The set of related responsibilities which depict the nature of the services health educators perform in society.
>
> *Role Delineation:* The process of clarifying the role performed by health educators through specifying responsibilities and functions and identifying requisite skills and knowledge.

Area of responsibility: A major aspect of the role which encompasses an aggregate of related functions.

Function: A collection of related activities that must be performed to fulfill an area of responsibility.

Skill: An ability to do or to apply something in order to carry out an activity.

Knowledge: Concepts, facts, and information which are the foundation for the role specified.

Competency: An acceptable level of skill proficiency required to carry out an activity.

The Role Delineation Project was intended to help establish minimum acceptable levels of competence to protect consumers of health education services. The format for identifying these competencies is from the general to the specific, as shown in Figure 10.1. The areas of responsibility identified by the project are:

1. Determining the appropriate focus for health education;
2. Planning health education programs in response to identified needs;
3. Implementing planned health education programs;
4. Evaluating health education;
5. Coordinating selected health education activities;
6. Acting as a resource for health and health education;
7. Communicating health and health education needs, concerns, and resources.

As an example, one of the seven areas of responsibility is presented in Table 10.1 in exactly the form it was presented by the Role Delineation Project in 1980.

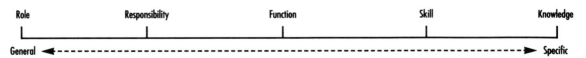

Source: W. H. Greene and B. G. Simons-Morton, *Introduction to Health Education* (Prospect Heights, IL: Waveland Press, 1984). Reprinted by permission from the publisher.

FIGURE 10.1. Relative Specificity of Facets of the Role Delineation Project

---

TABLE 10.1. Sample Area of Responsibility in Role Delineation Project.

Area of Responsibility V

The entry-level health educator, working with individuals, groups, and individuals, is responsible for:

EVALUATING HEALTH EDUCATION

The entry-level health educator, working with individuals, groups, and individuals, is responsible for:

Function: A. Participating in developing a design to assess achievement of education objectives.
Skill: 1. The health educator must be able to assist in specifying indicators of program success.
Knowledge: The health educator must be able to:
  a. differentiate between what can and cannot be measured (e.g., knowledge gained, changes in morbidity rates due to health education).
  b. translate objectives into specific indicators (e.g., knowledge gained, values stated, behaviors mastered).
  c. describe range of methods and techniques used for educational measurement (e.g., inventories, scales, competency tests).
  d. list steps involved in evaluative activities (e.g., setting standards, specifying objectives, developing criteria for achievement of objectives).

Skill: 2. The health educator must be able to help to establish the scope for program evaluation.
Knowledge: The health educator must be able to:
  a. define scope of evaluation efforts (e.g., match standards with goals, explain relationship between activities and outcomes).
  b. describe feasibility of evaluative activities (e.g., time availability, resources, setting, nature of the program).
  c. explain the beliefs and purposes behind health education activities (e.g., value to consumers, increase control over health matters, informed public).

Skill: 3. The health educator must be able to help develop methods for evaluating programs.
Knowledge: The health educator must be able to:
  a. identify various measures for determining knowledge, attitudes, and behavior (e.g., questionnaires, self-assessment inventories, knowledge tests).
  b. describe data available for evaluations (e.g., program attendance, reports of behaviors, survey data, letters from consumers and others, test scores).
  c. list strengths and weaknesses of various data, collection methods (e.g., value of self-report, expense of observing behavior).

Skill: 4. The health educator must be able to participate in the specification of instruments for data collection.
Knowledge: The health educator must be able to:
  a. describe advantages and disadvantages of "homemade" and commercial instruments (e.g., utility, cost, timeliness).
  b. identify sources of instruments (e.g., professional organizations, research organizations, consultants, textbook publishers).

Skill: 5. The health educator must be able to assist in the determination of samples needed for evaluation.
Knowledge: The health educator must be able to:
  a. define sample concepts (e.g., stratified, random, convenience, universe).
  b. identify strengths and weaknesses of sampling techniques (e.g., sampling error, skewed results, normal distributions, precision of estimates).

— Continued

TABLE 10.1.   **Sample Area of Responsibility in Role Delineation Project. — *Continued***

Skill:
Knowledge:
	6. The health educator must be able to assist in the selection of data useful for accountability analysis.
	The health educator must be able to:
	    a. describe the uses of cost-benefit analysis (e.g., amount of investment needed for program success, efficacy of health education).
	    b. describe uses of cost-effectiveness analysis (e.g., modify programs, select alternative(s) from competing choices).

The entry-level health educator, working with individuals, groups, and organizations, is responsible for:

Function:
Skill:
Knowledge:
	B. Assembling resources required to carry out evaluation.
	  1. The health educator must be able to acquire facilities, materials, personnel, and equipment.
	The health educator must be able to:
	    a. describe facilities, materials, and equipment needed (e.g., telephones, typewriters, computers).
	    b. identify required expertise and sources for expertise (e.g., survey methodology from universities, physician for clinical study, experts in evaluation).
	    c. identify ways of obtaining necessary facilities, materials, expertise, and equipment (e.g., personal visitations, formal requests, budgetary requisitions).

Skill:
Knowledge:
	2. The health educator must be able to train personnel for evaluation as needed.
	The health educator must be able to:
	    a. describe the process for assessing training needs (e.g., listing skills needed, reviewing skills of available personnel, comparing skills with program requirements).
	    b. describe steps for implementing training programs (e.g., specifying learning objectives, selecting instructional methods, carrying out methods, evaluating).

Skill:
Knowledge:
	3. The health educator must be able to secure the cooperation of those affecting and affected by the program.
	The health educator must be able to:
	    a. describe how to involve relevant parties in the evaluation process (e.g., explaining importance, answering questions, asking for cooperation).
	    b. identify importance of safeguarding rights of individuals involved (e.g., explanation of purposes of procedures, confidential record-keeping).

The entry-level health educator, working with individuals, groups, and organizations, is responsible for:

Function:
Skill:
Knowledge:
	C. Helping to implement the evaluation design.
	  1. The entry-level health educator must be able to collect data through appropriate techniques.
	The health educator must be able to:
	    a. identify the applicability of various techniques to a given situation (e.g., observations, interviews, questionnaires, written tests).
	    b. describe how to acquire data from existing sources (e.g., scan newspapers, review journal articles, scan morbidity and mortality data, health records).
	    c. distinguish between quantitative and qualitative data (e.g., counts vs. expressions of satisfaction, changes in physical indices vs. loss of interest).

— Continued

TABLE 10.1. *Sample Area of Responsibility in Role Delineation Project.*

Skill:	2. The health educator must be able to analyze collected data.
Knowledge:	The health educator must be able to:

     a. identify basic statistical measures (e.g., counts, means, median).

     b. describe processes of statistical analysis (e.g., selected analysis based on stated concern, collecting data, use of statistical techniques).

     c. explain the results of statistical analysis (e.g., report data, make inferences, draw conclusions).

     d. identify steps in analyzing qualitative data (e.g., developing categories, ascribing means to data, making inferences).

     e. explain how data may be kept and used as needed (e.g., record keeping system, computer storage, filing systems, progress reports).

Skill: 3. The health educator must be able to interpret results of program evaluation.

Knowledge: The health educator must be able to:

     a. identify relationships between analyzed data and program objectives (e.g., objectives met, reasons for lack of achievement, changes in program reflected in data).

     b. recognize importance of looking for unanticipated results (e.g., appearance of seemingly unrelated results, significant deviations from what was expected).

     c. identify variables necessary for interpretation of data (e.g., SES, sex, age, medical diagnosis).

     d. recognize risks of drawing conclusions not fully justified by the data (e.g., program's value to other fields, program successes, program failures).

The entry-level health educator, working with individuals, groups, and organizations, is responsible for:

Function: D. Communicating results of evaluation.

Skill: 1. The health educator must be able to report the processes and results of evaluation to those interested.

Knowledge: The health educator must be able to:

     a. describe how to organize, write, and report findings (e.g., objectives, activities, results, interpretation, conclusions).

     b. translate evaluation findings into terms understandable by others (e.g., professionals, consumers, administrators).

     c. explain various ways to depict findings (e.g., graphs, slides, flip charts).

Skill: 2. The health educator must be able to recommend strategies for implementing results.

Knowledge: The health educator must be able to:

     a. list strategies that can be used for implementation (e.g., involve those affected, explain results to given audiences, propose new or modified programs).

     b. identify implications from findings for future programs or other actions (e.g., alert others beyond programs, publish reports on programs and their evaluation).

Skill: 3. The health educator must be able to incorporate results into planning and implementation processes.

Knowledge: The health educator must be able to:

     a. describe how program operations can be modified based on evaluation results (e.g., discussions with personnel, proposed changes in objectives/methods/content).

     b. explain how evaluation results are part of the planning process (e.g., formative vs. summative evaluation, self-renewal of programs).

Source: Bureau of Health Education, U. S. Department of Health and Human Services, "Health education and Credentialing: The Role Delineation Project," *Focal Points,* (July 1980).

One can only marvel at the detail with which the example of Table 10.1 delineates the health educator's role in the area of program evaluation. Each of the seven competency areas identified by the Role Delineation Project are broken down in equal detail. This example illustrates the continuity of the processes of program development and improvement as, for example, in one knowledge item the evaluator must develop the capacity to put results of evaluation to work, and in another the health educator will have the capacity to explain how results of evaluation are part of planning.

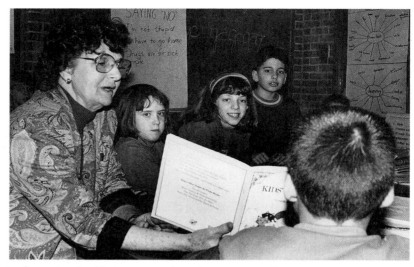

Implementing health instruction through a variety of strategies is an important competency for elementary teachers.

This level of detail provides a framework for health education professional preparation programs. The Role Delineation Project is being applied in the following significant ways in the preparation of health educators.

1. Program accreditation through the National Council on Accreditation of Teacher Education (NCATE) has adopted the competencies of the Role Delineation Project as its standards for health education.

2. Because of NCATE's adoption of the competencies, a number of institutions have revised their professional preparation curricula to come into compliance (McMahon, Bruess, and Lohrman, 1987).

3. In 1988, the National Task Force on the Preparation and Practice of Health Educators changed its incorporation papers and became the National Commission for Health Education Credentialing (NCHEC). The primary purpose of NCHEC is the certification of health educators. It has based its examination

and, therefore, its certification of individual health education specialists upon the competencies detailed by the National Task Force on the Preparation and Practice of Health Educators (1985), which were based on the Role Delineation Project. NCHEC's "Responsibilities and Competencies for Entry-Level Health Educators" is presented in the appendix.

AN APPROACH FOR CLASSROOM TEACHERS

Close examination of the "Responsibilities and Competencies for Entry-Level Health Educators" reveals that its orientation is probably more toward the responsibilities and competencies necessary for professionals in the public and community health settings. Many competencies required of the classroom teachers are missing.

During the 1980s and early 1990s, comprehensive school health education gained recognition as a national priority. This acknowledgment came from major health and education organizations such as the Carnegie Council on Adolescent

---

TABLE 10.2   Health Instruction Responsibilities for Elementary (K–6) Classroom Teachers

---

Responsibility I: Communicating the concepts and purposes of health education.

Competency A: Describe the discipline of health education within the school setting.
Subcompetencies:

    1) Describe the interdependence of health education and the other components of a comprehensive school health program.
    2) Describe comprehensive school health instruction, including the most common content areas.

Competency B: Provide a rationale for K-6 health education.

Competency C: Explain the role of knowledge, skills, and attitudes in shaping patterns of health behavior.

Competency D: Define the role of the elementary teacher within a comprehensive school health program.
Subcompetencies:

    1) Describe the importance of health education for elementary teachers.
    2) Summarize the kinds of support needed by the K-6 teacher from administrators and others to implement an elementary school health education program.
    3) Identify available quality continuing education programs in health education for elementary teachers.
    4) Describe the importance of modeling positive health behaviors.

Responsibility II: Assessing the health instruction needs and interests of elementary students.

Competency A: Utilize information about health needs and interests of students.

Competency B: List behaviors and how they promote or compromise health.

Responsibility III: Planning elementary school health instruction.

Competency A: Select realistic program goals and objectives.

Competency B: Identify a scope and sequence plan for elementary school health instruction.

Competency C: Plan elementary school health education lessons which reflect the abilities, needs, interests, developmental levels, and cultural backgrounds of students.

Competency D: Describe effective ways to promote cooperation with and feedback from administrators, parents, and other interested citizens.

Competency E: Determine procedures which are compatible with school policy for implementing curricula containing sensitive health topics.

Responsibility IV: Implementing elementary school health instruction.

Competency A: Employ a variety of strategies to facilitate implementation of an elementary school health education curriculum.
Subcompetencies:

    1) Provide a core health education curriculum.
    2) Integrate health and other content areas.
    3) Incorporate topics introduced by students into the health education curriculum.
    4) Utilize affective skill-building techniques to help students apply health knowledge to their daily lives.
    5) Involve parents in the teaching/learning process.

— Continued

TABLE 10.2   Health Instruction Responsibilities for Elementary (K–6) Classroom Teachers — *Continued*

Competency B: **Subcompetencies:**	Incorporate appropriate resources and materials.
	1) Select valid and reliable sources of information about health appropriate for K-6.
	2) Utilize school and community resources within a comprehensive program.
	3) Refer students to valid sources of health information and services.
Competency C:	Employ appropriate strategies for dealing with sensitive health issues.
Competency D:	Adapt existing health education curricular models to community and student needs and interests.
Responsibility V:	Evaluating the effectiveness of elementary school health instruction.
Competency A:	Utilize appropriate criteria and methods unique to health education for evaluating student outcomes.
Competency B:	Interpret and apply student evaluation results to improve health instruction.

Source: Joint Committee of the Association for the Advancement of Health Education and the American School Health Association, "Health Instruction Responsibilities and Competencies for Elementary (K-6) Classroom Teachers". *Journal of School Health*, 62 (2) (February 1992): 76-77. Reprinted by permission of American School Health Association, Kent, Ohio.

Development (Carnegie Corporation of New York, 1989); the American Medical Association and the National Association of State Boards of Education (National Commission on the Role of the School and the Community in Improving Adolescent Health, 1990); American Association of School Administrators (1990); and the U. S. Centers for Disease Control (U. S. Public Health Service, 1990).

National surveys identified lack of teacher training as one of the most significant obstructions to the effective implementation and delivery of school health education (ABT Associates, 1980; Metropolitan Life Foundation, 1985). This is particularly true in the elementary grades. A Joint Committee of the Association for the Advancement of Health Education and the American School Health Association (1992) was formed for the purpose of addressing this situation by delineating responsibilities and competencies for the health instruction preparation of elementary school teachers. The result of that effort is given in Table 10.2.

Even though the competencies detailed in Table 10.2 do not include those for teachers in grades 7-12, the work of the joint committee produced welcome results for school health educators. The responsibilities must be specified for entry-level teachers. The emphasis on classroom instruction, curriculum provision, planning lessons, and evaluation of instruction is the essense of classroom teaching. No doubt, the responsibilities and competencies are modeled after *A Framework for the Development of Competency-based Curricula for Entry Level Health Educators* (National Task Force on the Preparation and Practice of Health Educators, 1985). The work of the joint committee, however, recognizes that a specific set of competencies applicable to elementary classroom teachers is unlike competencies necessary in other health education settings.

SUMMARY

Evolution of the identification of competencies for entry-level health education took giant strides beginning in 1948. The process that began then eventually became the Role Delineation Project, which formed the basis for the Certified Health Education Specialist credential. The competencies identified also have become the basis for accrediting health education preparatory programs. Some professionals have found that competencies relating to school health instruction may have been deemphasized in the Role Delineation Project. The competencies no doubt will continue to evolve.

REFERENCES

ABT Associates. *School Health Education Evaluation*. Cambridge, MA: ABT Associates, 1980.

American Alliance of Health, Physical Education, and Recreation, School Health Division Task Force. *Professional Preparation in Safety Education and School Health Education*. Washington, DC: AAHPER, 1974.

American Association of School Administrators. *Healthy Kids for the Year 2000: An Action Plan for Schools*. Arlington, VA: American Association of School Administrators, 1990.

American School Health Association Committee on Professional Preparation and College Health Education. Professional preparation of the health educator. *Journal of School Health, 46* (September 1976): 418-421.

Bureau of Health Education, U. S. Department of Health and Human Services. Health education and credentialing: The Role Delineation Project. *Focal Points* (July 1980): 7-31.

Carnegie Corporation of New York, Carnegie Council on Adolescent Development, Task Force on Education of Young Adolescents. *Turning Points: Preparing American Youth for the 21th Century*. Washington, DC: Carnegie Council on Adolescent Development, 1989.

Henderson, A. C., D. V. McIntosh and W. E. Schaller. Progress report of the Role Delineation Project. *Journal of School Health, 51* (May 1981): 373-376.

Joint Committee of the Association for the Advancement of Health Education and the American School Health Association. Health instruction responsibilities and competencies for elementary (K-6) classroom teachers. *Journal of School Health, 62* (February 1992): 76-77.

McMahon, J. D., C. E. Bruess, and D. K. Lohrman. Three applications of the Role Delineation Project 1985 Curriculum Framework. *Journal of School Health, 57* (September 1987): 274-278.

Metropolitan Life Foundation. *Healthy Me—School Health Education Survey*. New York: Metropolitan Life Foundation, 1985.

National Commission on the Role of the School and the Community in Improving Adolescent Health. *Code Blue: Uniting for Healthier Youth*. Alexandria, VA: National Association of State Boards of Education, 1990.

National Task Force on the Preparation and Practice of Health Educators. *A Framework for the Development of Competency-based Curricula for Entry Level Health Educators*. New York: National Commission for Health Education Credentialing, 1985.

Neutens, J. J. Professional competencies of the health educator. In L. Rubinson and W. F. Alles, *Health Education: Foundations for the Future*. Prospect Heights, IL: Waveland Press, 1984.

Sliepcevich, E. M. *Proceedings of the Workshop on Commonalities and Differences, Preparation and Practice of Community, Patient, and School Health Educators* (Department of Health, Education and Welfare, Pub. No. 78-71). Washington, DC: Government Printing Office, 1978.

Society for Public Health Educators, Task Force on Professional Preparation and Practice of Health Education. *Guidelines for the Preparation and Practice of Professional Health Educators*. San Francisco: SOPHE, 1976.

U. S. Public Health Service. *Healthy People 2000: National Health Promotion and Disease Prevention Objectives*. Washington, DC: Government Printing Office, 1990.

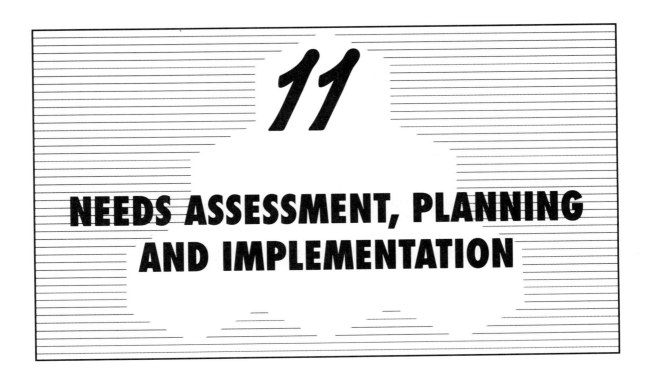

11

NEEDS ASSESSMENT, PLANNING AND IMPLEMENTATION

Developing a program of health education or health promotion can be a long and tedious endeavor. For most projects that at first seem insurmountable, a model for the process can be of enormous aid. Figure 11.1 presents a useful way to visualize the process of program development. The key elements in achieving the final desired product are *needs assessment, development of the program plan, implementation of the plan*, and *evaluation*.

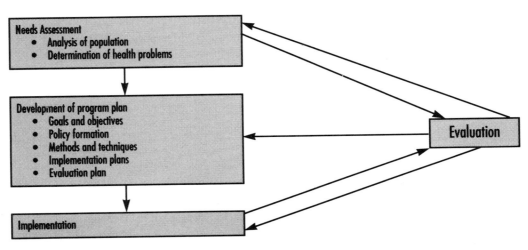

FIGURE 11.1. Planning Paradigm

As discussed in Chapter 10, the Role Delineation Project identified seven responsibilities defined by competencies and subcompetencies that entry-level health educators should possess. Among these competencies are needs assessment, planning, implementation, and evaluation. The separate identification of these responsibilities should not be construed as meaning they are independent of one another. To consider needs assessment, particularly the determination of health problems, as part of the planning process is completely logical. To envision implementation and evaluation as part of the planning process is equally logical. This text takes the approach that the lines separating the four competencies are not concrete and that the overall planning process consists of needs assessment, program planning, planning for implementation, and planning for evaluation. It also takes the position that as long as a program is active, these four responsibilities never end.

Although a detailed description of the four responsibilities is not within the scope of this book, the responsibilities of needs assessment, program planning, and implementation are introduced in this chapter and the responsibility of evaluation in the following chapter. The nature of these tasks can be so demanding that entire texts and courses are needed to completely confront these responsibilities comprehensively.

Reeves, Bergwall, and Woodside (1984) defined planning as "making current decisions in the light of their future effects." Ackoff (1974) even went so far as to describe a style of planning that attempts to create the future. At the very least, health educators should see their work as an effort to *improve* the future. Such an important task should not be undertaken without a well thought-out plan of action. Planning, however, is an endless process. As Reeves et al. (1984) pointed out, planning is designed to help the organization cope with a turbulent environment. Therefore, the successful planner must constantly seek information about new developments and incorporate these data into the plan. Flexibility is a major asset in planning.

Just as separating needs assessment and planning is difficult, so is affixing a point at which planning ends and implementation commences. Many experts see implementation as a continuation of the needs assessment/planning process. Certainly, selecting appropriate methods, media, and materials for carrying out a program can be viewed as an important part of the process of planning and implementation. Applying what is selected in meaningful ways to the learner/client is just as critical. Description of these competencies is more suitable to the many "methods" textbooks and, therefore, will not be addressed thoroughly here.

Planning for health education is contingent upon a number of factors including size of the population, results of the needs assessment process, and resources available. A number of paradigms have been advanced that help clarify the planning process.

Breckon, Harvey, and Lancaster (1984) set forth seven general principles of planning that serve as a useful way to introduce the topic.

1. *Plan the process.* Plan for planning, complete with timetable for planning and for the plan. Determine who is to be involved in planning, the best time to plan the program, what data are needed, where the planning should occur, what resistance is expected, and what will enhance the project's success.

2. *Plan with people.* Involve clients and consumers of the project to give them ownership in the activity and to avail the planning group of clients' knowledge of subtleties of the problem. Involve administrators and health educators to generate more ideas.

3. *Plan with data.* Seek out the necessary information on relevant diseases, disorders, and behaviors, and analyze those data by age, gender, and other applicable variables.

4. *Plan for permanence.* Plan for an ongoing, long-term program. Most health problems do not go away and require education for generations. Include planning for long-term staffing.

5. *Plan for priorities.* Spend your time developing programs of highest need *and* greatest opportunity for success. Prioritize your list of needs, and revise them periodically. This implies an overall assessment of community needs and agency opportunities.

6. *Plan for outcomes and impact.* Commit your energy to planning programs that will change undesirable behaviors to desirable actions. Plan to measure and evaluate behavior change and to measure and evaluate reduction of the major problem the behavior caused. Think in terms of both immediate and long-term results.

7. *Plan for evaluation.* Build evaluation into the program design. Develop a plan for evaluating the short- and long-term results. Plan to evaluate the planning process.

NEEDS ASSESSMENT

Needs assessment is the process of identifying the problems and needs of a target population. It is an attempt to understand a setting and its people in relation to each other and to the external environment. Needs assessment requires the ability to *analyze the population* and the ability to *determine the health problems* of that population. This is a vital responsibility for health educators, especially community or worksite health educators. Just as good physicians get to know their patients and make diagnoses before undertaking treatment, good planners must get to know the population under study and define its problems before recommending actions.

Health educators must have skills in obtaining information about people (called demographic information), such as education level, income level, ethnic background, average household size, and occupation. Planners also must be adept at obtaining health-related information about a group of people, such as live birth rate, infant mortality rate, death rate, causes of death, incidence of infectious diseases, hospital admissions, and access to health care. They also must

be skilled in gathering information about individuals' behavior, identifying those that foster well-being and those that hinder it, and inferring needs for health education from the data. Finally, the health education planner must be proficient in determining the resources within a community. The major criterion in choosing data to collect and analyze is the extent to which the data will help guide decisions about planning, implementation, and evaluation. Collection and analysis of data are not the ends in themselves; they are means to the ends.

Numerous sources of information about the people in a given population are available—for instance, census, school, health department, and hospital records. Of course, the planner may choose to generate the information.

The methods and technology of needs assessment can be simple and inexpensive or highly complex and costly, depending on the purpose of the data collection. Perhaps the best starting place in assessing needs is to determine how the problem has been measured in the past. Some characteristics associated with health may be difficult to measure in a functional way. Once the means to express the existence of a problem have been established, standards or other criteria can be determined to indicate the extent of the problem. The next step is to determine what information is desired, including where those data can be found and how they can best be collected. Data collection and analysis comprise the next step. Data should be collected from at least a representative sample of the population under study, preferably chosen at random. Depending on the type of data collected, their use, and the standard of accuracy desired, statisticians may be required to determine statistical significance. After analysis, the assessor should be able to describe the nature and extent of the health problem.

Sources of health-related data are readily available. For instance, each school district keeps records pertaining to factors such as immunization, chronic diseases and conditions, absenteeism, and ethnic makeup of the population.

Other public records contain information about social issues such as housing and average family income. The Centers for Disease Control, the National Institutes of Health, and other governmental offices provide these valuable data on request. Local community health organizations constitute an excellent source of information about specific health issues and problems.

In addition to locating existing data, the health educator must have skills in generating data. Some methods, such as medical examinations and surveys, require direct contact with the individual. Other methods, such as analysis of medical records, health department records, school nurse reports, or news articles do not require direct contact with individuals within the population. Information gathered during needs assessment may be either *quantitative* or *qualitative*.

Four essential characteristics of the data collection process are:

1. *Validity.* The instrument used to gather information reveals the information for which it is used or measures what it purports to measure.
2. *Reliability.* The instrument yields the same or similar results if it is administered to the same people again.
3. *Representativeness of the sample.* The properties measured are characteristic of the population at large. The most representative population has an equal chance of being included.
4. *Generalizability.* The conclusions drawn from the sample can be applied to the population at large.

Examples of Needs Assessment Methodologies

Mail survey

The mail survey or questionnaire is a low-cost method of gaining information about a community. The amount of staff time necessary to analyze the responses depends upon the number of items on the survey, the level of detail required of the analysis, and the number of returns. It can produce a large sample of the community at little cost and time. A major disadvantage of mail surveys is the low percentage of return. Another drawback is the possibility that the respondent does not understand the question. Although the mail survey may afford candid responses, people often respond only if the survey gives them an opportunity to express complaints. Therefore, the information sometimes is of low quality. Mail surveys usually produce quantitative data.

Face-to-face interview

Face-to-face interviews have several advantages. They usually produce a high response rate. They can be designed to be highly flexible. They also can be used as a morale builder in the community because they ask for individuals' input (League of California Cities, 1976). The person-to-person interview, however, has major disadvantages. First, it usually is costly because of expenses in training the interviewer and technical staff, the time required for interviewing, the necessity of a second contact for people missed the first time, and travel expenses. Also, even after training, the interviewer may be biased. Too, interviews can raise false expectations of individuals in depressed areas. Of all the interview techniques, however, the face-to-face interview produces the most representative results; of the survey methods, data are the most detailed and high quality. Results of person-to-person interviews may be either quantitative or qualitative.

Face-to-face interviews may contain simple questions that elicit yes or no responses or numbers such as the number of rooms in the dwelling. These questions, of course, are more likely to yield only quantitative information. Interviews also may be more open-ended, requiring the respondent to give explanations, perceptions, opinions, or comments. Open-ended questionnaires require more time and expense to administer and even more time to interpret. Considerable time may be required to train the analyzer. These instruments usually are designed to produce qualitative data.

Telephone Interview

In terms of cost, the telephone interview generally runs between the face-to-face interview and the mail-out questionnaire. It is easy to administer and, if not too lengthy, generates a fairly high response rate. The results usually are of high quality, although they can be contaminated by interviewer bias. Sometimes telephone interviews can raise community morale, and at other times they can raise expectations unjustifiably. One major negative aspect of telephone surveys is that the sample is not always representative of the entire community population. Telephone questionnaires can generate either quantitative or qualitative results.

Medical Examination

Medical exams are perhaps the most expensive method of gathering information about a population. They also take considerable time. A major advantage of medical exams is that they usually yield highly accurate information, although some tests require interpretation and may be subject to some difference of opinion among physicians. Medical exams reveal quantitative information about groups of people that, taken as a whole, can yield qualitative information.

Focus Groups

The focus group is a marketing technique that attempts to understand the behavior of consumers (Folch-Lyon and Trost, 1981). Frequently, the strategy is applied to gain introductory information to direct the design of more powerful research. It also can be used to identify attitudes related to the product being studied.

Members of the focus group are selected based upon their representativeness of a larger group. The session usually lasts about 2 hours. During this time, the moderator directs the session, focusing attention on a single area or issue. After the session is finished, the opinions, behaviors, and reactions of the group members are analyzed to draw conclusions about the attitudes and practices of the larger group represented by the focus group. Focus groups may require some expense if the participants are paid.

Examination of Existing Records

Existing records can generate considerable information at relatively low cost. If this is done on an ongoing basis, trends can be easily detected. If done on a one-time basis, a good deal of time may be invested to discern trends, but relatively little time to determine a condition at any given time. A good deal of health information is a matter of public record and is easily obtainable. Records from health departments, federal agencies, educational institutions and school systems, employment records, and medical sources can spawn quantitative data of relatively high quality. Major disadvantages include the absence of direct current community input and possible lack of cooperation from agencies.

Analysis of News Articles

Frequently, articles from local newspapers can help identify health problems and draw conclusions about their occurrence. This technique is relatively inexpensive and may yield qualitative information. Use of news articles, however, is a crude method and probably is useful only in obtaining general information. It is inferior to the other methods because validity is questionable. Newspapers tend to print sensational stories and frequently omit information about chronic disease, substandard housing, and other social problems.

These and other methods of gathering information produce data that can be analyzed to determine the needs that health education will strive to meet. The actual process of analyzing data and exposing specific needs depends upon many factors, including the nature of the information-gathering techniques and level of the data. To adequately discuss all of the possible means of analyzing information is not possible here.

DEVELOPMENT OF PROGRAM PLAN

The individuals who will be involved in the program also must be involved in planning the program. This necessitates the formation of a committee or planning team. Members of the committee should be people representing all facets of the population to be served, as well as professionals. A principle of education programming is that individuals are more likely to act when their needs are being met and when they are involved in decision making. A committee to develop a school health education program should include health educators, administrators, nurses, physicians, parents, community members (including those from community organizations), and possibly students. Development of a school health education instructional program is the process usually referred to as *curriculum development*. A committee to develop a community health education program should include citizens in the target population, health educators, physicians, members of community health organizations, and others interested in the targeted problem. Roles of the various members of the group should be discussed and agreed upon.

Planning requires understanding the parts of programs and how they are intended to interact to produce an outcome (Dignan and Carr, 1987). It also requires understanding how behavior is formed and changed. The power spawning the understandings inherent in these requirements is theory. Though mostly borrowed from other disciplines, theory is the unifying thread that explains the condition that exists and the action that can change that condition. Several theories of human behavior and learning are discussed in Chapter 9.

Goals and Objectives

Formulating goals and objectives is a major step in any planning process. The direction, day-to-day activities, and evaluation of a program are established by its goals and objectives. Designing goals and objectives is a major skill required of health educators.

Goals are broad statements of what is to be accomplished. They form the foundation of the remainder of the planning process. Therefore, they must be written in language that is so clear and so precise that all members of the planning committee, as well as other observers, understand clearly the exact intention and direction of the project. Goals must deal in real terms with the problems of the target population and realistic solutions to those problems.

Goal statements should have unanimous agreement. In the absence of consensus, the nature of the planning task should be reexamined, the composition of the planning group should be questioned, and a solution for the dilemma should be decided before any further activities take place (Dignan and Carr, 1987).

Some situations may be aided by developing *program goals*. These goals proclaim the program's intended achievements. Usually they do not describe the various program services. The goals that are most critical to health education are *educational goals*. According to Dignan and Carr (1987), educational goals may reflect the program's effect on the *agency* or on the *learner/client*. We are most concerned with goals relating to effects on the learner/client. These goals may reflect either anticipated changes in *health status* of the target population or changes in *behavior* of the target population. Goals may be long-term or short-term. In some instances, identifying both long- and short-term goals may be useful.

According to Mager (1962), an expert on preparing objectives, objectives are precise statements that map out the tasks necessary to reach a goal. Objectives are composed of two parts: *content* and *behavior*. They should be fashioned so as to make clear the content of the intervention, the type and direction of change facilitated in the target population, magnitude or degree of change, and a precise explanation of the way the change will be measured. Including the time-frame within which the change will take place is useful in most situations. The reader of an objective should have a clear understanding of the requirements for its successful completion. This type of objective is referred to as a *behavioral objective*.

Each objective should be written in a complete sentence with a precise verb. Examples of precise verbs are *list, discuss, define, diagram,* and *apply*. By using verbs such as these, the planner, implementer, and learner/client gain a clear understanding of how attainment of the objective will be measured.

Objectives should indicate how attainment will be measured. We are all familiar with knowledge tests. Other ways to measure knowledge include programmed texts, structured interviews, and self-reporting. Changes in attitudes, feelings, and emotions can be measured in similar ways, although these affective objectives are more difficult to state precisely and are harder to measure specifically. Behavioral changes can be measured by direct observation, self-reporting, and reports from others. Nonetheless, objectives for all three domains—cognitive, affective, and behavioral—should be developed.

Sometimes, constructing *educator objectives* is helpful. This type of objective can guide the teacher by describing what he or she hopes to achieve in the area of health being examined. Educator objectives should be written only after learner behavioral objectives have been developed. They speak to teaching methodology, techniques, informational content, and other aspects the instructor determines to be necessary. Examples of educator objectives are:

◆ To show a video on exercise.

◆ To assign students to list the major points of the video.

◆ To discuss the major points listed.

◆ To demonstrate proper methods of stretching and warm-up.

Educator objectives must reflect methodology within the teacher's competency.

Policy Formation

Once a clear statement of intent and direction has been established, the policies in place in the institutions and agencies that will be involved in effecting change must be analyzed. Policies are governing principles, usually accompanied by written limitations on behavior and organizational action. At this point, administrators may be added temporarily to the planning committee, or at least consulted. Policies should be examined so program plans can work within the existing policies when possible.

Establishing new policies or altering existing policies may become necessary. The planner should not assume that a policy is cast in stone and cannot be changed. The process may require educating administrators, but if the program is justifiable in terms of learner/client needs, change is usually possible.

Policies should have substantial support of the planning committee and the target population, should be fair and nondiscriminatory, and should be developed to allow flexibility and creativity on the practitioner's part. Flexibility will allow for unforeseen occurrences. Policies should include a mechanism for altering the policies themselves if they are found later to be detrimental to the program.

Methods and Techniques

The planning committee must determine how the objectives will be obtained. Once again the committee may be temporarily expanded to include consultants with special expertise in teaching methods or community organization. *Methods* are general descriptions of how change within the target population is to be accomplished. Examples of methods are classroom instruction, mass media, and community development. *Techniques* or *activities*, in contrast, are specific strategies, such as field trips, lectures, pamphlets, public service announcements, small-group discussions, debates, and simulations.

Deciding which methods and techniques will be most effective in reaching the program goals and objectives is the key element of the process. Members of the target population should be consulted in selecting the methods, when feasible. Obviously, to consult kindergarten pupils regarding the relative effectiveness of teaching methods would have questionable benefit. The success of the method, however, depends in large part on its acceptance by the target population. A good deal of information already exists discussing the advantages and disadvantages of several methods and activities. Selection and application of teaching methods and techniques is not within the scope of this text.

Implementation plan

The logistics for implementing the program vary according to the scope of the program, characteristics of the target population, number of institutions or organizations involved, resource requirements, and a number of other factors. Implementation of a new program or service should be well-planned, and the roles of the various organizations and individuals carefully delineated.

Frequently, a pilot project in which the program is implemented on a small scale, is helpful as a part of the implementation plan. A small-scale beginning can reveal gaps in service and other deficiencies that can be corrected before the entire project is put in place. For instance, school health education instructional programs can be tried out in one or two grades or in a single school before implementating them in the entire school district. Community or worksite health education/promotion programs might be tried out in a single site or department before implementation in its entirety.

Development of the strategies for implementing the program can be as critical as the program itself. Care should be taken to develop a thorough plan.

At some point, it must be determined if the program is actually plausible. According to Smith (1989), a program is plausible if:

— it intends to bring about some change;

— its intentions are clear;

— its planned activities are reasonable—that is, they are of the right nature to influence the expected outcomes;

— its activities are sufficient in quantity and quality to exert that influence;

— its resources are present in sufficient amount and type for the activities to be implemented as planned.

These items may be addressed at various points during the planning process and require some rudimentary evaluation. To commit resources, however, any program requires some appraisal of the plan, in terms of these requirements, for plausibility.

Evaluation Plan

Evaluation means comparing something to a preset standard. For instance, suppose you were to measure the height of every person in your class. How would you determine which individuals are "tall," "short," "medium?" To make this determination, you must have a preset standard defining these three classifications. For instance, you might say that a male whose height is more than 6 feet is "tall," and a male whose height is less than 5½ feet is "short." Anyone between these two points is considered to be "medium" height.

Have you ever regarded one person as tall and another person as medium height only to observe them as the same height when they are standing together? Maybe you have seen a basketball player on television and evaluated his height as "short" only to learn that he is 6½ feet tall. Certain *extraneous* variables, such as body type, shoe sole or heels, or context can lead to mistaken evaluations. Similarly, evaluation of the effect of programs and curricula can be contaminated by variables we do not wish to be a part of our evaluation. This is why a well-conceived plan of evaluation is so important.

Development of the evaluation plan should include those who will be conducting the evaluation and those whose work will be evaluated. Employing consultants with specific expertise in evaluation, to assist in formation of the plan, is certainly acceptable.

The actual processes that take place in the program should be evaluated. Likewise, the short- and long-term outcomes of the program should be evaluated. The ultimate standards by which performance of the program is evaluated are its goals and objectives. Program evaluation will be discussed in more detail in the next chapter.

IMPLEMENTATION

Putting a program or curriculum into action takes a good deal of preparation. Needs have been identified, goals and objectives finalized, and requirements of the program delineated. At this point, the people involved in the program must employ and train staff, as well as obtain facilities, equipment, materials, and other resources. This involves contracts, purchasing decisions, budgeting, and a multitude of other preliminary actions.

Green and Kreuter (1991) left some interesting food for thought with the statement:

> In the final analysis, textbooks can offer little on implementation that will improve upon a good plan, an adequate budget, good organizational and policy support, good training and supervision of staff, and good monitoring in the process evaluation stage . . . . The key to success in implementation beyond these six ingredients is experience, sensitivity to people's needs, flexibility in the face of changing circumstances, an eye on long-term goals, and a sense of humor.

The selection of quality staff is epitomized in this statement.

Workshops or training sessions often are conducted to acquaint staff with the plan and methods. This is especially useful when new school curricula are implemented. Of course, if teachers participate in the design and are kept abreast of developments as they occur, this is much easier. Nonetheless, workshops usually are a fruitful part of the implementation process.

At the implementation stage of the process and throughout the program's operation, individuals from the target population should be included. People are more likely to act when they can relate the educational situation to their own lives, and they should be involved in carrying out programs designed to address their needs.

No matter how carefully the plan is developed, the program or curriculum likely will have to be changed as it is implemented. This should be expected.

PLANNING MODELS
PRECEDE-PROCEED Model

PRECEDE is an acronym for *p*redisposing, *r*einforcing, and *e*nabling *c*auses in *e*ducational *d*iagnosis and *e*valuation. The PRECEDE framework, developed by Green et al. (1980), provides a highly focused target of intervention and renders insights concerning evaluation. PRECEDE was enriched and expanded in PROCEED, an acronym for *p*olicy, *r*egulatory, and *o*rganizational *c*onstructs in *e*ducational and *e*nvironmental *d*evelopment. PRECEDE and PROCEED work in tandem, providing a continuous series of steps or phases in planning, implementation, and evaluation. Identifying priorities and setting objectives in the PRECEDE phases provide the objectives and criteria for policy, implementation, and evaluation in the PROCEED phases (Green and Kreuter, 1991). The framework starts with the final consequences of behavior and conditions and works backward to the original causes. This forces the planner to begin the planning process from the outcome end, asking the *why* before the *how*. Figure 11.2 presents the PRECEDE-PROCEED framework.

In *Phase 1*, the social diagnosis, the quality of life of the population is assessed, producing a picture of some of the general problems of concern to people. Quality of life concerns must be considered before assigning priority to problems because planning is enhanced if goals are known, it conserves resources, it informs the client (learner) of expected outcomes in advance, and it strengthens evaluations. General social problems—for instance, unemployment, hostility, and crime—are strong indicators of the quality of life. Many quality of life indicators and factors associated with them can be expressed numerically as population density, crime rates, and dropout rates. These are readily obtainable from government offices, behavioral sciences literature, and similar sources. Others are

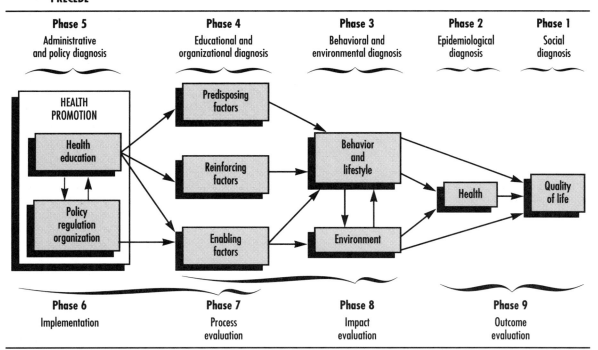

FIGURE 11.2.   PRECEDE-PROCEED Model for Health Education Planning

Source: L. W. Green, and M. W. Kreuter. *Health Promotion Planning: An Educational and Environmental Approach* (Mountain View, CA: Mayfield Publishing, 1991). Reprinted by permission of the publisher.

perceived needs and can be identified through open-ended interviewing.

Phase 2, the epidemiological diagnosis, involves identifying health problems associated with the unsatisfactory quality of life. In this phase, the planner must (a) identify the specific problems contributing to the social problems, and (b) select the specific health problems most deserving of attention. The epidemiological data can show, for instance, the total number of active cases of a disease (its *prevalence*); the number of new cases of a disease in a certain period of time (its *incidence*); or how health problems are distributed in a population. These types of information can suggest their importance in relation to quality of life. This is essentially needs assessment.

Green et al. (1980) explained two approaches to identifying health problems: the reductionist approach and the expansionist approach. The *reductionist approach* is commonly used because a planner is rarely in a position to survey the overall quality of life in a community as a formal antecedent to specifying which health problems deserve attention. In real life situations, we usually must rely on surveys that various agencies conduct routinely. A review of professional and scientific literature is necessary for an adequate professional response. Therefore, in a reductionist approach we work from the broader social problem toward a diagnosis of its health components or causes. Usually we do not intervene in nonhealth matters. The reductionist approach allows us to arrive at manageable, important, few means when problems seem too large to attack.

Health educators often are assigned to a narrow, oversimplified problem, such as hypertension or obesity. To merely identify a problem such as hypertension does not offer much direction toward its solution. Examining the situation from a broader perpective, usually through current literature, is useful. This is the *expansionist approach*. Perhaps further investigation may indicate that the population under study has a family history of hypertension, which *may*

suggest hereditary causation. On the other hand, analysis may indicate that large numbers of the population consume diets high in saturated fat, suggesting dietary education as a possible solution. Frequently, viewing the situation from a broader perspective can clarify the direction of the program.

After separating the health problems from the nonhealth problems affecting quality of life, health problems are described in detail. Although this can serve a number of functions, perhaps the most significant is the clarification of responsibilities among professionals, agencies, and departments.

When several health problems are identified, priorities have to be set. This requires a full description of each problem and how it is manifested. For instance, if large numbers of the population are hypertensive, obese, and smoke cigarettes, it may be necessary to determine which problems and their causes should receive the most of the program resources. This requires full description of each health problem, its manifestations, and possible causal overlaps among the health problems. Health education usually is part of a larger community action, so detailing the problem helps the various individuals and groups involved coordinate and blend their work. It also helps in developing specific objectives. Effective objectives are critical, as they give a program direction.

Phase 3, the behavioral diagnosis, identifies specific health-related behaviors linked to the health problem selected. This phase is essential because health education is effective only to the extent to which it influences health practices. The first step is to establish cause-and-effect relationships between behavior and health. Target behaviors are selected, and an approach to changing them is stated in the form of behavioral objectives. Nonbehavioral factors such as age, genetics, climate, residence, mental impairment, and gender were identified in the PRECEDE framework as possible contributors to health problems. In the PROCEED revision, nonbehavioral factors were replaced by environmental factors, those external to the individual, which can be changed to support the health, quality of life, or behavior of that person or others affected by that person.

Health educators should not ignore these factors, because they allow us to maintain a perspective on the multiple determinants of the health problem identified. Often these factors are addressed through political and environmental strategies rather than health education. Behavioral diagnosis is a five-step process:

1. Differentiating between behavioral and non-behavioral causes of the health problem.
2. Developing an inventory of behaviors: that is, preparing a list of highly specific behaviors that can be used as the basis for specifying the behavioral objectives of the program.
3. Rating behaviors in terms of importance based upon availability of data demonstrating a clear link between the behavior and the health problem, and frequency of occurrence.
4. Rating behaviors in terms of changeability.
5. Choosing behavioral targets based upon importance and changeability.

After completing the five-step process, the final procedure for the health education planner in the behavioral diagnosis is to prepare precise behavioral objectives.

In *Phase 4*, educational and organizational diagnosis, factors that have the potential for affecting behavior are identified. The three kinds of factors most responsive to health education are:

1. *Predisposing factors*, antecedents to behavior that provide a rationale or motivation for the behavior. They include knowledge, beliefs, attitudes, and values.
2. *Enabling factors*, antecedents to behavior that allow motivation or aspiration to be realized or hindered. They include personal skills, personal resources, health-related skills, and community resources.

3. *Reinforcing factors*, subsequent to behavior, that provide the continuing reward, incentive, or punishment for the behavior and contribute to its continuation or discontinuation. Reinforcing factors include the social and physical benefits of the action and may be tangible or imagined. They may be delivered by self, family, peers, teachers, or others.

At the center of educational diagnosis is selection from among the predisposing, enabling, and reinforcing factors those that, if modified, will help to bring about the desired behavior. This involves identifying and sorting factors into the three categories, setting priorities among the categories, establishing priorities within the categories, and writing learning and resource objectives. It also includes separating the factors as negative or positive.

Phase 5, the administrative and policy diagnosis, involves assessing organizational and administrative capabilities and resources for the development and implementation of a program. Administrative diagnosis is a three-step process:

1. Assessment of resources needed, including time, personnel and money.
2. Assessment of available resources.
3. Assessment of barriers to implementation, including attitudinal and political ones, as well as those relating to power.

Policy diagnosis is the appraisal of conditions that are "givens" because of policy, regulations, and organization. It includes: (a) assessment of policies, regulations, and organizations, including flexibility and professional discretion; and (b) assessment of political forces. Policies and regulations can be used to implement programs, or they can stand as impenetrable barriers. Utilizing political forces and understanding the system can greatly enhance the chances of successfully implementing a program.

At some point in the process, educational strategies must be selected to affect the predisposing, reinforcing, and enabling factors. In the

PRECEDE framework, this task is addressed after educational diagnosis. In the revised framework, it is mentioned after Phase 5. Obviously, a wide selection of methodologies is available from which to choose. Some examples are simulations and games, programmed learning, educational television, audiovisual aids, and mass media. A variety of educational strategies is preferable to a single method. All three categories of factors should receive attention. The more complex the cause of the behavioral problem, the greater is the range of strategies required.

Implementation, Phase 6, and Planning are functionally merged. This is the point at which PRECEDE and PROCEED meet.

Three types or "levels" of evaluation comprise Phases 7, 8, and 9. Green et al. (1980) defined evaluation as the comparison of an object of interest against a standard of acceptability. *Process evaluation* is that of professional practices. *Impact evaluation* assesses the immediate result of the program on knowledge, attitudes, and behavior. *Outcome evaluation* may not be completed for years. It is the evaluation of long-term effects of the program—the outcome as measured by the change in quality of life. Although it seems to be near the end of the PROCEED framework, evaluation should be continuous, an integral part of the model from the outset.

The PRECEDE-PROCEED framework is founded upon two fundamental propositions (Green and Kreuter, 1991):

1. Health and health risks are caused by multiple factors.

2. Because health and health risks are determined by multiple factors, efforts to effect behavioral, environmental, and social change must be multidimensional or multisectoral.

All health educators would be wise to hold these two propositions in the forefront of their planning and execution of their art.

Mico's Model for Health-Education Planning

Mico's (Ross and Mico, 1980) model for health education planning is designed in two dimensions, as shown in Table 11.1. The horizontal dimension is composed of six phases:

1. Initiation of the planning activity
2. Needs assessment
3. Goal setting
4. Planning or programming the activity
5. Implementing the activity
6. Evaluation of the activity's effectiveness

The three vertical dimension identify the:

— activity's content or subject matter;

— steps and techniques (methods) associated with each horizontal phase;

— the process or interactions involved.

The success or failure of the activity often depends upon what happens in Phase 1 (Initiation). The key elements are understanding the clients' problems and the clients' system, an entry strategy, making an initial contract, and making the clients aware that a problem exists so they are ready to change. Obviously, the health educator's credibility is pivotal to the initial success of the project.

The contract is an initial commitment from the client and does not necessarily have to be in writing. It is used to build trust and to develop readiness in the client. It also clarifies what is expected of each party, describes the scope and conditions of the activity, identifies the resources needed, and carries provisions for change if conditions warrant.

Leaders in the community or organization must be identified in Phase 1. The leadership's knowledge of health education must be adequate to ensure success. Values of those involved— leaders, consumers, and providers—must be clarified to lessen the possibility of later conflict.

TABLE 11.1.   Mico's Model for Health Education Planning

	Content Dimension	Method Dimension	Process Dimension
Phase 6: Evaluation	4. Knowledge of problem and client systems	4. Redefine problem and standards	4. Consensus of new definitions
	3. Technology of feedback systems	3. Feedback to activity, reporting accountability	3. Communication, threat reduction
	2. Language and systems	2. Data collection and analysis	2. Learning assimilation
	1. Nature of evaluation	1. Clarify evaluation measures	1. Agreement
Phase 5: Implementation	4. Writing skills	4. Reporting	4. Communications
	3. Dynamics of problem solving	3. Problem solving	3. Creative conflict resolution, win-win
	2. Knowledge of subject and content T & TA[3] being provided for	2. Training and technical assistance	2. Skill development, helping
	1. Knowledge of plan, how it is to work	1. Initiate activity	1. Communications, orientations
Phase 4: Planning/ Programming	3. Nature of political process	3. Negotiate commitments, MOAs[2]	3. Negotiation
	2. Systems analysis and management science	2. Design management systems and tools	2. Role clarification, communications
	1. Techniques of planning	1. Develop implementation plan	1. Understanding and commitment
Phase 3: Goal Setting	5. Theory of change	5. Determine strategies for implementation	5. Consensus
	4. MBO[1] technology	4. Select goals and objectives	4. Decision making, consensus
	3. Forecasting	3. Alternative goals statement, force-field analysis	3. Reality testing, creative problem solving
	2. Nature of policy	2. Link to policy development	2. Understanding of process and rules
	1. Role of goals, how to set them, measure	1. Establish criteria for goals	1. Agreement
Phase 2: Needs Assessment	4. Relevance of data	4. Describe nature and extent of problem	4. Reduce fantasy by fact
	3. Language of systems	3. Data collection and analysis	3. Open communications, sensitivity to data sources
	2. Data sources	2. Determine data to be collected	2. Agreement
	1. Standards and criteria	1. Identify and review present criteria	1. Agreement on starting point
Phase 1: Initiate	3. Power and influence structures community organization, culture	3. Organize concerned	3. Involvement, leadership, values clarification
	2. Contract terminology and resources	2. Develop initial contract	2. Legitimacy, commitment, trust, readiness
	1. Knowledge of problem and client system	1. Entry or intervention strategy, force-field analysis, interviewing	1. Unfreezing, threat reduction, credibility, awareness of need

Source: H. S. Ross, and P. R. Mico, *Theory and Practice in Health Education* (Palo Alto, CA: Mayfield Publishing, 1980). Reprinted by permission.

[1] MBO: Management by objective   [2] MOA: Memoranda of agreement   [3] T & TA: Training and technical assistance

Phase 2 of the model is Needs Assessment. Mico has pointed out that the technology for needs assessment can be simple and inexpensive or highly refined and costly, depending on the purpose. This phase has four steps.

The first step is to identify how the problem has been measured in the past. This can help bring the problem into focus. All the major performers should agree on the starting point of the assessment, the standards and criteria, and the nature and extent of the problem. The second step is to determine what data to collect and how to collect them. The planning committee must agree on approaches and on why each is important. Step three involves collecting and analyzing the data. Planning for this step requires becoming familiar with the technical approaches and methods, costs, practicality, and effectiveness of various data collection and analysis methods so sensible decisions can be made. The approach taken by the committee must be agreed upon. Therefore, open communication among the committee, the health educator, and the client (learner) is essential. The final step is to describe the nature and extent of the problem, based upon accurate data and expert analysis of those data.

Phase 3 is Goal Setting. Mico defined *goal* as a future event toward which a committed endeavor is directed. He defined *objectives* as steps to be taken in pursuit of a goal. Phase 3 entails a five-step operation.

The first step is to establish criteria for goals. As an example of criteria, goals must be measurable events and they must be framed in a reasonable time. The second step is to ensure that goal setting is linked to the organizational or community policy development. This is important because policy is the key driving force behind the organization of systems necessary to carry out the plan. The third step necessitates making a comprehensive statement of alternative goals and the effects or consequences of each. This requires the ability to project into the future to anticipate changes that are likely to occur. In the fourth step, goals to pursue are selected from the list of alternatives. Several models of decision making can be applied to this step. Mico strongly recommended total group support in decision making. The fifth step is to develop strategies for implementing goals.

In Phase 4 of the Mico model, Planning/Programming, an implementation plan is established, systems and tools for managing the activity are designed, and commitment from those involved is negotiated. This is a three-step phase.

In the first step, written plans are developed. This may take concentrated study of planning methods and requires understanding and commitment. In the second step, management systems and tools are designed. The design must: (a) assure continuity of effort as an activity proceeds toward its goal, (b) monitor the activity's implementation, (c) keep communication open among the plan's elements and people, and (d) institute a prevention/intervention system to determine if a problem is developing. If a problem is apparent, the problem can be prevented by dealing with its indicators. Mico endorses *management by objectives* (MBO), a system of management based on establishment of specific actions to be carried out or end results to be attained. MBO includes information regarding the resources and timeframes necessary to carry out the tasks, as well as the identity of those responsible for implementation. The final step in Phase 4, negotiating commitments, can be done through written documents called *memoranda of agreement* (MOA) or through the contract mentioned in Phase 1. Sometimes this requires considerable political and negotiating skills.

In the first step in Phase 5, Implementation, the activity is initiated. This involves providing assistance to participants, problem solving, and reporting progress. (One could argue that the actual initiation began with the first entry or intervention by a health educator or the planning committee.) The second step provides for ongoing training, technical assistance, and consultation. This is referred to as *training and technical assistance* (T&TA). By helping people to do a better job, the learning value of the activity is enhanced. Frequently, training courses and technical manuals must be developed. The third step requires constructively dealing with problems as they arise. The fourth step entails reporting or documenting the activity's ongoing progress so everyone is informed.

Phase 6, Evaluation, is a four-step procedure that is crucial to the success of the new program.

The evaluation measures are clarified in the first step. If the objectives initially had built-in measurement indicators, evaluation can begin by identifying and reviewing those measures. This step includes accountability for funds and other resources. Some members of the team may have expertise in interpreting measurement indicators and results: others may not. The measures must be understood by all. The second step, data collection and analysis, reveals the results of the activity and the reasons for them. The next step is reporting the evaluation so participants have feedback on the extent of success of the activity. The fourth step entails using what was learned in evaluation to redefine the problem and refine measures and standards to determine its nature and extent. Well-planned and well-executed evaluation can contribute to the self-renewal of a program and give it continual energy.

Department of Health, Education, and Welfare Guidelines

Passage of Public Law 93–641, the National Health Planning and Resources Development Act (1974), evoked an immediate need for guidelines for planning programs relating to public health. Following are highlights (not exact quotes) from statements in the law, as well as guidelines (Bureau of Health Planning and Resources Development, 1976, 1977) concerning functions of areawide and state health planning agencies:

◆ Assemble and analyze data concerning health status, the health care delivery system, effect

of the system, resources, use of resources, and environmental and occupational exposure factors.

◆ Establish health plans that include long-range goals, objectives, recommended actions, and resource requirements.

◆ Implement the plans—to the extent practicable, with sponsorship by other appropriate individuals and public and private entities.

Public education is an implicit part of the law.

The Department of Health, Education, and Welfare (now the U. S. Department of Health and Human Services) guidelines divided the planning process into five phases: defining problems, setting goals, designing plans, implementing plans, and evaluating programs. Although lack of funding has made implementation of PL 93–641 much less effective than hoped, the DHEW planning guidelines are worthy of attention because they can be transferred to the work of health education program planners.

Defining problems

The guidelines listed seven problem-definition steps.

1. *Determine health status gaps and trends caused by personal (individual and community) actions.*

   This is a needs assessment step that results in comparision between the current status and the desired status of health. A number of techniques may yield relevant data. Once gaps in health status are identified, those caused entirely or partly by personal actions should be determined. Health status gaps related to deficiencies in the physical environment, social environment, and health and medical care services should be identified.

2. *Determine gaps and trends in personal (individual and community) health actions.*

This is another comparison between current or projected status and goals or desired status. Among other types of action, it should include personal practices aimed at promoting vigorous well-being and preventing avoidable disability and premature death. This step reflects both the values and the knowledge about health of the people in the target group.

3. *Determine characteristics of affected persons, and trends in these characteristics.*

Knowing what population groups have the greatest gaps in personal actions related to actual or potential shortcomings in health status is useful. Differences in gaps may be linked to characteristics such as age, gender, income, cultural group, education, or residence, or some combination. Data on trends—for example, increasing smoking among teenage girls—could affect planning decisions.

4. *Determine positive and negative forces affecting personal (individual and community) health actions.*

Many forces may cause gaps in actions or operate as barriers against actions from current status toward desired status. Others tend to support favorable change. Knowing these forces may strengthen and create dynamic educational and supportive activities that build on positive forces and weaken negative forces.

5. *Determine gaps, trends, and forces regarding health education practices.*

If health education activities are in place, they should be identified and analyzed. Whenever possible, all settings and services should be included. Health education activities should be analyzed in terms of availability, accessibility, continuity, acceptability, quality, and cost. Consumers and providers of health education alike should take part in setting goals or standards of practice. These standards serve as a guide for the kinds of data to collect and as benchmarks in analyzing performance.

The DHEW identified three classifications of standards pertaining to health education practice: (a) standards for educating the individual in healthful behavior; (b) standards for education within the health care system; and (c) standards for education for citizen participation. Comparison of data on current health education practices against these standards could identify deficiencies in health education practice. Data on positive and negative forces affecting health education practices can lead to specific strategies of helping professionals who want to improve their health education performance.

6. *Determine gaps, trends, and forces regarding health education resources.*

Attention is focused here on financing, personnel, organizational arrangements, facilities, equipment, supplies, technical assistance, and legislation. Professionals and consumers should determine standards for health education resources and compare actual status with the standards.

7. *Determine aspects of problems that should be tackled regarding health, action, education, resources, and forces.*

Findings of the previous problem-definition steps should be reviewed to select areas that offer the greatest promise for favorable change. Priorities may be set based upon criteria such as public concern for the problem, likelihood that a large proportion of the population will improve its health substantially if the problem is reduced, probability that the benefits of significantly reducing the problem will justify the costs, and chances of obtaining necessary resources.

Setting goals

Setting goals gives direction to program development. Goals are expected results, ends, outcomes, or products rather than methods, activities, or processes. The DHEW model (Bureau of Health

Planning and Resources Development, 1976) indicated that:

> Goals are expressions of the desired conditions of health status and health systems expressed as quantifiable, timeless aspirations. Goals should be both technically and financially achievable, and responsive to community ideals.

Thus, according to DHEW, goals are intended states that are considered preferable to the current situation. Health goals describe proposed changes in health status or in factors that directly affect health status. The phrase "technically and financially achievable" means the knowledge and resources are sufficient and available for success. Various indicators may be applied to produce the "quantifiable" aspect, including those relating to accessibility, disability, premature death, disease, or capacity to participate. To be quantifiable, goals must be specific and clear concerning time, direction of change, measure of the characteristic to be changed, magnitude of change, and definition of measure (Health Resources Administration, 1976).

Figure 11.3 exhibits the relationship of program development to health goals. The planning process moves roughly from top to bottom of the chart. The actual goals for health focus on Level II, health status; Level III, forces affecting health; and the portion of Level IV that includes personal action. Arguably, from a practical point of view, individual, group, and community participation in health program development should be included as a goal.

Designing plans

The National Health Planning and Resources Development Act required each areawide health systems agency to establish, review annually, and amend as necessary a health systems plan (HSP) and an annual implementation plan (AIP). Although all requirements under the original act may not now be current, the sequence of steps used to design health education plans is of interest to health education program developers. The six steps in the design process follow.

1. Set objectives.

Objectives specify the status of individual health behavior and of health education services desired during a specific time period. Each objective indicates how much of the relevant goal will be achieved by a certain time. Many consumer groups and provider groups should be represented in fashioning objectives.

2. Choose recommended actions and projects.

Deciding on a general approach before trying to list specific recommended actions is helpful at times. Brainstorming sessions and focus groups may be useful in considering various courses of action. The DHEW model indicates that special attention be given at this stage of the program to action that will facilitate consumer participation in the pursuit of all goals.

Educational methods should fit the people, problems, goals, and objectives in each situation. In this model, educational methods are divided into three categories: (a) information giving, with recipients being largely passive; (b) problem solving, with active involvement of recipients; and (c) a combination of the two.

After alternative general approaches have been identified, the effectiveness of each approach in meeting the project's goals and objectives should be analyzed. This may require soliciting expert opinion or consulting educational and behavioral research.

A series of recommended actions should be developed for the approaches given the highest priority. After the actions have been discussed and critiqued, a revised statement of recommended actions may be prepared. Expected impact on population groups, geographic areas, health, and health systems should be estimated.

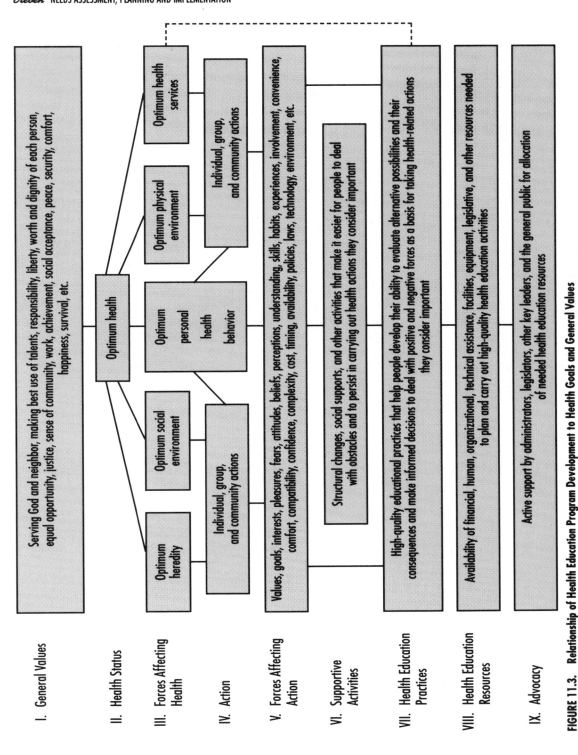

FIGURE 11.3.   Relationship of Health Education Program Development to Health Goals and General Values

I. General Values

II. Health Status

III. Forces Affecting Health

IV. Action

V. Forces Affecting Action

VI. Supportive Activities

VII. Health Education Practices

VIII. Health Education Resources

IX. Advocacy

Serving God and neighbor, making best use of talents, responsibility, liberty, worth and dignity of each person, equal opportunity, justice, sense of community, work, achievement, social acceptance, peace, security, comfort, happiness, survival, etc.

Optimum health

Optimum health services

Optimum physical environment

Optimum personal health behavior

Optimum social environment

Optimum heredity

Individual, group, and community actions

Individual, group, and community actions

Values, goals, interests, pleasures, fears, attitudes, beliefs, perceptions, understanding, skills, habits, experiences, involvement, convenience, comfort, compatibility, confidence, complexity, cost, timing, availability, policies, laws, technology, environment, etc.

Structural changes, social supports, and other activities that make it easier for people to deal with obstacles and to persist in carrying out health actions they consider important

High-quality educational practices that help people develop their ability to evaluate alternative possibilities and their consequences and make informed decisions to deal with positive and negative forces as a basis for taking health-related actions they consider important

Availability of financial, human, organizational, technical assistance, facilities, equipment, legislative, and other resources needed to plan and carry out high-quality health education activities

Active support by administrators, legislators, other key leaders, and the general public for allocation of needed health education resources

Bureau of Health Planning and Resources Development, *Guidelines Concerning the Development of Health Systems Plans and Annual Implementation Plans* (Washington, DC: U. S. Department of Health, Education and Welfare, 1976).

3. Identify resource requirements.

Resources such as personnel, financing, organizational mechanisms, facilities, equipment, supplies, and technical assistance should be determined. Establishing a health education center to provide leadership in developing and coordinating health education resources may be helpful.

4. Develop specific evaluation procedures.

The specific procedures to be implemented in the evaluation step should be delineated.

5. Develop pretest plans.

To the extent possible, pretesting all aspects of proposed plans is recommended. This provides the opportunity to revise objectives, actions, resource requirements, evaluation procedures, and timetables. It also can help eliminate undesirable components and facilitate more promising features.

6. Obtain approvals and commitments.

All appropriate organizations and individuals at all relevant levels should be asked to endorse the health education plans. Commitments should be obtained regarding the needed resources and responsibility for carrying out recommended actions.

Implementing plans

Putting the plan into motion means putting people to work. They may have to gain technical assistance from outside agencies, secure grants, and award contracts. It means each member of the team carrying out his or her responsibilities toward reaching the goals of the health education program. Because fragmentation of effort is one of the common deficiencies of health education, attempts should be made to foster coordination and cooperation. Encouraging collaboration in operating programs is important.

Sharing resources, preventing unnecessary duplication, promoting continuity of services, and establishing central sources from which people may obtain information about health and health services are all crucial.

Evaluating programs

In the DHEW framework, representatives of all affected organizations and populations should participate in deciding why, what, how, where, and by whom health education programs should be evaluated. An evaluation task force might include representatives of participating agencies, funding agencies, professional peers, health planning agencies, consumers, and outside consultants.

Plans for evaluation should be developed before the program is carried out. Plans should indicate what information will be collected, how and when it will be obtained, how it will be analyzed, and who will be responsible for each of these activities. The DHEW guidelines propose seven evaluation steps.

1. Determine extent to which objectives have been achieved.

The success of this step depends upon the clarity and measurability of the objectives of the program as well as the relevance and accuracy of the data collected before, during, and after the implementation phase. More than one method of gathering data could be employed in this step.

2. Determine extent to which recommended actions and activities were carried out and resources used as planned.

This step requires accurate record keeping of actions and when they are carried out, the numbers of different types of paid and volunteer personnel utilized, the amount of time they worked on various parts of the program, and dollars spent. The greater the expenditure, the more detailed the record keeping should be. Reasons for changes in actions and resources also should be recorded and analyzed.

3. *Determine relationships between achievement of objectives, carrying out of recommended actions and activities, and use of resources.*

Although this is one of the most difficult parts, it is also one of the most important elements of evaluation. The aim here is to ascertain the degree of success in achieving objectives and whether that success is the result of program activities or other factors. The complexity of that determination may vary, but, some sort of carefully controlled study should be implemented for that purpose.

4. *Determine strengths and weaknesses of program development processes.*

Decisions and predictions made and processes used at all stages of program development should be reviewed. This includes involvement, problem definition, goal setting, plan design, plan implementation, and program evaluation. Effectiveness, efficiency, and appropriateness of each procedure should be analyzed carefully.

5. *Determine favorable and unfavorable by-products.*

Most health education programs produce some effects that were unplanned. Examining these "side effects," both negative and positive, is useful in evaluating the overall impact of the program.

6. *Review importance of this program compared with others.*

This review should include a look at any significant new developments, such as shift in public values, additional data on needs, or change in availability of resources, that may suggest a change in the current program or even a different one. This comparison also considers fairly the effectiveness and benefits in relation to costs.

7. *Decide whether to continue; if so, recommend ways to improve program.*

Once the decision is made to continue a program, it should be revised according to the evaluation findings.

The DHEW guidelines were developed for the purpose of implementing community health education programs under Public Law 93–641. They were not produced specifically for planning school-based health education programs. Regardless of this, and of their age, these guidelines can provide much insight to health educators and health education planners who are involved in their initial planning experience in many settings.

SUMMARY

The literature offers a number of excellent structures for planning a health education or health promotion program. Some of those structures, in the form of guidelines, models, and frameworks are outlined in this chapter. All of these structures contain several key elements: needs assessment, goals and objectives as foundations for planning, planning for implementation, and evaluation. These elements are necessary in the planning process whether the setting is a school, community, worksite, or elsewhere. Evaluation, although a part of planning, is a continuous part of the process requiring special attention and competencies. It is addressed in the next chapter.

REFERENCES

Ackoff, R. L. *Redesigning the Future.* New York: John Wiley and Sons, 1974.

Breckon, D. J., J. R. Harvey, and R. B. Lancaster. *Community Health Education: Settings, Roles, and Skills.* Rockville, MD: Aspen Systems Corporation, 1984.

Bureau of Health Planning and Resources Development. *Guidelines Concerning the Development of*

Health Systems Plans and Annual Implementation Plans. Washington, DC: U. S. Department of Health, Education, and Welfare, 1976.

Bureau of Health Planning and Resources Development. *Draft Guidelines for the Development of the State Health Plan.* Washington, DC: U. S. Department of Health, Education, and Welfare, 1977.

Dignan, M. B. and P. A. Carr. *Program Planning for Health Education and Health Promotion.* Philadelphia: Lea & Febiger, 1987.

Folch-Lyon, E., and J. F. Trost. Conducting focus group sessions, Part I. *Studies in Family Planning,* 12 (December 1981): 443–449.

Green, L. W., and M. W. Kreuter. *Health Promotion Planning: An Educational and Environmental Approach.* Mountain View, CA: Mayfield Publishing, 1991.

Green, L. W., M. W. Kreuter, S. G. Deeds, and K. B. Partridge. *Health Education Planning: A Diagnostic Approach.* Palo Alto, CA: Mayfield Publishing, 1980.

Health Resources Administration, U. S. Department of Health, Education, and Welfare. *Papers on the National Health Guidelines: Baselines for Setting Health Goals and Standards.* Washington, DC: Government Printing Office, 1976.

League of California Cities. *Social Needs Assessment Handbook.* Sacramento: League of California Cities, 1976.

Mager, R. F. *Preparing Instructional Objectives.* Belmont, CA: Fearon, 1962.

National Health Planning and Resources Development Act of 1974, Public Law 93–641, 93rd Congress, 1975.

Reeves, P. N., D. F. Bergwall, and N. B. Woodside. *Introduction to Health Planning* (3d ed.). Arlington, VA: Information Resources Press, 1984.

Ross, H. S. and P. R. Mico. *Theory and Practice in Health Education.* Palo Alto, CA: Mayfield Publishing, 1980.

Smith, M. F. *Evaluability Assessment: A Practical Approach.* Boston: Kluwer Academic Publishers, 1989.

12

EVALUATION

Evaluation is probably the most misunderstood part of the planning and implementation of health education. Students often view evaluation as a test for which they must cram to get a good grade. Health educators sometimes see evaluation as the laborious task of filling out forms for which the only outcome is meetings with supervisors to discuss their deficiencies. Supervisors, planners, and teachers may see evaluation as a way of enforcing discipline on employees and students. Evaluation is none of these.

The purpose of evaluation is not to prove or disprove but to improve (Creswell and Newman, 1989). Practiced appropriately, evaluation can provide feedback to professionals about the strengths and weaknesses of their programs. It can be a means to improve service and instructional delivery. It also can alert parents and students to problems before they become impossible to avert or difficult to correct. When recognized as a part of the planning process, evaluation can be a method of determining if objectives are being met and can provide feedback relevant to changes that may enhance the attainment of objectives. Hindsight, after all, is usually more accurate than foresight. Although evaluation appears at the end of the process of health education in many schematic depictions, it should encourage revisions throughout the implementation phase and excite professionals toward new beginnings. In short, evaluation should be a nonthreatening, positive force on health education regardless of setting.

Evaluation has a number of purposes. According to Bedworth and Bedworth (1992), evaluation is conducted to determine:

- the value of learning experiences.
- the value of learning aids and the ways in which they have been used or are being used.
- the effectiveness of methods, techniques, and strategies.
- the speed at which learning is taking place.
- the quality of learning for each individual as well as for the group.

◆ the changes that must be made in any element of the program (e.g., goals, objectives, processes).

In addition, program evaluation is conducted to:

◆ determine if a prospective program is plausible.

◆ assess attainment of desired outcomes, goals, and objectives.

◆ assess accomplishments of the program.

◆ identify limitations or weaknesses of the program.

◆ identify strengths of the program.

◆ identify areas to emphasize in staff development.

◆ justify the program and its expenditure of resources.

Evaluation can be made clear and precise by carefully planning the evaluation itself. Instruments for measuring various characteristics must be designed or selected so they yield complete and accurate information. To be useful, the data obtained from those measurements should be organized in the most helpful way.

MEASUREMENT AND EVALUATION

Green et al. (1980) defined evaluation as the *comparison of an object of interest against a standard of acceptability.* The standard of acceptability is expressed in well-written objectives. The comparison must be based upon some data. These data are collected by the process of measurement. Measurement is the *determination of quantity or quality of an object of interest.* It provides a means for learning something about a program that can be used for evaluation (Veney and Kaluzny, 1991). Therefore, measurement is the basic tool of evaluation.

Recall the example given in the previous chapter. The task was to evaluate the height of a person or persons as tall, medium, or short. The

standards of acceptability for each level are: 6 feet tall or taller is "tall"; 5½ feet tall and shorter is "short"; and between 5½ feet and 6 feet is "medium." To apply these standards of acceptability, one must measure—that is, determine the quantity of feet and inches of each individual whose height is being evaluated.

Similarly, the objective for a 6-month health education program may be to reduce to 5% the number of male teens who dip snuff. To evaluate our program, we must measure the percentage of male teens who dip snuff prior to implementation of the program and also the percentage who use snuff 6 months after implementation of the program. This can be done in a number of ways. One possibility is a self-report questionnaire of a random sample of male teens in the population. We can evaluate our program effectiveness as satisfactory if it meets the standard of acceptability: 5% or less of male teens in the sample dip snuff after the 6-month program.

Many instruments may be available for measuring an entity. And measuring may be of different types. For instance, the price of the jar of ketchup on the grocer's shelf may be expressed in cents per ounce or in cents per quarts. Because ounces and quarts are different units of measure, we may be frustrated and confused shoppers (evaluators). In a similar vein, we may choose to measure the success of a program by increased knowledge, number of observed behaviors, or many other ways. Dignan and Carr (1987) stated, "The type of measurement chosen depends on the criteria selected for evaluation, the need for precision, and the opportunity to collect information."

We cannot overemphasize the role of objectives in pointing to evaluation. They establish the criteria upon which measurement and evaluation are based. Oberteuffer, Harrelson, and Pollock (1972) stated:

> Specification of instructional objectives in behavioral terms not only facilitates but assumes the validity of related evaluation procedures. . . . Objectives provide a blueprint for what is to be evaluated and how it might be done.

Frequently, we measure and evaluate only the cognitive domain. This is because the cognitive domain is easier to measure than either the affective or the action domain. Just as objectives should emphasize all three domains, however, all three domains should be included in measurement and evaluation.

Evaluation involves the collection and analysis of information to determine the relevance, progress, efficiency, and effectiveness of program activities (Veney and Kaluzny, 1991). *Relevance* is the issue of whether the service is needed. *Progress* refers to tracking program activities and assessing whether program implementation complies with the plan. The *efficiency* question asks whether the program results could be obtained less expensively. *Effectiveness* refers to meeting predetermined needs.

MEASUREMENT INSTRUMENTS

Measurement instruments are the tools we use to collect data. Among the many examples of measurement instruments are written exams, observation, searches through existing records, and self-report questionnaires.

Measurement may be qualitative or quantitative. *Qualitative* measurement attempts to provide statements that describe processes or experiences resulting from exposure to a program or an activity. Being descriptive, it may refer to how well something is done. Qualitative information usually is grouped according to similar characteristics, such as drinkers/nondrinkers, male/female, or different age groups.

Analyzing qualitative data such as that gained from interviews is a creative process; different people may approach it in different ways. It is based more on the examiner's experience and knowledge of a given subject than on tried-and-true analysis methods (Patton, 1980). It can produce results showing how much or, sometimes, how many. One of the goals of qualitative evaluation is to develop an understanding of the processes by which programs reach their intended audiences, the impact produced, and the changes that may take place thereafter (Patton, 1982).

Quantitative measurement yields numerical values such as how many questions were answered correctly, how often a person engaged in a specific behavior, how many pounds a person weighed, or how many people comprised a household. It usually is easily explained and defensible.

Measurement instruments may be objective or subjective. Both can be serviceable to health educators in evaluating the fulfillment of specific objectives. *Objective instruments* are consistent in scoring regardless of who is doing the measurement. The user must demonstrate little judgment in interpreting responses procured with the instrument. These instruments are good at measuring recall, recognition of facts, or at counting observations. Quantitative measures are more likely to be objective than qualitative measures are. They frequently fail at measuring comprehension, application, or attitudes.

Subjective instruments, on the other hand, require training and skill at interpreting responses obtained with the instrument. Two or more people may arrive at different determinations or scores from a subjective instrument. Therefore, establishing validity and reliability of subjective instruments is more difficult. Qualitative measures more frequently are subjective than quantitative measures are.

For measurement instruments to be useful, they must have a number of important qualities: validity, reliability, sensitivity, objectivity, discrimination, and administrability. The first of these is validity.

Validity

Validity is the tendency to measure what the test is intended to measure. It is of different types:

1. *Content validity* indicates how well the instrument samples the unit being measured (Creswell and Newman, 1989).

2. *Predictive validity* is the degree to which a test can predict how well a student will do in a particular situation (Anspaugh and Ezell, 1990). For example, if students who score well on a written test of skills to resist social and peer pressure to drink alcohol are actually less likely to drink, the test has good predictive validity for future drinking behavior.

3. *Concurrent validity* is the degree to which the scores on the test in question relate to scores on another accepted performance criterion. This is a central control issue in health education. The consideration is how well the measures of knowledge, attitude, and practice obtained with the test actually compare to behavior.

4. *Construct validity* is the degree to which an instrument measures some hypothetical entity such as intelligence or appreciation of health. It is based upon logical inferences indicating that the instrument actually measures what it is designed to measure.

Reliability

Reliability is the ability to yield consistent results each time the instrument is used. A reliable instrument employs the same processes and generates the same types of information every time it is used. An instrument that is valid is always reliable, but a reliable instrument is not always valid. For example, a poorly callibrated scale may yield the same incorrect weight repeatedly. Similarly, a poorly worded action questionnaire may produce the same or similar responses. These may be the answers that the respondent thinks the teacher wants rather than true and accurate responses. If the scale is properly callibrated, and the questionnaire is worded properly, however, they will provide valid results repeatedly. Of course, total accuracy and total consistency are theoretical and do not exist in the real world.

Sensitivity

Sensitivity is the ability to reflect changes in the state or amount of the phenomenon being measured. Can the test really measure changes in a student's attitudes or an increase in his or her knowledge?

Objectivity

Objectivity is the ability to not only yield similar scores on successive occasions but also to yield similar scores when administered by different people. This implies elimination of personal bias and self-interest. It also implies fairness in both the way it is constructed, such as its reading level, and in the way in which it is scored. Instruments that yield qualitative information tend to be less objective, and analysis of their information by different people is less consistent than that of quantitative instruments.

Discrimination

A test discriminates if it accurately provides different scores between the students who possess the quality being measured, such as knowledge, and those who do not.

Administrability

Administrability means that instruments must meet time and resource requirements. If a test requires sophisticated scoring technology or several hours to administer, it may be impractical for a given situation.

LEVELS OF EVALUATION

A comprehensive evaluation of programs consists of four levels of evaluation. In health education/promotion we refer to the levels as diagnostic evaluation, process evaluation, impact evaluation, and outcome evaluation.

Resources, time, complexity, and the program's dominant goal may make it difficult to evaluate well at all levels.

Diagnostic Evaluation

Diagnostic evaluation is a component of needs assessment. Its function is to analyze health problems and issues to determine which groups or individuals most need knowledge, attitude change, behavior change, or skill development. It provides specific knowledge of the health conditions that exist and suggests actions to correct them.

Process Evaluation

Process evaluation focuses on the functioning elements of the program or curriculum, including teaching methods, content, materials, time allotments, steps of implementation, achievement of the enabling objectives, and instructor performance. It is associated with ongoing operations of the program and helps to improve the program and its management. This ongoing type of program evaluation is directed at what about the program is working and what is not, and whether it is being carried out as intended, so that changes can be made to increase its probability of success (Smith, 1989).

Process evaluation helps to explain the causes of a program's strengths or weaknesses and to indicate modifications that are needed to improve the program (National Task Force, 1985). Perceptions of the participants (clients or students) are an important indicator of process success. Process evaluation frequently leads to change in methods, activities, techniques, and instructor performance. It should be continuous.

Impact Evaluation

Impact evaluation is based on measures of the immediate effects of the program or curriculum. These effects usually are indicated by changes in knowledge, attitudes, and skill development.

Impact evaluation is highly dependent upon the quality of the measurement instrument and does not necessarily indicate that long-term goals have been attained.

Outcome Evaluation

Outcome evaluation is based on measures of the long-term or ultimate changes that take place as a result of the program or curriculum. They may include indications of behavioral change or changes in quality of life, morbidity, or mortality. Outcome evaluation can be difficult and expensive because of the obstacles involved in following large groups of people for a long time. Hochbaum (1982) observed:

> Such problems stem from 1) the usual inability to observe and measure behavioral outcomes when these do not manifest themselves until long after the program has ceased, for example in school health education, and, 2) the difficulty of identifying the role played by health education in producing behavioral outcomes when other interventions, conditions, or events may have influenced such outcomes as much or more, either by adding to or by counteracting the educational efforts.

Tracking individuals to determine the permanence of behavior change is equally problematic. For these reasons, most evaluations conclude at the impact level.

Traditionally, evaluation has been divided into two levels: formative and summative (Scriven, 1967). In health education, we refer to process evaluation as formative and differentiate summative evaluation into impact and outcome evaluation.

EVALUATION OF THE LEARNER

Most of the discussion of evaluation thus far has centered on program evaluation, mostly because of the emphasis the Role Delineation Project placed on program evaluation. Teachers, however, evaluate students regularly, if not daily. Perhaps the outstanding omission of the Role

Delineation Project is specific emphasis on the competencies and skills necessary to evaluate students.

Teachers must be skilled at evaluating students' progress. One of the most popular methods is through pretests and posttests. *Pretests* by definition are tests given before instruction to determine the specific knowledge, attitudes, behaviors, and skills the learner possesses. They are diagnostic in nature and can tell the teacher what learning activities are necessary and which can be omitted. They provide baseline information that is useful in evaluating both the learner's progress and the effectiveness of the learning experience. Posttests provide data relative to change in the learner's knowledge, attitudes, behaviors, and skills. Posttest score minus pretest score on the same test may be an indication of change. Basically, pretest-posttest is diagnostic evaluation followed by impact evaluation. Pretest-posttest methodology can provide effective evaluation of program methodology as well as student performance.

Classroom measurement instruments may be standardized or teacher-made. *Standardized tests* are those that have been published after careful development and refinement. Standardized tests, however, may not include the items necessary to measure the qualities required to evaluate a specific teacher's lessons. They also may have been normed with a target population somewhat different from the class being tested. If this is the case, comparisons of students' performance will be of poor quality, as they are not comparisons with the students' peers.

For these and other reasons, teacher-made tests are the most commonly used tests in the classroom evaluation. Although they can be constructed to fit specific purposes and students, they may lack qualities such as validity and reliability. Teachers should make an effort to improve their skills at generating tests by attending workshops and taking courses on test construction. Test construction and testing are competencies that every teacher should strive to improve. Although standardized tests have some

attractive qualities, they probably will never replace teacher-made tests.

Self-inventories, questionnaires, checklists, interviews, sociodramas, small-group discussions, informal essays, observations, and anecdotal records usually produce subjective measurement. Objective teacher-made instruments frequently take the form of tests composed of multiple choice, true-false, matching, completion, or essay items.

The following are some practical ideas for developing and using these instruments:

Essay questions

◆ Use essay questions to measure objectives, such as critical thinking skills, that cannot be measured well through other questions types.

◆ Limit and define the scope of learner responses to essay questions by phrasing the questions specifically enough so students know the kind of response that is intended.

◆ Elicit reactions to a situation, not a description of it.

◆ Instead of eliciting a restatement of facts, construct questions to elicit the how, why, or significance of a piece of information.

◆ Use several brief essays rather than one or two extended essays.

◆ Write model answers with specific points that should be included in students' responses. Do not concentrate so narrowly that a listing of facts or items is required.

◆ When grading the papers, read the first question on all papers, then the second on all papers and so on, to increase uniformity and objectivity in grading.

Completion items

◆ Make the missing word or phrase a significant one that, if answered incorrectly, would invalidate the entire statement.

◆ Do not require the learner to make more than one or two completions in any one item.

◆ Write items in language and vocabulary appropriate to the students' reading level.

◆ Minimize reliance on rote memorization that occurs by simply lifting items from the text with blanks inserted for key words.

◆ In general, place the blank near or at the end of the statement.

◆ Avoid using "a" or "an" before the blank, as this can tip off the correct answer.

◆ Try to provide blanks that have only one correct answer by avoiding ambiguous items.

◆ Avoid extraneous clues to the correct answers.

True-false items

◆ Avoid loosely worded and ambiguous statements—for example, those that use qualifiers such as "many" and "few."

◆ Make the important element of the statement readily apparent to the student.

◆ Avoid using terms such as "usually," "always," "no," "never," and "all." These provide extraneous clues.

◆ Make approximately half of the items true and approximately half false.

◆ Base true-false items on statements that are absolutely true or false without qualification or exception.

◆ Do not take sentences directly from the textbook.

◆ Do not make true statements consistently longer than false statements and vice versa.

◆ Avoid statements that are partly true and partly false.

◆ Avoid long and involved statements with many qualifying clauses.

◆ Do not use trick questions.

◆ Avoid negative questions wherever possible, and double-negatives in any case.

Multiple-choice items

◆ Use clear and precise language with unambiguous meaning and vocabulary appropriate to the age group and maturity of the students.

◆ Use either a direct question or an incomplete statement, whichever seems more appropriate and effective. If an incomplete statement is used, the responses should come at the end of the sentence.

◆ Make sure each item has one and only one correct or best answer.

◆ Base each item on a single central problem that is clearly and completely stated in the stem.

◆ Avoid negative statements whenever possible. If they must be included, underline or capitalize the negative word so the student will not overlook it.

◆ Whenever possible, make all choices approximately the same length. In no case should the correct answer become obvious by its length.

◆ Keep the choices short whenever possible.

◆ Be sure all of the responses are plausible, with no obviously incorrect choices.

◆ Make responses grammatically consistent with the stem and parallel to one another in form.

◆ Arrange the responses in logical order, if one exists.

◆ Whenever there is no reason for the answers to be arranged in order, randomly position the correct answers throughout the test.

◆ Make the responses independent and mutually exclusive.

◆ Use the "none-of-the-above" and "all of the above" options with caution.

◆ Avoid using lists of options such as "A, B, and C, but not D" and "C and D only."

◆ Make all responses plausible and attractive to learners who lack the information or ability the item tests.

◆ For future tests, change incorrect responses that attract no or few answers.

Matching items

◆ Explain clearly in the instructions the basis on which items are to be matched and the procedure to be followed.

◆ Limit the test to one subject area or topic.

◆ Word the items and responses clearly and precisely.

◆ Keep the lists of items to be matched relatively short, especially for young children.

◆ Arrange the list of items for maximum clarity and convenience to the learner.

◆ Place all items and responses on a single page.

◆ Avoid extraneous clues.

◆ Provide for extra responses to reduce guessing.

◆ Provide only one possible correct response for each item.

◆ If responses can be used more than once, make this clear to the student in the oral and written instructions.

◆ Arrange the responses in random order.

Regardless of whether the evaluation is objective or subjective, the measurement techniques should be designed or selected on the basis of their capacity to measure qualities or entities that are relevant to the objectives. Each type of test item has its strengths and weaknesses. Knowledgeable educators select the test item on the basis of its applicability to the learners, content, objectives, and setting. A few advantages and disadvantages of the various types of test items are provided in the accompanying box.

An unfortunate weakness of most teacher-made tests is the lack of ability to assess attitudes or behavior. Essay exams provide better means for assessing attitudes than do the other items mentioned. Some attitude scales that have been developed are quite effective. These frequently are based upon either the *forced-choice* format or the *Likert scale*.

The forced-choice format might contain items such as those in Figure 12.1. A disadvantage of the forced-choice instrument is its often obvious presentation of the response the teacher prefers. Students who are interested in pleasing the teacher may make this choice rather than expressing their true feelings.

The Likert scale provides a greater range of choices than the typical forced-choice scale does. Likert scales for young children should provide only a few choices, such as those in Figure 12.2. For children who are more mature, several choices can be utilized, such as those in Figure 12.3. Responses may be weighted. For instance, in items 1 and 2 in Figure 12.3, "Strongly Agree" may be given a value of 5, "Agree" a 4, "Undecided" a 3, "Disagree" a 2, and "Strongly Disagree" a value of 1. Depending on the wording of the item, the values may be reversed for some items, such as items 3 and 4 in Figure 12.3. The total numerical score provides a rough measure of attitude. Just as with the forced-choice, students may respond in ways that reflect their perceptions of the teacher's wishes.

Evaluating health attitudes and their associated values also may be done by self-reporting. This requires students to be able and willing to realize what their true feelings are about a given issue, concept, or concern. These requirements are not often met by young children and adolescents. The student may respond only in ways that seem positive and popular.

Behavior can be measured by behavior inventories, personal interviews, or self-report questionnaires. All of these eventually boil down to self-report instruments. They all ask respondants

Figure 12.1. Forced-Choice Attitude Scale Items

		Agree	Disagree
1.	Regular exercise is important to good health.	_____	_____
2.	Smiling makes me feel good.	_____	_____
3.	Drinking alcohol can result in problems with the law.	_____	_____
4.	A few minutes of quiet time to myself every day makes me feel good.	_____	_____

Figure 12.2. A Likert Scale with Three Choices

		Agree	Not Sure	Disagree
1.	It helps to talk to someone about my problems.	_____	_____	_____
2.	Smoking can lead to serious illness.	_____	_____	_____
3.	I try to eat a lot of different foods.	_____	_____	_____
4.	Flossing my teeth takes too much time.	_____	_____	_____

Figure 12.3. A Likert Scale with Five Choices

		Strongly Agree	Agree	Undecided	Disagree	Strongly Disagree
1.	Cigarettes contain an addictive drug.	_____	_____	_____	_____	_____
2.	Regular exercise is good for the heart.	_____	_____	_____	_____	_____
3.	I would rather watch TV than play outside.	_____	_____	_____	_____	_____
4.	Marijuana is a harmless drug.	_____	_____	_____	_____	_____

to report their own behavior, such as how many times you exercised last week or how many cigarettes you smoked today. Self-report questionnaires are especially useful in evaluating the effects of a program in meeting its goals if the answers are given confidentially or anonymously. Unfortunately, students may not be totally honest if they can be identified, especially if the behavior is illegal. Therefore, determining behavior of an identified individual often is difficult.

Teacher observation sometimes can be an effective method of gauging behavior. This method often is clouded because teachers can observe students only in the school environment, when children may be on their best behavior or may not have the freedom to engage in some behaviors, such as drinking and smoking.

An emerging trend in student evaluation is the *mastery approach*. This approach can take many forms, but the central idea is that certain skills or competencies must be mastered to achieve an acceptable level of proficiency. The student and teacher often cooperatively decide what actions the student must take to master the skills and what level of proficiency is acceptable. For instance, the student may be required to

Advantages and Disadvantages of Types of Test Items

ESSAY-QUESTION TESTS

Advantages:

1. Essay tests are relatively easy to prepare.

2. Essay questions can be written on the chalkboard or even dictated, eliminating the expense of duplicating materials.

3. Originality and creativity on the student's part are encouraged.

4. Essay questions stimulate students to organize their thinking.

5. Chances of cheating are minimized because of the amount of writing involved.

6. Answers to essay questions help reveal students' individuality. Questions can invoke a variety of responses that reflect personal attitudes, values, habits, and differences.

7. Guessing at answers is reduced to a minimum.

8. Essay questions are the best-known way of evaluating an individual student's ability to express herself or himself.

Disadvantages

1. Determining reliability is difficult because different teachers score essay answers in different ways.

2. Scoring is rather subjective and is unconsciously influenced by factors such as legibility, neatness, grammar, spelling, word choice, and bluffing.

3. Scoring is time-consuming.

4. Students with poor writing skills are at a disadvantage.

5. Writing essay answers is time-consuming, and students may feel pressured by this type of test. Slow writers are not necessarily slow thinkers, but this may be the impression they give.

6. Younger children have particular difficulty in formulating and writing answers to essay questions.

7. An essay-question test can sample only a limited amount of the material covered.

COMPLETION ITEMS

Advantages:

1. Completion items are easy to construct.

2. Completion items have wide applications to testing situations presented in the form of charts or diagrams.

3. Completion tests minimize guessing because the answers must come from the student.

4. Completion items do not require student writing ability as a major factor.

5. Completion tests allow for objective and fairly quick scoring.

Disadvantages:

1. Completion items stress factual information. The result may be a collection of items calling for unrelated facts or isolated bits of information.

2. Completion tests place a premium on rote memory rather than on real understanding.

3. Phrasing an item so only one correct response is elicited is often difficult. Alternative answers students provide may be close to correct, making scoring problematic.

4. In a poorly formatted completion test, answers may be scattered all over the page, as on a diagram, making scoring time-consuming.

5. Clues within an item can allow students to respond correctly without understanding the concept being assessed.

TRUE-FALSE ITEMS
Advantages:

1. The true-false format is familiar to students.
2. This type of test is easy to construct.
3. True-false items can sample a wide range of subject matter. Because the items can be answered in a short time, a large number can be included on a simple test.
4. True-false tests are easy to score, and the score is quite objective.
5. The true-false test can be used effectively as an instructional test to promote interest and introduce points for discussion.
6. True-false is versatile and can be employed for short quizzes, lesson reviews, and end-of-chapter tests.
7. Tests can have items constructed either as simple factual statements or as questions that require reasoning.
8. Tests can have items that are especially useful when only two options exist concerning an issue.

Disadvantages:

1. A simple true-false item is of doubtful value for measuring achievement.
2. The true-false test encourages guessing. Even without any knowledge of the subjective matter, a student can pick many correct answers by random choice.
3. Constructing items that are completely true or completely false without making the correct response choice obvious can be difficult.
4. Avoiding ambiguities, irrelevant details and clues is difficult.
5. Unless the test consists of a large number of items, reliability is likely to be low.
6. Items that test for minor details receive as much credit as items that test for major points.
7. If the material is controversial in any way, true-false items are difficult to construct.
8. Sometimes the relative degree of truth in an item is debatable. These items should be avoided because students will try to guess what is in the teacher's mind instead of making their own decisions.

MULTIPLE-CHOICE ITEMS
Advantages:

1. Items can be written to measure inference, discrimination, and judgment.
2. Items can be constructed to measure recall as well as recognition.
3. Guessing is minimized with three or four alternative choices.

4. Sampling of material covered can be extensive. Many questions can be included on a test because a response can be made quickly.

5. Scoring is objective.

6. Scoring is rapid.

Disadvantages:

1. Developing a multiple-choice test is time-consuming.

2. Items too often are factually based, unduly stressing memory.

3. More than one response may be correct or nearly correct.

4. To exclude clues as to the correct response is difficult.

5. Incorrect, but plausible, alternative answers often are difficult to develop.

6. Items can take up a considerable amount of space.

7. The student must do a lot of reading.

8. The format does not allow students to express their own thoughts.

MATCHING TESTS

Advantages:

1. Matching items are adaptable to many subject areas.

2. Matching tests are especially useful for maps, charts, or pictorial representations.

3. Matching tests can be developed fairly quickly.

4. The matching test is a format that uses space economically.

5. The matching test is easy to score.

Disadvantages:

1. Matching items do not assess the extent to which the student has grasped the meaning.

2. The test becomes more difficult as the number of items to be matched increases.

3. The items test only factual information.

4. Matching permits guessing.

5. Matching tests are likely to include clues to correct answers.

Source: D. J. Anspaugh, and G. O. Ezell, *Teaching Today's Health* (3d ed.) (Columbus, OH: Merrill Publishing, 1990). Reprinted by permission of Macmillan.

answer a certain number of questions on an examination, write a paper that satisfactorily expresses feelings about an issue, collect and analyze television advertisements for food products, and monitor his or her own diet for 3 weeks to demonstrate achievement of a certain minimal level of calories derived from fat. All materials showing actions taken to demonstrate mastery are collected in a portfolio, which the teacher evaluates in light of the agreed-upon standards.

When evaluating students' performance or change, grading is usually the result. The following principles always should be paramount:

◆ Make evaluations relevant to objectives.

◆ Use only the behaviors that reflect academic achievement to determine grades.

◆ Evaluate fairly and consistently.

◆ Make it clear to the students how they will be evaluated.

◆ Allow students access to grade progress throughout the term.

◆ Use more than one method of evaluation.

◆ Never use grades as a tool for discipline.

Students and parents expect classroom evaluation to result in grades. Student grades may have different meanings, depending upon the referencing framework within which it has been assigned. Three referencing frameworks (Nitko, 1983) are common:

1. *Task-referenced* or *criterion-referenced grades* are based upon absolute standards of achievement—for example, the requirement that a student answer 80% of the test questions correctly, or to do six pull-ups.

2. *Group* or *norm-referenced grades* are based upon relative standards in that the student's grade reflects his or her ranking compared with everyone else in the group. A common example of norm-referenced grades is the "curving" of test scores.

3. *Self-referenced grades* reflect a comparison between a pupil's performance and the teacher's perception of that individual's capability. For example, in classrooms with students who have a wide range of abilities, standards may be higher for some students than for others, allowing even students of low academic talent opportunities for positive feedback.

Although published almost 30 years ago, Diederich's (1964) words still ring clear:

> Teachers should not be in a position merely to declare that students are improving or not improving. . . . They should approach the task of evaluation not with the arrogance of a judge, but with the humility of an enquirer. The proper frame of mind for evaluation is fear and trembling. Then, if everything turns out all right, the relief of the teachers should be even more stupendous than that of the students!

SUMMARY

Evaluation is an integral part of planning and implementating health education programs. Evaluation is the principal component of planning. Evaluation is a positive aspect of programs in that it can provide feedback to professionals about the strengths and weaknesses of programs. Program evaluation has many specific purposes, most of which enhance the likelihood of a positive outcome. Health education program evaluation is conducted on four levels: diagnostic, process, impact, and outcome.

Measurement is a tool of evaluation, providing data upon which evaluation should be based. Measurement instruments may be subjective or objective, qualitative or quantitative. They should be valid, reliable, and, when possible, objective. They also should discriminate among those who possess the quality being measured and those who do not. Further, instruments should conform to the conditions of the administrative situation.

Student evaluation is an activity classroom teachers carry out regularly. Student progress can be determined using a pretest-posttest format. Instruments for measuring performance can be standardized or teacher-made. The most common teacher-made tests contain essay questions, completion items, true-false items, multiple-choice items, or matching lists, in some combination. Each has its advantages and disadvantages, and each can be enhanced by following some practical rules. Although these test formats are most useful in measuring knowledge, other instruments can be developed and implemented to assess attitudes and behaviors. These include forced-choice, Likert scales, behavior inventories, and self-report questionnaires. They, too, have strengths and weaknesses.

In schools, evaluation of students eventually results in grading. Grading can be task-referenced, criterion-referenced, norm-referenced, or self-referenced. Each of these may be useful in given situations. Whatever method is followed, evaluation should be a serious endeavor that, by adhering to some basic rules and principles, will have a positive outcome by pointing the way to improvement.

REFERENCES

Anspaugh, D. J. and G. O. Ezell. *Teaching Today's Health* (3d ed.). Columbus, OH: Merrill Publishing, 1990.

Bedworth, A. E. and D. A. Bedworth. *The Profession and Practice of Health Education.* Dubuque, IA: Wm. C. Brown Publishers, 1992.

Diederich, P. B. The classroom teacher and the teacher-made test. *Education Horizons,* 43 (Fall 1964): 20.

Creswell, W. H., Jr., and I. M. Newman. *School Health Practice.* St. Louis: Times Mirror/Mosby College Publishing, 1989.

Dignan, M. B. and P. A. Carr. *Program Planning for Health Education and Health Promotion.* Philadelphia: Lea & Febiger, 1987.

Green, L. W., M. W. Kreuter, S. G. Deeds, and K. B. Partridge. *Health Education Planning: A Diagnostic Approach.* Palo Alto, CA: Mayfield Publishing, 1980.

Hochbaum, G. Certain problems in evaluating and their implications for test development. *Health Values,* 6 (January/February 1982): 14–21.

National Task Force for the Preparation and Practice of Health Educators. *A Guide for the Development of Competency-Based Curricula for Entry-Level Health Educators.* New York: National Task Force, 1985.

Nitko, A. *Educational Tests and Measurements: An Introduction.* New York: Harcourt, Brace, Jovanovich, 1983.

Oberteuffer, D., O. A. Harrelson and M. B. Pollock. *School Health Education* (5th ed.). New York: Harper and Row, 1972.

Patton, M. Q. *Qualitative Evaluation.* Beverly Hills, CA: Sage, 1980.

Patton, M. Q. *Practical Evaluation.* Beverly Hills, CA: Sage, 1982.

Scriven, M. The methodology of evaluation. In R. E. Stare, editor. *Perspectives of Curriculum Evaluation.* Chicago: Rand McNally, 1967.

Smith, M. F. *Evaluability Assessment: A Practical Approach.* Boston: Kluwer Academic Publishers, 1989.

Veney, J. E. and A. D. Kaluzny. *Evaluation and Decision Making for Health Services* (2d ed.). Ann Arbor, MI: Health Administration Press, 1991.

13

FEDERAL PRIORITIES FOR HEALTH

In the United States, government often sets priorities related to health issues, which lead to decisions and ultimately action to reverse health problems. These decisions affect our everyday lives in subtle and sometimes dramatic ways. They often set the tone and direction of health education and can justify programs and funding for health education initiatives.

Historically, we have been a nation that addresses its health concerns primarily as a response to crises. The states offer some excellent examples of this. For instance, the boards of health in New York and Massachusetts were established in 1797, and the state health department of Louisiana was formed in 1855 to combat yellow fever epidemics. Outbreaks of diseases such as smallpox, tuberculosis, and AIDS also have prompted governmental action at state and federal levels.

The health of early American seamen was deplorable, and they had extreme difficulty obtaining competent medical care. This led to passage of the Marine Hospital Service Act of 1798, the first ingress by the federal government into the health care system. The Marine Hospital Service, which later evolved into the U. S. Public Health Service, was the first prepaid medical and hospital insurance in the United States. For 20 cents per month, sailors could purchase coverage. The act also authorized the President to appoint physicians in each port to furnish medical and hospital care for seamen.

Not until the middle of the 19th century did a true landmark in the history of American public health emerge: publication of Lemuel Shattuck's (1948) *Report of the Sanitary Commission of Massachusetts: 1850*. Although it was not a federal report, it provided insights for generations to follow, giving recommendations for public health and governmental action that still are not fully implemented. The following is a sample of those recommendations:

◆ Establish state and local boards of health.

◆ Collect and analyze vital statistics.

◆ Develop sanitation programs for towns.

◆ Maintain a system of sanitary inspections.

◆ Study the health of children.

◆ Study and supervise health conditions of immigrants.

◆ "Supervise" mental disease.

◆ "Control" alcoholism.

◆ Control and reduce food adulteration.

◆ Control smoke nuisances.

◆ Preach health from the pulpit.

◆ Teach the science of sanitation in medical schools.

◆ Include prevention as a part of medical practice.

◆ Support routine health examinations.

The Nation's Health, published in 1948 by the Federal Security Agency, is one of the most important documents in the history of health planning. It made recommendations and established goals related primarily to resources and financing of a health care system and a national health insurance program. It accentuated community coordination of action, programs of rehabilitation of people with handicaps, mental health services, and sufficient numbers of hospitals.

HEALTHY PEOPLE

Healthy People: The Surgeon General's Report on Health Promotion and Disease Prevention (U. S. Department of Health, Education, and Welfare, 1979), submitted to President Jimmy Carter, identified real risks to the health of the American people. Preparation of *Healthy People* was essentially a process of formulating objectives through building consensus among experts, professionals, and national advocacy organizations. The report identified five age-related population groups: infants, children, adolescents and young adults, adults, and older adults.

The 1979 report demonstrated striking gains in the nation's health since the turn of the century. It also verified that any further notable improvement in the health of Americans would require adoption of health promotion and disease prevention strategies and coordinated action in their implementation.

Healthy People established health goals for each of the five population groups and recommended actions necessary for attaining the goals in three categories: preventive health services, health protection, and health promotion. The goals and subgoals were:

Infant Health

Goals: To continue to improve infant health; to reduce infant mortality by at least 35%, to fewer than nine deaths per 1,000 live births by 1990

Subgoals: a. Reducing the incidence of low birthweight

b. Reducing the number of birth defects

Children

Goals: To improve child health, foster optimal childhood development; to reduce deaths among children ages 1 to 14 by at least 20%, to fewer than 34 per 100,000 by 1990

Subgoals: a. Enhancing childhood growth and development

b. Reducing childhood accidents and injuries

Adolescents and Young Adults

Goals: To improve the health and health habits of adolescents and young adults; to reduce deaths among people ages 15 to 24 years by at least 20%, to fewer than 93 per 100,000 by 1990

Subgoals: a. Reducing fatal motor vehicle accidents

b. Reducing alcohol and drug misuse

Adults

Goals: To improve the health of adults; to reduce deaths among people ages 25 to 64 by at least 25%, to fewer than 400 per 100,000 by 1990

Subgoals: a. Reducing heart attacks and strokes
b. Reducing death from cancer

Older Adults

Goals: To improve the health and quality of life for older adults; by 1990, to reduce the average annual number of days of restricted activity because of acute and chronic conditions by 20%, to fewer than 30 days per year for people aged 65 years and older

Subgoals: a. Increasing the number of older adults who can function independently
b. Reducing premature death from influenza and pneumonia

Healthy People also contained an inventory of 15 priority areas grouped into three categories. These priority areas are outlined below.

Preventive Health Services

1. Family planning.
2. Pregnancy and infant care.
3. Immunizations.
4. High blood pressure control.
5. Sexually transmissible diseases services.

Health Protection

1. Toxic agent control.
2. Occupational safety and health.
3. Accidental injury control.
4. Fluoridation of community water supplies.
5. Infectious agent control.

Health Promotion

1. Smoking cessation.
2. Reducing misuse of alcohol and other drugs.
3. Improved nutrition.
4. Exercise and fitness.
5. Stress control.

With the exception of the older adult group, the emphasis is on decrease in deaths. Little mention is made of the quality of life, the ability to self-actualize, high level of wellness, or the ability to enjoy one's life. Thus, though government seemed to recognize generally that health education must play a significant role in attaining the goals of *Healthy People*, the tendency was to overlook the very ideals that health educators hold dear.

OBJECTIVES FOR THE NATION

The U. S. Department of Health and Human Services (1980) published another report titled *Promoting Health/Preventing Disease: Objectives for the Nation*. This document produced measurable and quantifiable objectives for each of the 15 priority areas contained in *Healthy People*. It also identified sources of national, state, and local data used to monitor progress toward the objectives but stopped short of specifically identifying the governmental agencies that would have principal responsibility for attaining individual portions of the objectives. The objectives were placed within the following relevant priority areas:

1. Improved health status.
2. Reduced risk factors.
3. Increased public or professional awareness.
4. Improved services or protection.
5. Improved surveillance/evaluation systems.

MIDCOURSE REVIEW

The U. S. Public Health Service (1986) published *The 1990 Health Objectives for the Nation: A Midcourse Review*, a review, indicating that a good deal of tangible progress was being made toward meeting the objectives. An overall summary (Bedworth and Bedworth, 1992) of progress according to the general categories discussed earlier indicated that:

◆ Infant mortality dropped from 14.1 per 1,000 live births to 10.6 per 1,000 live births.

◆ The national goals for healthy children showed a reduction from 42 deaths per 100,000 to 32 deaths per 100,000.

◆ Deaths per 100,000 for healthy adolescents and young adults fell from 115 to 99.

◆ The death rate per 100,000 for healthy adults was reduced from 533 to 447.

The midcourse evaluation was optimistic for the progress made to that point but suggested that lack of data to measure the status of many objectives indicated that they are unlikely to be achieved. Further analysis revealed that by 1985, 14% of the objectives for preventive services were achieved, with an additional 32% likely to be achieved by 1990. Only 11% of the objectives for health promotion were achieved, and more than 35% were likely to be achieved by 1990.

When the objectives are analyzed according to the five categories or priority areas, we find that in 1985 only 23% were achieved for health status; 2% were achieved for risk reduction; 10.5% for public and professional awareness; 16% for improved services or protection; and 13% for improved surveillance/evaluation services. Specific priority areas showing the greatest progress included high blood pressure control, immunization, control of infectious disease, and smoking. Priority areas showing the least progress included pregnancy and infant health, family planning, and physical fitness and exercise (McGinnis and DeGraw, 1991).

By the end of the 1980s, the states had shown considerable acceptance of the necessity to establish and pursue health objectives. In 1989, 90% of the states and territories had established objectives for at least some of the priority areas in the 1990 national objectives. About 40 states had established centralized units within the state health agency to promote and coordinate health promotion/disease prevention operations.

Although the objectives for 1990 set in motion a 10-year plan for disease prevention and health promotion and contributed greatly to a new sense of purpose and focus for public health, school health education, and preventive medicine, they were not without serious flaws. In 1980, those objectives were met with a good deal of skepticism by people representing the concerns of special populations, such as ethnic and racial minorities and the elderly. In setting objectives related to health and mortality of the whole American population, the objectives ignored and hid the wide variations among distinctive populations. These discrepancies are particularly evident among black and white, old and young, and rich and poor.

Most of the objectives pertaining to increased services and protective measures were stated generally as target averages for the nation rather than as specific objectives for subpopulations (U. S. Department of Health and Human Services, 1992). This situation was rectified partially when representatives of five special populations in separate federally sponsored conferences set separate health promotion priorities and identified specific barriers and resources for disease prevention and promotion in each of those populations (U. S. Department of Health and Human Services, 1981).

Although the work represented consensus among experts, professionals, and advocacy groups and about 3,000 organizations were invited to comment and review the document before its final publication, many viewed it as a top-down, science-driven, professionally dominated set of objectives. They saw it as giving too little weight to social concern and real quality of life issues and too much emphasis to bureaucratic and technocratic criteria such as morbidity, mortality, and cost-containment.

Consistency of funding for programs to address the objectives and goals and priority areas was lacking. With the Reagan administration came the New Federalism, a philosophy that would reduce large-scale public sector spending on domestic activities. The main proposition of the New Federalism was to return power and responsibilities to the states. Critics see President Reagan's New Federalism and Economic Recovery Act as a mechanism to reduce federal expenditures for key domestic activities and as an abandonment of the national commitments to certain costly social programs, including some of those that have served to guard the health of the citizens.

The resulting transfer of responsibility to the states and their political subdivisions without adequate funding forced a struggle at state and local levels to provide for human services in the face of diminishing financial resources. A shift in executive branch emphasis to national defense and the world events of the 1980s, including the unrest in the Middle East, did nothing to enhance funding for programs that could have been directed toward meeting the *Healthy People* objectives.

YEAR 2000 OBJECTIVES FOR THE NATION

The Office of Disease Prevention and Health Promotion (ODPHP) of the U. S. Public Health Service coordinated the national effort to develop Year 2000 Objectives. In 1989, the draft copy of *Promoting Health/Preventing Disease: Year 2000 Objectives for the Nation* was circulated, and many of those involved in work related to improving and preserving the health of Americans had their first glimpse of the Year 2000 Objectives. In style, it bears some resemblance to the 1990 Objectives, breaking down

the population by age group: infants, children, adolescents and young adults, adults, and older adults. It proposed three overarching public health goals that permeate the structure and content of the document. Those goals are:

1. To increase the span of healthy life for Americans.
2. To reduce health disparities among Americans.
3. To achieve access to preventive services for all Americans.

The Year 2000 Objectives in *Healthy People 2000* (U. S. Department of Health and Human Services, 1991) also listed priorities for health promotion and disease prevention under three main goals: health promotion, health protection, and preventive services. Each of the three principal goals is further broken down into 22 specific priority areas, 21 of which are grouped in the three principal goals. The other, surveillance and data systems, stands alone. The accompanying box lists the principal goals and their respective priority areas. All of the 22 specific priority areas, with the exception of surveillance and data systems, group the objectives into health status objectives, risk reduction objectives, and services and protection objectives. There are 298 specific objectives.

McGinnis and DeGraw (1991) provided the following excellent explanation of the three principal goals:

1 Health promotion strategies are related to individual lifestyle—personal choices made in a social context—that can have a powerful influence over one's health prospects. These priorities include physical activity and fitness, nutrition, tobacco, alcohol and other drugs, family planning, mental health, and violent and abusive behaviors. Educational and community-based programs can address lifestyle in a cross-cutting fashion.

2. Health protection strategies are related to environmental or regulatory measures that

Priorities for Health Promotion and Disease Prevention
From *Healthy People 2000*

Health Promotion

Physical Activity and Fitness
Nutrition
Tobacco
Alcohol and Other Drugs
Family Planning
Mental Health and Mental Disorders
Violent and Abusive Behavior
Educational and Community-Based Programs

Health Protection

Unintentional Injuries
Occupational Safety and Health
Environmental Health
Food and Drug Safety
Oral Health

Prevention Services

Maternal and Infant Health
Heart Disease and Stroke
Cancer
Diabetes and Chronic Disabling Conditions
HIV Infection
Sexually Transmitted Diseases
Immunization and Infectious Diseases
Clinical Preventive Services

Surveillance and Data Systems

Surveillance and Data Systems

Source: U. S. Department of Health and Human Services, *Healthy People 2000: National Health Promotion and Disease Prevention Objectives* (Public Health Service Publication No. 91-50212) (Washington, DC: Government Printing Office, 1991).

confer protection on large population groups. These strategies address issues such as unintentional injuries, occupational safety and health, environmental health, food and drug safety, and oral health. Interventions addressing these issues are not exclusively protective in nature. They must have a substantial health promotion element as well.

3. Preventive services strategies include counseling, screening, immunization, or chemoprophylactic interventions for individuals in the clinical setting. Priority areas for these strategies are maternal and infant health, heart disease and stroke, cancer, diabetes and chronic disabling conditions, HIV infection, sexually transmitted diseases, and infectious diseases. Obviously, overlap exists among these three broad categories.

To assure participation of groups with specific expertise and to increase the likelihood of

achieving the objectives, ODPHP provided funding and cooperated with various organizations that work with certain high-risk groups in specific settings. In cooperation with the Public Health Service, the American School Health Association (1991) published a compilation of the *Healthy People 2000* objectives related to school health, in the *Journal of School Health*. The Public Health Service, under a cooperative agreement with the American Association of School Administrators, worked with school administrators nationwide to increase awareness of the Year 2000 Objectives as they relate to schools and to promote adoption of school health programs. ODPHP worked through the Maternal and Child Health Bureau of the Health Resources and Services Administration to publish *Healthy Children 2000*, a compilation of the Year 2000 Objectives that relate to mothers, infants, children, adolescents, and youth.

The American Medical Association was identified to receive funding to focus on the adolescent population through the Healthier Youth by the Year 2000 Project. The AMA produced a document titled *Healthy Youth 2000*, which included objectives from *Healthy People 2000* that relate to the 10- to 24-year age group (McGinnis, 1992). Table 13.1 presents selected objectives that apply to youth. The objectives are organized by priority areas identified in *Healthy People 2000* (e.g., physical activity and fitness, nutrition, tobacco). Objectives in each priority area are grouped into objectives related to health status, risk reduction, and services and protection. At the end of several sections are related objectives, those pertaining to populations that include but are not limited to youth.

Table 13.1 illustrates the enormity of health problems facing the youth of America. It also portrays the task ahead for educators and health professionals who are committed to addressing these problems. Examining only one priority area serves as an example of the work ahead. The Physical Activity and Fitness priority area shows the need for planned programs of physical education and other activity-related programs. Daily physical education is still not a reality for most school children, even though the benefits of exercise are well documented. Even when physical education is in place, Objective 1.9 illustrates the need for more class time in real physical activity. Objective 1.5 suggests that leisure-time activity is overlooked in our youth. One major implication of this priority area is the importance of cooperation and integration of

---

TABLE 13.1.   YEAR 2000 OBJECTIVES FOR YOUTH

PHYSICAL ACTIVITY AND FITNESS

   Risk Reduction

   Objective 1.4
   Increase to at least 20% the proportion of aged 18 and older, and to at least 75% the proportion of children and adolescents aged 6–17, who engage in vigorous physical activity that promotes development and maintenance of cardiorespiratory fitness, 3 or more days per week for 20 or more minutes per occasion.
   (Baseline: 12% for people aged 18 and older in 1985; 66% for youth aged 10–17 in 1984)

   Services and Protection

   Objective 1.8
   Increase to at least 50% the proportion of children and adolescents in first through twelfth grades who participate in daily school physical education.
   (Baseline: 36% in 1984–86)

   Services and Protection

   Objective 1.9
   Increase to at least 50% the proportion of school physical education class time that students are being physically active, preferably engaged in lifetime physical activities.
   (Baseline: Students spent an estimated 27% of class time being physically active in 1984)

— *Continued*

TABLE 13.1.　YEAR 2000 OBJECTIVES FOR YOUTH — *Continued*

RELATED OBJECTIVES

Risk Reduction

Objectives 1.3, 15.11 (Heart Disease and Stroke), *17.3* (Diabetes and Chronic Disabling Conditions)
Increase to at least 30% the proportion of people aged 6 and older who engage regularly, preferably daily, in light to moderate physical activity for at least 30 minutes per day.
(Baseline: 22% of people aged 18 and older were active for at least 30 minutes 5 or more times per week and 12% were active 7 or more times per week in 1985)

Risk Reduction

Objective 1.5
Reduce to no more than 15% the proportion of people aged 6 and older who engage in no leisure-time activity.
(Baseline: 24% for people aged 18 and older in 1985)

Risk Reduction

Objective 1.6
Increase to at least 40% the proportion of people aged 6 and older who regularly perform physical activities that enhance and maintain muscular strength, muscular endurance, and flexibility.
(Baseline available in 1991)

Risk Reduction

Objectives 1.7 and 2.7 (Nutrition)
Increase to at least 50% the proportion of overweight people aged 12 and older who have adopted sound dietary practices combined with regular physical activity to attain appropriate body weight.
(Baseline: 30% of overweight women and 25 percent of overweight men for people aged 18 and older in 1985)

NUTRITION

Health Status

Objectives 1.2, 2.3 (Physical Activity and Fitness), *15.10* (Heart Disease and Stroke), *17.11* (Diabetes and Chronic Disabling Conditions)
Reduce overweight to a prevalence of no more than 20% among people aged 20 and older and no more than 15% among adolescents aged 12–19.
(Baseline: 26% for people aged 10–74 in 1976-80, 24% for men and 27% for women; 15% for adolescents aged 12–19 in 1976–80)

Risk Reduction

Objective 2.8
Increase calcium intake so at least 50% of youth aged 12–24 consume three or more servings daily of foods rich in calcium.
(Baseline: 7% of women and 14% of men aged 19–24 consumed three or more servings in 1985–86)

— Continued

TABLE 13.1.   YEAR 2000 OBJECTIVES FOR YOUTH — *Continued*

Related Objectives
Risk Reduction

Objective 2.10
Reduce iron deficiency to less than 3% among children aged 1–4 and among women of childbearing age.
(Baseline: 5% for women aged 20–44 in 1976–80)

Risk Reduction
Objective 2.13
Increase to at least 85% the proportion of people aged 18 and older who use food labels to make nutritious food selections.
(Baseline: 74% used labels to make food selection in 1988)

TOBACCO
Risk Reduction

Objective 3.5
Reduce the initiation of cigarette smoking by children and youth so that no more than 15% have become regular cigarette smokers by age 20.
(Baseline: 30% of youth had become regular cigarette smokers by ages 20–24 in 1987)

Risk Reduction

Objective 3.9
Reduce smokeless tobacco use by males aged 12–24 to a prevalence of no more than 4%.
(Baseline: 6.6% among males aged 12–17 in 1988; 8.9% among males aged 18–24 in 1987)

Related Objectives
Risk Reduction

Objective 3.6
Increase to at least 50% the proportion of cigarette smokers aged 18 and older who stopped smoking cigarettes for at least one day during the preceding year.
(Baseline: In 1984, 34% of people who smoked in the preceding year stopped for at least one day during that year.)

Risk Reduction

Objective 3.7
Increase smoking cessation during pregnancy so at least 60% of women who are cigarette smokers at the time they become pregnant quit smoking early in pregnancy and abstain for the remainder of their pregnancy.
(Baseline: 30% of white women aged 20–44 quit at any time during pregnancy in 1985)

— Continued

TABLE 13.1.   YEAR 2000 OBJECTIVES FOR YOUTH — *Continued*

ALCOHOL AND OTHER DRUGS
Health Status

Objective 4.1b
Reduce deaths among people aged 15–24 caused by alcohol-related motor vehicle crashes to no more than 18 per 100,000.
(Baseline: 21.5 per 100,000 in 1987)

Risk Reduction

Objective 4.5
Increase by at least 1 year the average age of first use of cigarettes, alcohol, and marijuana by adolescents aged 12–17.
(Baseline: Age 11.6 for cigarettes, age 13.1 for alcohol, and age 13.4 for marijuana in 1988)

Risk Reduction

Objective 4.6
Reduce the proportion of young people who have used alcohol, marijuana, and cocaine in the past month as follows:

Substance/Age	1988 Baseline	Target 2000
Alcohol/aged 12–17	25.2%	12.6%
Alcohol/aged 18–20	57.9%	29%
Marijuana/aged 12–17	6.4%	3.2%
Marijuana/aged 18–25	15.5%	7.8%
Cocaine/aged 12–17	1.1%	0.6%
Cocaine/aged 18–25	4.5%	2.3%

Risk Reduction

Objective 4.7
Reduce the proportion of high school seniors and college students engaging in recent occasions of heavy drinking of alcoholic beverages to no more than 28% of high school seniors and 32% of college students.
(Baseline: 33% of high school seniors and 41.7% of college students in 1989)

Risk Reduction

Objective 4.8
Reduce the consumption by people aged 14 and older to an annual average of no more than 2 gallons of ethanol per person.
(Baseline: 2.54 gallons of ethanol in 1987)

— Continued

TABLE 13.1.   YEAR 2000 OBJECTIVES FOR YOUTH — *Continued*

Risk Reduction

Objective 4.9
Increase the proportion of high school seniors who receive social disapproval associated with the heavy use of alcohol, occasional use of marijuana, and experimentation with cocaine, as follows:

Behavior	1988 Baseline	2000 Target
Heavy use of alcohol	56.4%	70%
Occasional use of marijuana	71.1%	85%
Trying cocaine once or twice	88.9%	95%

Risk Reduction

Objective 4.10
Increase the proportion of high school seniors who associate risk of physical or psychological harm with the heavy use of alcohol, regular use of marijuana, and experimentation with cocaine, as follows:

Behavior	1988 Baseline	2000 Target
Heavy use of alcohol	44%	70%
Regular use of marijuana	77.5%	90%
Trying cocaine once or twice	54.9%	80%

Risk Reduction

Objective 4.11
Reduce to no more than 3% the proportion of male high school seniors who use anabolic steroids.
(Baseline: 4.7% in 1989)

Related Objective

Health Status

Objective 4.3
Reduce drug-related deaths to no more than 3 per 100,000.
(Age-adjusted baseline: 3.8 per 100,000)

FAMILY PLANNING

Health Status

Objective 5.1
Reduce pregnancies among girls 17 and younger to no more than 50 per 1000 adolescents.
(Baseline: 71.7 pregnancies per 1000 girls aged 15–17 in 1985)

— Continued

TABLE 13.1.   YEAR 2000 OBJECTIVES FOR YOUTH — *Continued*

Special Target Populations

Pregnancies (per 1000)	1985 Baseline	2000 Target
Black adolescent girls 15–19	186*	120
Hispanic adolescent girls 15–19	158	105

*Nonwhite adolescents

Risk Reduction

Objectives 5.4, 18.3 (HIV Infection), *19.9* (Sexually Transmitted Diseases)
Reduce the proportion of adolescents who have engaged in sexual intercourse to no more than 15% by age 15 and no more than 40% by age 17.
(Baseline: 27% of girls and 33% of boys by age 15; 50% of girls and 66% of boys by age 17; reported in 1988)

Risk Reduction

Objective 5.5
Increase to at least 40% the proportion of ever sexually active adolescents aged 17 and younger who have abstained from sexual activity for the previous three months.
(Baseline: 26% of sexually active girls aged 15–17 in 1988)

Risk Reduction

Objective 5.6
Increase to at least 90% the proportion of sexually active, unmarried people aged 19 and younger who use contraception, especially combined method contraception that both effectively prevents pregnancy and provides barrier protection against disease.
(Baseline: 78% at most recent intercourse and 63% at first intercourse; 2% used oral contraceptives and the condom at most recent intercourse; among young women aged 15–19 reporting in 1988)

Services and Protection

Objective 5.8
Increase to at least 85% the proportion of people aged 10–18 who have discussed human sexuality, including values surrounding sexuality, with their parents and/or have received information through another parentally endorsed source, such as youth, school, or religious programs.
(Baseline: 66% of people aged 13–18 have discussed sexuality with their parents; reported in 1986)

Services and Protection

Objectives 5.10 and *14.12* (Maternal and Child Health)
Increase to 60% the proportion of primary care providers who provide age-appropriate preconception care and counseling.
(Baseline data available in 1992)

— *Continued*

TABLE 13.1.   YEAR 2000 OBJECTIVES FOR YOUTH — *Continued*

Related Objective
Health Status
Objective 5.2
Reduce to no more than 30% the proportion of pregnancies that are unintended.

Special Target Populations

Unintended Pregnancies	1988 Baseline	2000 Target
Black women	78%	40%

MENTAL HEALTH AND MENTAL DISORDERS
Health Status
Objectives 6.1a and *7.2a* (Violent and Abusive Behavior)
Reduce suicides among youth aged 15–19 to no more than 8.2 per 100,000 people.
(Baseline: 10.3 per 100,000 in 1987)

Health Status
Objective 6.1b and *7.2b* (Violent and Abusive Behavior)
Reduce suicides among men aged 20–34 to no more than 21.4 per 100,000 people.
(Baseline: 25.2 per 100,000 people in 1986)

Health Status
Objectives 6.2 and *7.8* (Violent and Abusive Behavior)
Reduce by 15% the incidence of injurious suicide attempts among adolescents aged 14–17.
(Baseline: Baseline data available in 1991)

Health Status
Objective 6.3
Reduce to less than 10% the prevalence of mental disorders among children and adolescents.
(Baseline: An estimated 12% among youth younger than 18 in 1989)

Related Objectives
Health Status
Objective 6.5
Reduce to less than 35% the proportion of people aged 18 and older who experienced adverse health effects from stress within the past year.
(Baseline: 42.6% in 1985)

— Continued

TABLE 13.1.   YEAR 2000 OBJECTIVES FOR YOUTH — *Continued*

	Special Population Target	
	1985 Baseline	**2000 Target**
People with disabilities	53.5%	40%

Risk Reduction

Objective 6.8
Increase to at least 20% the proportion of people aged 18 and older who seek help in coping with personal and emotional problems.
(Baseline: 11.1% in 1985)

	Special Population Target	
	1985 Baseline	**2000 Target**
People with disabilities	14.7%	30%

Risk Reduction

Objective 6.9
Decrease to no more than 5% the proportion of people aged 18 and older who report experiencing significant levels of stress who do not take steps to reduce or control their stress.
(Baseline: 21% in 1985)

VIOLENT AND ABUSIVE BEHAVIOR

Health Status

Objective 7.1
Reduce homicides to no more than 7.2 per 100,000 people.
(Age-adjusted baseline: 8.5 per 100,000 in 1987)

	Special Population Targets	
Homicide Rate (per 100,000)	**1987 Baseline**	**2000 Target**
Children aged 3 and younger	3.9	3.1
Black men aged 15–34	90.5	72.4
Hispanic men aged 15–34	53.1	42.5
Black women aged 15–34	20.0	16.0

Health Status

Objective 7.3
Reduce weapon-related deaths to no more than 12.6 per 100,000 people from major causes.
(Age-adjusted baseline: 12.9 per 100,000 by firearms, 1.9 per 100,000 by knives, in 1987)

— *Continued*

TABLE 13.1.   YEAR 2000 OBJECTIVES FOR YOUTH — *Continued*

Health Status

Objective 7.4
Reverse to less than 25.2 per 1000 children the rising incidence of maltreatment of children younger than age 18.
(Baseline: 25.2 per 1,000 in 1986)

Type-Specific Targets

Incidence of Types of Maltreatment (per 1,000)	1986 Baseline	2000 Target
Physical abuse	5.7	<5.7
Sexual abuse	2.5	<2.5
Emotional abuse	3.4	<3.4
Neglect	15.9	<15.9

Health Status

Objective 7.7a
Reduce rape and attempted rape of women aged 12–34 to no more than 225 per 100,000.

Special Population Target

Incidence of Rape and Attempted Rape (per 100,000)	1986 Baseline	2000 Target
Women aged 12–34	250	225

Risk Reduction

Objective 7.9
Reduce by 20% the incidence of physical fighting among adolescents aged 14–17.
(Baseline data available in 1991)

Risk Reduction

Objective 7.10
Reduce by 20% the incidence of weapon-carrying by adolescents aged 14–17.
(Baseline data available in 1991)

Related Objective
Health Status

Objective 7.6
Reduce assault injuries among people aged 12 and older to no more than 10 per 1,000 people.
(Baseline: 11.1 per 1,000 in 1986)

— *Continued*

TABLE 13.1.   YEAR 2000 OBJECTIVES FOR YOUTH — *Continued*

EDUCATIONAL AND COMMUNITY-BASED PROGRAMS
Risk Reduction

Objective 8.2
Increase the high school graduation rate to at least 90%, thereby reducing risks for multiple problem behaviors and poor mental and physical health.
(Baseline: 79% of people aged 20–21 had graduated from high school with a regular diploma in 1989)

Services and Protection

Objective 8.10
Establish community health promotion programs that separately or together address at least three of the Healthy People 2000 priorities and reach at least 40% of each State's population.
(Baseline data available in 1991)

Related Objectives
Services and Protection

Objective 8.9
Increase to at least 75% the proportion of people aged 10 and older who have discussed issues related to nutrition, physical activity, sexual behavior, tobacco, alcohol, other drugs, or safety with family members on at least one occasion during the preceding month.
(Baseline data available in 1991)

UNINTENTIONAL INJURIES
Health Status

Objective 9.3b
Reduce deaths among youth aged 15–24 by motor vehicle crashes to no more than 33 per 100,000 people.
(Baseline: 36.9 per 100,000 people in 1987)

Health Status

Objective 9.5
Reduce drowning deaths to no more than 1.3 per 100,000.
(Age-adjusted baseline: 2.1 per 100,000)

Drowning Deaths Per 100,000	Special Population Targets	
	1987 Baseline	2000 Targets
Children aged 4 and younger	4.2	2.3
Men aged 15–34	4.5	2.5
Black males	6.6	3.6

— Continued

TABLE 13.1.   YEAR 2000 OBJECTIVES FOR YOUTH — *Continued*

Related Objectives

Health Status

Objective 9.10
Reduce nonfatal spinal cord injuries so that hospitalizations for this condition are no more than 5.0 per 100,000.
(Baseline: 5.0 per 100,000 in 1988)

Special Population Targets

Nonfatal Spinal Cord Injuries (per 100,000)	**1988 Baseline**	**2000 Target**
Males	8.9	7.1

Risk Reduction

Objective 9.13
Increase use of helmets to at least 80% of motorcyclists and at least 50% of bicyclists.
(Baseline: 60% of motocyclists in 1988 and an estimated 8% of bicyclists in 1984)

ENVIRONMENTAL HEALTH

Health Status

Objective 11.1
Reduce asthma morbidity, as measured by a reduction in asthma hospitalizations, to no more than 160 per 100,000 people.

Special Population Targets

Asthma Hospitalizations (per 100,000)	**1987 Baseline**	**2000 Targets**
Blacks and other nonwhites	334	265
Children	284*	225

*Children aged 14 and younger

ORAL HEALTH

Health Status

Objective 13.1
Reduce dental caries (cavities) so that the proportion of children with one or more caries . . . is no more than 60% among adolescents aged 15.
(Baseline: 78% of adolescents aged 15 in 1986–87)

Special Population Targets

Dental Caries Prevalence	**1986-87 Baseline**	**2000 Targets**
American Indian/Alaska Native adolescents aged 15	93%*	70%

*In permanent teeth in 1983–84

— *Continued*

TABLE 13.1.   YEAR 2000 OBJECTIVES FOR YOUTH — *Continued*

Health Status

Objective 13.2
Reduce untreated dental caries so that the proportion of children with untreated caries . . . is no more than 15% among adolescents aged 15.
(Baseline: 23% of adolescents aged 15 in 1986–87)

	Special Population Targets	
Untreated Dental Caries	**1986–87 Baseline**	**2000 Targets**
Adolescents aged 15 whose parents have less than a high school education	41%	25%
American Indian/Alaska Native adolescents aged 15	84%*	40%
Black adolescents aged 15	38%	20%
Hispanic adolescents aged 15	31–47%**	25%

*1983–84 baseline
**1982–84 baseline

Risk Reduction

Objective 13.8
Increase to at least 50% the proportion of children who have received protective sealants on the occlusal (chewing) surfaces of permanent molar teeth.
(Baseline: 11% of children aged 8 and 8% of adolescents aged 14 in 1986–87)

MATERNAL AND INFANT HEALTH

Related Objectives

Although not age specific, the following objectives are especially pertinent to pregnant adolescents.

Health Status

Objective 14.3
Reduce the maternal mortality rate to no more than 3.3 per 100,000 live births.
(Baseline: 6.6 per 100,000 in 1987)

	Special Population Target	
Maternal Mortality	**1987 Baseline**	**2000 Target**
Blacks	14.2*	5*

*Per 100,000 live births

— *Continued*

TABLE 13.1.   YEAR 2000 OBJECTIVES FOR YOUTH — *Continued*

Health Status

Objective 14.4
Reduce incidence of fetal alcohol syndrome to no more than 0.12 per 1,000 live births.
(Baseline: 0.22 per 1,000 live births)

Special Population Targets

Incidence Per 1,000 Births	1987 Baseline	2000 Targets
American Indians and Alaska Natives	4	2
Blacks	0.8	0.4

Risk Reduction

Objective 14.5
Reduce low birthweight to an incidence of no more than 5% of live births and very low birthweight to no more than 1% of live births.
(Baseline: 6.9 and 1.2%, respectively, in 1987)

Special Population Targets

	1987 Baseline	2000 Targets
Blacks—low birthweight	12.7%	9%
Blacks—very low birthweight	2.7%	2%

Risk Reduction

Objective 14.6
Increase to at least 85% the proportion of mothers who achieve the minimum recommended weight gain during their pregnancies.
(Baseline: 67% of married women in 1980)

Risk Reduction

Objective 14.7
Reduce severe complications of pregnancy to no more than 15 per 100 deliveries.
(Baseline: 22 hospitalizations [prior to delivery] per 100 deliveries in 1987)

Risk Reduction

Objective 14.10
Increase abstinence from tobacco use by pregnant women to at least 90% and increase abstinence from alcohol, cocaine, and marijuana by pregnant women by at least 20%.
(Baseline: 75% of pregnant women abstained from tobacco use in 1985)

Services and Protection

Objective 14.11
Increase to at least 90% the proportion of all pregnant women who receive prenatal care in the first trimester of pregnancy.
(Baseline: 76% of live births in 1987)

— Continued

TABLE 13.1.   YEAR 2000 OBJECTIVES FOR YOUTH — *Continued*

Special Population Targets

Proportion of Pregnant Women Receiving Early Prenatal Care	1987 Baseline	2000 Targets
Black	61.1*	90*
American Indian/Alaska Native	60.2*	90*
Hispanic	61.0*	90*

*Percent of live births

Services and Protection

Objective 14.14
Increase to at least 90% the proportion of pregnant women and infants who receive risk-appropriate care.
(Baseline data available in 1991)

HIV INFECTION

Risk Reduction

Objectives 18.4a and *19.10b* (Sexually Transmitted Diseases)
Increase to at least 60% the proportion of sexually active, unmarried women aged 15–19 who used a condom at last sexual intercourse.
(Baseline: 26% of sexually active, unmarried women aged 15–19 reported that their partners used a condom at last sexual intercourse in 1988)

Risk Reduction

Objective 18.4b and *19.10b* (Sexually Transmitted Diseases)
Increase to at least 75% the proportion of sexually active, unmarried young men aged 15–19 who used a condom at last intercourse.
(Baseline: 57% of sexually active, unmarried young men reported that they used a condom at last sexual intercourse in 1988)

Related Objectives

Risk Reduction

Objective 18.5
Increase to at least 50% the estimated proportion of all intravenous drug abusers who are in drug abuse treatment programs.
(Baseline: An estimated 11% of opiate abusers were in treatment.)

Risk Reduction

Objective 18.6
Increase to at least 50% the estimated proportion of intravenous drug abusers not in treatment who use only uncontaminated drug paraphernalia (works).
(Baseline: 25 to 35% of opiate abusers in 1989)

— *Continued*

TABLE 13.1.   YEAR 2000 OBJECTIVES FOR YOUTH — *Continued*

SEXUALLY TRANSMITTED DISEASES

Health Status

Objective 19.1b
Reduce gonorrhea among adolescents aged 15–19 to no more than 750 cases per 100,000.
(Baseline: 1,123 per 100,000 in 1989)

IMMUNIZATION AND INFECTIOUS DISEASES

Related Objective

Health Status

Objective 20.1
Reduce indigenous cases of vaccine-preventable diseases as follows:

Disease	1988 Baseline	2000 Targets
Diphtheria among people aged 25 and younger	1	0
Tetanus among people aged 25 and younger	3	0
Polio (wild-virus type)	0	0
Measles	3,058	0
Rubella	225	0
Congenital rubella syndrome	6	0
Mumps	4,866	500
Pertussis (whooping cough)	3,450	1,000

CLINICAL PREVENTIVE SERVICES

Risk Reduction

Objective 21.2c
Increase to at least 50% the proportion of adolescents aged 13–18 who have received, as a minimum within the appropriate interval, all of the screening and immunization services and at least one of the counseling services appropriate for their age and gender as recommended by the U. S. Preventive Services Task Force.
(Baseline data available in 1991)

---

the disciplines of health education, recreation, and physical education. Study of Table 13.1 can lead health educators to a number of significant conclusions about the role of professionals in the health of the nation's children.

Many of the objectives in *Healthy People 2000* are directly related to performance of schools. In fact, successful schools are the key to many of the objectives. The risks of adolescence and childhood can be reduced by a planned and sequential health education program. In addition, comprehensive health education can affect future decisions about the self, the family, and the community. More than one-third of the Year 2000 Objectives can be achieved directly by schools or the schools can significantly affect their attainment. The objectives that schools can achieve directly are presented in Table 13.2.

Healthy People 2000 has offered both the opportunity and the challenge to schools, and particularly to health educators, to improve the health of young Americans. Schools offer the most efficient means available to improve the health of young people and to enable them to avoid risks to their health. Objective 8.4—increase to at least 75% the proportion of the nation's elementary and secondary schools that provide planned and sequential, quality school health education kindergarten through 12th grade—supplies the federal foundation for a truly national initiative in health education. The American Public Health Association (1975) noted that the school provides an educational setting in which the child's total health during the impressionable years is a priority concern. No other community setting even approximates the magnitude of the grades K–12 school education enterprise. By its sheer numbers—46 million students each year and more than 5 million instructional and noninstructional staff—the school dwarfs any other setting in touching the lives of our citizens. Perhaps its greatest contribution to the health of young people and to comprehensive school health education is the language used in *Healthy People 2000* (U. S. Department of Health and Human Services, 1992) to describe school health:

> Health education in the school setting is especially important for helping children and youth develop the increasingly complex knowledge and skills they will need to avoid health risks and maintain good health throughout life. Quality school health education that is planned and sequential for students in kindergarten through 12th grade, and taught by educators trained to teach the subject, has been shown to be effective in preventing risk behaviors. Quality school health education addresses and integrates education, skills development, and motivation on a range of health problems and issues (e.g., nutrition, physical activity, injury control, use of tobacco, alcohol and other drugs, sexual behaviors that result in HIV infection, other sexually transmitted diseases, and unintended pregnancies) at developmentally appropriate ages (see Objective 8.4). The content of the

education is determined locally by parents, school boards, and other members of the community.

> Other aspects of the school environment can also be important to school health. State and local health departments can work with schools to provide a multi-dimensional program of school health that may include school health education, school-linked or school-based health services designed to prevent, detect, and address health problems, a healthy and safe school environment, physical education, healthful school food service selections, psychological assessment and counseling to promote child development and emotional health, school site health promotion for faculty and staff, and integrated school and community health promotion efforts.

Because the content of education is determined at the local level by parents, school boards, and community members, coalition building and partnership development are greatly needed if a truly comprehensive health program is to exist. To build these coalitions and partnerships, serious efforts must be made to educate parents, community members, school administrators, teachers in other disciplines, and governmental officials.

The effectiveness of properly designed and implemented school health education programs is backed by a great deal of documentation (see Chapter 7). Evidence and experience indicates that the effectiveness of these programs is influenced by the amount of classroom time devoted to the program, the extent to which school administrators support the program, and the extent to which teachers are prepared and motivated to implement the program.

To implement Objective 8.4, as well as the others listed in Table 13.2, all school districts and states must mandate and support planned and sequential, high-quality school health education throughout the educational experience. Presently, this is far from the case. A survey by the National Association of State Boards of Education and the Council of Chief State School Officers reported that 42 states require health education to be offered in schools, and 35 of these require it both for elementary and for secondary school students. Only 28 of the 42 states actually specify that they require "comprehensive school health education" (Corry, 1992). Exactly what these 28 states consider to be comprehensive health education has not been established. National data sources give varying estimates regarding the actual proportion of schools currently offering comprehensive school health education curricula.

Lest we assume that the Year 2000 Objectives were universally accepted and supported with no criticism, we examine some of the misgivings expressed. Green (1992) detailed some of the criticisms that were widely heard. One was that the final version of the objectives departed significantly in some instances from the objectives that had achieved consensus in the scientific, professional, and organizational review procedures. Political issues that had been brought to bear on the wording forced changes in the meaning of several of the objectives. Examples

---

Table 13.2. Objectives for Schools for the Year 2000

Objectives that appear in more than one area of the school health program are indicated with an asterisk (*).

I. School Health Instruction

NUTRITION

Objective 2.17*
Increase to at least 90% the proportion of school lunch and breakfast services and child care food services with menus that are consistent with nutrition principles in the *Dietary Guidlines for Americans.*
(Baseline data available in 1993)

Objective 2.19
Increase to at least 75% the proportion of the nation's schools that provide nutrition education from preschool through 12th grade, preferably as part of quality school health education.
(Baseline data available in 1991)

TOBACCO

Objective 3.10*
Establish tobacco-free environments and include tobacco use prevention in the curricula of all elementary, middle, and secondary schools, preferably as part of quality school health education.
(Baseline: 17% of school districts totally banned smoking on school premises or at school functions in 1988; 78% of school districts provided antismoking education at the high school level, 81% at the middle school level, and 75% at the elementary school level in 1988)

ALCOHOL AND OTHER DRUGS

Objective 4.10
Increase the proportion of high school seniors who associate risk of physical or psychological harm with the heavy use of alcohol, regular use of marijuana, and experimentation with cocaine, as follows:

Behavior	1989 Baseline	2000 Targets
Heavy use of alcohol	44%	70%
Regular use of marijuana	77.5%	90%
Trying cocaine once or twice	54.9%	80%

— Continued

Table 13.2.   Objectives for Schools for the Year 2000 – – *Continued*

Objective 4.13
Provide to children in all school districts and private and secondary school educational programs on alcohol and other drugs, preferably as a part of quality school health education.
(Baseline: 63% provided some instruction, 39% provided counseling, and 23% referred students for clinical assessment in 1987)

FAMILY PLANNING

Objective 5.8
Increase to at least 85% the proportion of people aged 10–18 who have discussed human sexuality, including values surrounding sexuality, with their parents or have received information through another parentally endorsed source, such as youth, school, or religious programs.
(Baseline: 66% of people aged 13–18 have discussed sexuality with their parents; reported in 1986)

VIOLENT AND ABUSIVE BEHAVIOR

Objective 7.16
Increase to at least 50% the proportion of elementary and secondary schools that teach nonviolent conflict resolution skills, preferably as a part of quality school health education.
(Baseline data available in 1991)

EDUCATIONAL AND COMMUNITY-BASED PROGRAMS

Objective 8.4
Increase to at least 75% the proportion of the nation's elementary and secondary schools that provide planned and sequential, quality school health education kindergarten through 12th grade.
(Baseline data available in 1991)

UNINTENTIONAL INJURIES

Objective 9.18
Provide academic instruction on injury prevention and control, preferably as part of quality school health education in at least 50% of public school systems (grades K–12).
(Baseline data available in 1991)

Objectives 9.19* and 13.16 (Oral Health)
Extend requirement of the use of effective head, face, eye, and mouth protection to all organizations, agencies, and institutions sponsoring sporting and recreation events that pose risks to injury.
(Baseline: Only National Collegiate Athletic Association football, hockey, and lacrosse; high school football; amateur boxing; and amateur ice hockey in 1988)

Table 13.2.   Objectives for Schools for the Year 2000 — *Continued*

HIV INFECTION

Objective 18.10

Increase to at least 95% the proportion of schools that have age-appropriate HIV education curricula for students in 4th through 12th grade, preferably as part of quality school health education.

(Baseline: 66% of school districts required HIV education, but only 5% required HIV education in each year for 7th through 12th grade in 1989)

SEXUALLY TRANSMITTED DISEASES

Objective 19.12

Include instruction in sexually transmitted disease transmission prevention in the curricula of all middle and secondary schools, preferably as part of quality school health education.

(Baseline: 95% of schools reported offering at least one class on sexually transmitted diseases as part of their standard curricula in 1988)

II. School Health Services
NUTRITION

Objective 2.17*

Increase to at least 90% of school lunch and breakfast services and child care food services with menus that are consistent with the nutrition principles in the *Dietary Guidelines for Americans.*
(Baseline data available in 1993)

ORAL HEALTH

Objective 13.12

Increase to at least 90% the proportion of all children entering school programs for the first time who have received an oral health screening, referral, and follow-up for necessary diagnostic, preventive, and treatment services.
(Baseline: 66% of children aged 5 visited a dentist during the previous year in 1986)

IMMUNIZATION AND INFECTIOUS DISEASES

Objective 20.11

Increase immunization levels as follows:

Basic immunization series among children under age 2: at least 90%.
(Baseline 70–80% estimated in 1989)

Basic immunization series among children in licensed child care facilities and kindergarten through post-secondary education institutions: at least 95%.
(Baseline: For licensed child care, 94%; 97% for children entering school for the 1987–1988 school year; and for postsecondary institutions, baseline data available in 1992)

Table 13.2.   Objectives for Schools for the Year 2000 — *Continued*

III. School Health Environment

TOBACCO

Objective 3.10*
Establish tobacco-free environments and include tobacco use prevention in the curricula of all elementary, middle, and secondary schools, preferably as part of quality school health education.
(Baseline: 17% of school districts totally banned smoking on school premises or at school functions in 1988; 78% of school districts provided antismoking education at the high school level, 81% at the middle school level, and 75% at the elementary school level in 1989)

UNINTENTIONAL INJURIES

Objective 9.19*
Extend requirement of the use of effective head, face, eye, and mouth protection to all organizations, agencies, and institutions sponsoring sporting and recreation events that pose risks of injury.
(Baseline: Only National Collegiate Athletic Association football, hockey, and lacrosse, high school football; amateur boxing; and amateur ice hockey in 1988)

---

of the differences between the consensus version of specific objectives and the edited versions after White House and Office of Management and Budget clearance follow.*

◆ The original Chapter 5, titled "Sexual Behavior," was retitled "Family Planning," and specific objectives were altered. For example, a specific objective for achieving age-appropriate sex education in schools disappeared.

◆ Throughout the document, the term "comprehensive school health" was replaced by the term "quality school health," apparently to avoid any suggestion of support for sex education, school contraceptive services, and other controversial subjects or services.

◆ The chapter on "Violent and Abusive Behavior" replaces the term "firearm injury-death" with the more ambiguous term "weapon-related violent death," obscuring the role of handgun control.

◆ The chapter on "Tobacco" weakened the force of Objective 3.15 with the addition of a few words: "Eliminate *or severely restrict . . .* tobacco product advertising and promotion to which youth younger than age 18 *are likely to be exposed* (italics indicate added words).

◆ The consensus version of Objective 21.4 was "Increase to at least 60% the proportion of people with health insurance coverage for the screening, counseling, and immunization services recommended by the U. S. Preventive Services Task Force." The "official" version is now: "Improve financing and delivery of clinical preventive services so that virtually no American has a financial barrier to receiving, at a minimum, the screening, counseling, and immunization services recommended by the U. S. Preventive Services Task Force." The administration's wording avoids a commitment to providing insurance coverage and puts the burden of coverage on those delivering services.

---

*Source: Green, L.W. Preface, U. S. Department of Health & Human Services, *Healthy People 2000: Summary Report*, 1992, Boston: Jones and Bartlett Publishers. Reprinted by permission.

Advocacy groups for racial and ethnic populations also criticized the Year 2000 Objectives for not including a separate category for minority-specific objectives. These groups saw a need for such a spotlight that would encourage state and local public health agendas toward specific actions regarding minority concerns. They wished to use the objectives as an authoritative source for building a case for minority health policies. Although consideration for minority-specific objectives was given early in the process, they were not included in the final issue.

Funding for programs to address the initiatives implied in the objectives has been sporadic and frequently immersed in political bickering, domestic agendas, and foreign affairs. The political changes in eastern Europe, the Persian Gulf conflict, prolonged recession, change in administration, and Congressional budget battles have resulted in a state of flux in federal fiscal matters.

HEALTHY KIDS FOR THE YEAR 2000

The American Association of School Administrators (AASA) was chosen as one of the nine national groups to help promote the Healthy People 2000 initiative. AASA organized two task forces of superintendents, health education teachers, principals, curriculum and personnel directors, and other educational leaders from various parts of the country. All of the participants were noted for their involvement in outstanding health education programs.

Participants in the task forces quickly recognized that education is the key to helping people make informed, healthy choices; and, to learn, children need to be healthy. They also appreciated the fact that we must invest now in comprehensive school health education programs or bear the consequences of more crime, welfare dependency, delinquency, and continued escalating health costs. Ten benefits of comprehensive health education programs were identified:

1. Less school vandalism.
2. Better attendance by students and staff.
3. Reduced health care costs.
4. Reduced substitute teaching costs.
5. Better family communication, even on sensitive issues such as sexuality.
6. Stronger self-confidence and self-esteem.
7. Noticeably fewer students using tobacco.
8. Improved cholesterol levels for students and staff.
9. Increased seatbelt use.
10. Improved physical fitness.

AASA identified a 12-step action plan for developing a comprehensive health education program (American Association of School Administrators, 1990). Recognizing that situations vary, the task force members were careful to acknowledge that many of the steps can occur simultaneously, in different order, or be tailored to individual districts' needs and timeliness. The 12 steps appear in Chapter 5.

OTHER FEDERAL INITIATIVES

Federal efforts in enhancing the health of the nation historically have been fragmented, and ventures frequently have tended to overlap. Within the executive branch, at least seven cabinet departments and two independent agencies play important roles in adolescent health. A particularly disturbing illustration of governmental inefficiency is that in fiscal year 1989, the National Institute of Child Health and Human Development, National Institutes of Health, spent only 6.9% of its budget on projects specifically related to adolescents (Dougherty et al., 1992). Given the mass of bureaucratic entanglements, however, some positive initiatives have emerged in the areas of health and health education. The following, though not intended to be complete, describes some important federal programs in child and adolescent health and health education.

U. S. Public Health Service

The U. S. Public Health Service (PHS) conducts a wide range of health promotion activities. For instance, the PHS, in cooperation with the American School Food Service Association, conducts activities and develops materials to improve nutrition in school breakfasts and lunches. The materials provide inservice training for school food service employees in menu planning, recipe development, nutrition education, and student involvement activities.

The Office of Adolescent Pregnancy Prevention Programs manages the Adolescent Family Life Demonstration Grants Program. In this program, "care projects" have been carried out in schools to provide services associated with adolescent pregnancy. The office also has conducted prevention projects that have tested Family Life Education curricula in schools.

The Indian Health Service (IHS) works directly with tribes and schools in planning and implementing school health education activities for Native American children. Educational efforts have included HIV prevention; dental health, including fluoridation of water and dental screenings; and nutrition programs. Many IHS programs have taken place in the context of comprehensive school health education.

The Office of Substance Abuse Prevention (OSAP) funds projects and develops materials relevant to the school setting related to preventing alcohol and other drug abuse. OSAP also funds demonstration programs for prevention, treatment, and rehabilitation of drug abuse and alcohol abuse by high-risk youth.

The National Cancer Institute (NCI) supports studies aimed at implementation, evaluation, and dissemination of cancer prevention curricula in schools. The institute also has supported school-based smoking prevention trials. In addition, NCI has published educational materials related to smoking prevention and cancer education programs.

The National Institute of Child Health and Human Development coordinates a coalition of private and federal agencies to sponsor a national Child Health Day each year. A symposium in Washington, DC, augmented by satellite community meetings and workshops sponsored by local organizations in practically every state, is the centerpiece of Child Health Day. Videotapes on adolescent health and childhood injury prevention produced for Child Health Day have been distributed widely to school systems, PTA's, and other child health organizations (McGinnis, 1992).

U. S. Department of Agriculture

The Food and Nutrition Service, U. S. Department of Agriculture, provides food and dietary guidance for children and adults (Nelsen, 1992). Programs include the National School Lunch and School Breakfast Program, the Food Distribution Programs, and the Special Supplemental Food Program for Women, Infants, and Children (WIC). These food assistance programs attempt to ensure that all needy people, especially children, have access to a healthy, nutritious diet. Many programs provide nutrition education to ensure that participants make informed decisions about the food they eat. In an effort to educate people about the 1990 *Dietary Guidelines for Americans*, the Food and Nutrition Service distributes without charge thousands of copies of the Nutrition Guidance for the Child Nutrition Programs to schools and child care workers.

The Nutrition Education and Training (NET) program helps to develop positive food habits by teaching the fundamentals of nutrition to children, parents, educators, and school food service personnel through grants to state agencies. NET coordinates learning experiences in the classroom, the school cafeteria, and the community. Teachers and school food service employees receive instruction about nutrition, education, and food service management. The NET program also heavily involves parents.

The Cooperative Extension System (CES) provides a nationwide educational network. One example of the educational programs developed by CES is *Nutrition for Life*, a comprehensive nutrition education program for young people in New York State schools, grades K–12. In this participatory program, realistic nutrition situations develop problem solving, decision making, and resource management skills, as well as valuing the wise use of personal and community resources. The Indiana *Have a Healthy Baby* program works with pregnant adolescents in friendly environments, their own schools, or homes. Utilizing videotapes, discussion, personalized contracts, and other activities, the program includes topics such as decisions affecting the baby, desirable amount of weight to gain during pregnancy, what to eat during pregnancy, effects of drug use and abuse on the baby, and what to feed the baby.

Division of Adolescent and School Health

The division, part of the national Centers for Disease Control (CDC), established a coordinated national system involving eight components specifically designed to help young people avoid behaviors that result in HIV infection (Kolbe, 1992). The eight components are:

1. Epidemiological surveillance program.
2. National organizations.
3. State and city departments of education.
4. Materials development and dissemination.
5. Training and demonstration centers.
6. Colleges and universities.
7. Youth in high-risk situations.
8. Evaluation.

This system is designed to enable CDC to work collaboratively with other federal agencies and with many national, state, and local education and health agencies. It allows for assessment of prevalence of youth risk behaviors that cause the most mortality and morbidity of HIV

and other causes. These behaviors are broken into six broad areas:

1. Sexual behaviors that result in HIV infection, other STD's and unintended pregnancies.
2. Drug and alcohol use.
3. Tobacco use.
4. Dietary patterns that contribute to disease.
5. Insufficient physical activity.
6. Behaviors that result in unintentional and intentional injuries.

It also monitors the extent to which the nation's schools provide health education to prevent risk behaviors in the six categorical areas, as part of a planned and sequential, kindergarten–12th grade, comprehensive school health education program. CDC also provides fiscal and technical support for 23 national organizations and the Indian Health Service, to help schools and other agencies that serve youth to implement effective HIV education within comprehensive school health education programs.

The system also facilitates development and dissemination of HIV education materials for youth, including "Guidelines for Effective School Health Education to Prevent the Spread of AIDS." The system supports three national training and demonstration centers that help state and local officials learn how to implement current HIV education programs in their respective states and cities. It extends services to colleges and universities to prevent HIV infection in students. CDC currently is evaluating the extent to which schools are implementing HIV education and the extent to which students consequently are reducing behaviors that result in HIV transmission.

U. S. Department of Education

The Department of Education plays an important role in encouraging health education in the schools (Ravitch, 1992). The Comprehensive

School Health Education Program under the Fund for Innovation in Education provides assistance in the form of grants to state and local education agencies for various activities related to improving comprehensive school health education. Activities include training programs for school personnel in health education; development of a comprehensive school health program; assessment of school health programs; dissemination of information to schools related to nutrition, personal health and fitness, disease prevention, and other urgent health problems affecting students. The Drug-Free Schools and Communities Act programs support alcohol and other drug abuse education and prevention activities. Educational materials are disseminated for children beginning before kindergarten.

National School Health Education Coalition (NaSHEC)

NaSHEC (Corry, 1992) encompasses more than 60 national organizations, associations, voluntary health agencies, corporations, and federal agencies. The goal of the coalition is to ensure that every student in grades K–12 receives a comprehensive rather than categorical or inconsistent health education. NaSHEC believes that comprehensive health education is essential to ensuring that children achieve their full health potential and that delivery and coordination of federal health education programs are vital to a comprehensive approach to health education. NaSHEC has been an advocate for legislation to assure coordination and prevent duplication of effort in school health programs and for the reestablishment of Office of Comprehensive School Health Education in the U. S. Department of Education.

STATE AND LOCAL ROLES

Policy making and the real work of educating youth and providing health services take place at state and local levels. The states have broad legal authority for a wide variety of programs. Although a federal program may elevate an issue to the state's active policy agenda, the federal influence tends to be secondary to the state's political agenda (Litman, 1990). As a result the states' roles in health can take a number of forms. They can:

— authorize or order that certain programs or content be included in public education;
— financially support the care and treatment of poor and chronically disabled people, including administration of federal and state Medicaid programs;
— give quality assurance and oversight of health care practitioners and facilities;
— regulate health care costs;
— regulate insurance carriers;
— authorize local government health services.

Some states seized the opportunity the 1990 Objectives presented and began mandating comprehensive health education in schools. As mentioned earlier, more than 40 states have mandated health education programs. Some state governments recognized that, in the 1990 Objectives, they had a blueprint for statewide planning for health promotion and disease prevention. A few state governments, such as those in California, Colorado, Texas, and Virginia, developed their own individual objectives for 1990, building on the national objectives. Some states organized their data-gathering and surveillance activities around their commitment to monitor their progress toward achievement of the 1990 Objectives.

On the local level, the 1990 Objectives provided a good deal of inspiration and direction to health professionals and people working on health problems (McGinnis, 1990). Local health educators had something upon which to hang their hats. Efforts toward coalition building and curriculum change gained momentum. The momentum only accelerated with the Year 2000

Objectives. At the same time states were mandating comprehensive school health education and local boards of education were involved in designing curriculum, another phenomenon was gaining strength. An organized effort by a vocal minority of citizens has attempted to derail the comprehensive health education train. Ultraconservatives and people who are fearful of what is unfamiliar to them are becoming organized in some communities to fight the concept of comprehensiveness in school health. In some instances, nonlocals have been transported to school board meetings to shout and protest comprehensive school health education.

Most of this opposition originated in education regarding sexuality, but it carries over to the entire program. For example, some groups oppose the development of decision-making skills within the school health curriculum because they view the world in absolute terms of right and wrong. They contend that separating the right from the wrong will dictate children's actions. The real world, however, does not often lend itself to such a clear dichotomy, and that philosophy does little to help children cope with the challenges of their world. Health educators should be aware of this type of opposition and be ready to confront it. This has become an integral part of the challenge to develop comprehensive school health education.

SUMMARY

Through documents such as *Healthy People: The Surgeon General's Report on Health Promotion and Disease Prevention*, and *Healthy People 2000: National Health Promotion and Disease Prevention Objectives* the federal government has established the nation's priorities in terms of improving people's health. The objectives provide both opportunity and challenge to schools, parents, and communities to enhance the health of Americans. Health education is recognized as a means to attaining the objectives.

Federal, state, and local governments have developed and are implementing ambitious programs to educate people of all ages about their health and how their behavior affects their health. Many programs provide direct services while educating. One avenue that has not been fully developed is a comprehensive health education program for our schools. Health educators, parents, and community leaders must take the lead in implementating comprehensive school health education as a means to reach the Year 2000 Objectives.

REFERENCES

American Association of School Administrators. *Healthy Kids for the Year 2000: An Action Plan for Schools.* Arlington, VA: AASA, 1990.

American Medical Association Healthier Youth by the Year 2000 Project. *Healthier Youth 2000: National Health Promotion and Disease Prevention Objectives for Adolescents.* Chicago: American Medical Association, 1991.

American Public Health Association. Resolutions and position papers: Education for health in the community setting. *American Journal of Public Health,* 65 (February 1975): 201–209.

Bedworth, A. E., and D. A. Bedworth. *The Profession and Practice of Health Education.* Dubuque, IA: Wm. C. Brown Publishers, 1992.

Corry, M. The role of the federal government in promoting health through the schools: Report from the National School Health Education Coalition. *Journal of School Health,* 62 (April 1992): 143–145.

Dougherty, D., J. Eden, K. B. Kemp, K. Metcalf, K. Rowe, G. Ruby, P. Strobel, and A. Solarz. Adolescent health: A report to the U. S. Congress. *Journal of School Health,* 62 (May 1992): 167–174.

Federal Security Agency, U. S. Office Of Education. *The Nation's Health.* Washington, DC: Government Printing Office, 1948.

Green, L. W. Preface. *Healthy People 2000: Summary Report.* Boston: Jones and Bartlett Publishers, 1992.

Kolbe, L. J. The role of the federal government in promoting health through the schools: Report from the Division of Adolescent and School Health, Centers for Disease Control. *Journal of School Health*, 62 (April 1992): 135–137.

Litman, T. J. Government and health: The political aspects of health care—a sociopolitical overview. In P. R. Lee and C. L. Estes, *The Nation's Health* (3d ed.). Boston: Jones and Bartlett Publishers, 1990.

McGinnis, J. M. Setting objectives for public health in the 1990s. *Annual Review of Public Health, 11* (1990): 231–249.

McGinnis, J. M. The role of the federal government in promoting health through the schools: Report from the Office of Disease Prevention and Health Promotion. *Journal of School Health*, 62 (April 1992): 131–134.

McGinnis, J. M. and C. DeGraw. Healthy schools 2000: Creating partnerships for the decade. *Journal of School Health*, 61 (September 1991): 292–297.

Nelsen, B. J. The role of the federal government in promoting health through the schools: Report from the Department of Agriculture. *Journal of School Health*, 62 (April 1992): 138–140.

Ravitch, D. The role of the federal government in promoting health through the schools: Report from the Department of Education. *Journal of School Health*, 62 (April 1992): 141–142.

Shattuck, L. *Report of the Sanitary Commission of Massachusetts, 1850.* New York: Cambridge University Press, 1948.

U. S. Department of Health, Education, and Welfare. *Healthy People: The Surgeon General's Report on Health Promotion and Disease Prevention.* Public Health Service Publication No. 79–55071). Washington, DC: Government Printing Office, 1979.

U. S. Department of Health and Human Services. *Promoting Health/Preventing Disease: Objectives for the Nation.* Washington, DC: Public Health Service, 1980.

U. S. Department of Health and Human Services. *Strategies for Promoting Health for Specific Populations.* Public Health Service Publication No. 81–50169). Washington, DC: Office of Health and Health Promotion, 1981.

U. S. Department of Health and Human Services. *The 1990 Health Objectives for the Nation: A Midcourse Review* (Public Health Service Publication No. 191–691/70228). Washington, DC: Government Printing Office, 1986.

U. S. Department of Health and Human Services. *Healthy People 2000: National Health Promotion and Disease Prevention Objectives.* (Public Health Service Publication No. 91–50212). Washington, DC: Government Printing Office, 1991.

U.S. Department of Health and Human Services. *Healthy People 2000: National Health Promotion and Disease Prevention Objectives* (Summary Report). Boston: Jones and Bartlett Publishers, 1992.

14

CURRENT AND FUTURE ISSUES IN HEALTH EDUCATION

Even though health education has been part of children's educational experience for many years, in many ways the profession is still in its own childhood. Like a child, it must continue to mature, establishing its role in the school systems of tomorrow, the health care system, work-sites, and other venues. Technology, as well as world and national health problems, will shape its development.

Although we have improved our ability to predict the health problems of tomorrow, we are met with surprising challenges. Who would have predicted 20 years ago that a "new" disease such as AIDS could have such a profound effect on American life, altering sexual attitudes and behaviors and threatening to bankrupt the insurance and health care industries? Predicting the future is always difficult. Still we can examine current issues and draw conclusions about approaching needs and coming events.

The future is careening toward us, bringing changes in our society and in the world. Hundreds of species become extinct each year. Our lifestyles change in sometimes imperceptible ways, which add up to huge cumulative change over time. The stress of change takes its toll.

Health educators must be willing and prepared to take their place in the world of tomorrow. The social issues will change, forcing the content of courses to change. Health educators can control the future to some extent and to a larger extent help individuals adjust to it. We must be prepared to act in both proactive and reactive ways.

CREDENTIALING

Perhaps the single topic receiving the most discussion among health educators, in papers presented at conferences and in private conversations, is professional credentialing. Credentialing is a formal process applied to assure that those practicing a profession meet acceptable standards. The process can have a number of mechanisms and can result in a number of methods of recognition. It has been applied at the state and national levels and is administered by state governments, independent organizations, and professional associations.

Credentialing has a number of benefits. If properly applied, it can:

— attest to the individual's knowledge and skills deemed essential to the field of practice as delineated by the profession;
— assist employers to identify qualified professionals;
— assist the public in recognizing the basic competencies of those who are credentialed;
— recognize a commitment to professional standards;
— enhance the profession;
— provide recognition to individual practitioners;
— facilitate geographic mobility of qualified practitioners.

State-Level Credentialing

Teacher Certification

Teacher certification is a process of legal recognition authorizing the individual holder of the certificate to perform specific services, usually teaching, in the public schools of the state. Some states require certification for administrative positions and some for teaching in colleges. The traditional method of attaining certification is to complete a college degree program of teacher education that meets the state certification requirements. Several states require applicants for certificates to pass the National Teachers Exam. Delaware has designated its own examination as a requirement for certification. In most states, a structure is in place requiring continual professional development, including college courses, workshops, seminars, and inservice programs. In short, to maintain their certification, teachers must anticipate taking courses continually, earning inservice credits and being observed and evaluated (Campbell, 1990). Certification for teachers is similar to licensure for other professions on the state level.

Competency Testing

A fairly recent innovation—and one that seems to be losing its momentum—is competency testing for experienced teachers. A few states, notably Arkansas, Georgia, Florida, and Texas, have implemented competency testing. No new states have been added to this list since 1985. Teachers and their unions generated a good deal of criticism and resistance to the tests. The cost of the tests was viewed in some quarters as too high for their benefits. In Arkansas, Georgia, and Texas, more than $9 million of school funds were spent on competency tests, which more than 99% of teachers passed (Needham, 1987). Minorities' performance on the Florida test threatened to worsen the existing shortage of minority teachers (Smith, Miller and Joy, 1988).

Many experienced teachers resisted being tested, and a few resigned rather than take the test. Some of those who resigned were considered to be excellent teachers and a significant loss to their communities. On the other hand, the tests identified a number of teachers whose levels of basic skills were extremely low. Regardless, for the present, state-level competency testing seems to have lost its steam. Some of the states that adopted the practice probably will drop it in the near future.

Credentialing at the National Level

National Board for Professional Teaching Standards

The NBPTS was initiated by the Carnegie Corporation and funded by private and public sources. It is governed by teachers, teacher educators, business people, and state and local officials. NBPTS proposes to offer teachers the opportunity to become nationally certified. The certificate will attest to highly accomplished practice as an educator. The following assumptions (National Board for Professional Teaching Standards, 1991) will be the basis for the certificates and the assessment approaches:

◆ All teachers should possess a core of professional knowledge and skills regardless of whom they teach or what they teach.

◆ Teachers should have knowledge and skills specific to the developmental stages of the children under their care.

◆ Teachers in each subject area should command a core of subject- and discipline-specific knowledge.

◆ Teachers should demonstrate depth as well as breadth of knowledge in disciplines they teach, as well as skill in conveying that knowledge to their students.

The first standards assessment instruments were to be implemented in 1993. They are expected to contain new forms of teacher assessment, other than paper-and-pencil tests, in recognition of the scientific and equity deficiencies of multiple-choice tests. Assessment forms are expected to include a structured portfolio composed of colleagues' comments, samples of students' work, and videotapes of classroom instruction (Beaudry, 1990; Laws, 1991). Individual teachers may be called upon to perform educational simulations to demonstrate their competence. Research into the new forms of assessment is proceeding. The new forms have been endorsed by the powerful National Council on Accreditation of Teacher Education (NCATE), the National Education Association, and the American Federation of Teachers (Cleary, 1992).

A number of criticisms of the NBPTS plan have been voiced. Perhaps the most valid is that an undergraduate degree in education, or health education for that matter, is not a prerequisite for assessment or for certification. Thus, a person could gain national certification in health

education without completing an academic major in the discipline.

Critics (Murphy, 1990; Cleary, 1991, 1992) also address problems with portfolio assessment. Extensive time would be required to train assessors and to do the actual evaluation. The cost of the assessment also is a drawback. The fairness of portfolio assessment and the validity of simulation exercises also have been called into question. Critics further point out that the board does not specify how portfolios and simulation exercises will have to be adapted to meaningfully assess the new roles of teachers in restructured schools. Behind-the-scenes planning, coordination, and advocacy might never be evaluated. Development of interdisciplinary health education curriculum would be difficult to evaluate in this way.

Regardless of the criticism, some form of national credentialing for teachers seems to be in our future, with the NBPTS playing a role. Other national organizations may also offer national teacher certification. How national certification will be utilized remains to be seen. To predict that it will begin as voluntary and eventually become a requirement is fair.

National Commission for Health Education Credentialing, Inc.

In 1988, the National Task Force on the Preparation and Practice of Health Education changed its incorporation papers and became the National Commission for Health Education Credentialing (NCHEC). This voluntary professional certification purports to establish a national standard for health education practice. It awards the Certified Health Education Specialist (CHES) credential. The purposes of NCHEC are to:

— certify health education specialists.

— promote professional development.

— strengthen professional preparation.

The certificate is awarded to those who pass an examination composed of 150 multiple-choice items. As Green (1991) attested, the test is good but far from perfect. Beginning in 1992, only individuals who have a degree from an accredited institution of higher education having a health education emphasis are eligible for certification. The seven major areas of responsibility tested are (National Commission for Health Education Credentialing, 1991):

1. Assess individual and community needs for health education.
2. Plan effective health education programs.
3. Implement health education programs.
4. Evaluate the effectiveness of health education programs.
5. Coordinate provision of health education services.
6. Act as a resource person in health education.
7. Communicate health and health education needs, concerns, and resources.

Recertification, required every 5 years, is based upon continuing education criteria developed by the Commission.

The Commission was organized in 1988, evolving from the work of the National Task Force on the Preparation of Health Educators. The Task Force, initiated in 1978, was charged with developing a credentialing system. During the charter certification phase, 1,558 CHES certificates were awarded without testing. In 1990, the first certification examination was given and 644 more health education specialists were certified. The number of CHESs has continued to grow rapidly.

CHES seems to be taking root as the major certification for individual health educators. In fact, there is some hope that it will be recognized as the certifying body in health education for NBPTS. This, of course, would solve the dilemma of NBPTS's not requiring a degree in health education. Other alternatives do exist. If the NBPTS is fully implemented, CHES could be considered equivalent to or additional to the NBPTS certification. The Commission is touting the certification as a future requirement for employment as a health educator, particularly in higher education. Whether this will come to pass remains to be seen.

Some health educators have found fault with the Commission and the CHES. Gold (1989) questioned the voluntary nature of the process in the quote:

> What began as voluntary is now often touted as mandatory. Even if the words on paper say "voluntary," the message being given by some of the proselytizers is that certification is a must. They are told if they do not become credentialed, it demonstates lack of support for the profession. Students and employers alike are led to believe that they must acquire and hire only these professionals. How is that voluntary? More importantly, how do we know that the certified health education specialist is better than a health educator who is not? And how do we know that this has not created an arena in which people become credentialed for defensive rather than professional reasons?

Early exams tended to emphasize community health and deemphasize school health education. The argument also is made that the 150-item multiple-choice examination does not measure an individual's competence or the generic competencies developed by the Role Delineation Project. The exam also does not seem to discriminate, as indicated by a high "pass" ratio. The charges incurred with registering for the examination, obtaining continuing education hours at designated NCHEC providers, and recertification place a heavy financial load on those who are just entering the profession.

Finally, there is the issue of perception of the generic homogenous health educator. The Role Delineation Project concluded that health educators, regardless of setting, have responsibilities in common and, therefore, competencies in common. This tends to produce the perception that health educators, whether teaching in an elementary school, conducting a program at a YMCA or a senior citizens center, or planning and supervising educational programs for a state public health department, are all the same, performing the same functions. The CHES credential perpetuates this idea, as the exam is based upon the seven Responsibilities and Competencies for Entry-Level Health Educators. Even though many health educators agree with this perception, many others see a difference in the roles, competencies, and functions of professionals in different settings.

Institutional Accreditation

Institutional accreditation is a voluntary process that is part of the private sector. Begun by individual professional associations as a way of achieving collective status, accreditation has evolved over the years into an organized, but not necessarily orderly, process. In 1975, the Council on Postsecondary Accreditation (COPA) was developed as an umbrella organization to recognize, review, and coordinate existing accrediting bodies of all types. COPA represents six regional accreditors, 44 groups that accredit various college programs, and six that accredit specialized institutions such as seminaries and proprietary schools. It has provided a forum for these accreditors and for college presidents.

COPA's power is illustrated by the fact that the U. S. Department of Education officially recognizes accrediting agencies and associations for determining eligibility for federal assistance, and Education uses COPA as one means to establish public recognition (U.S. Department of Health and Human Services, 1980). This recognition is translated into fiscal and administrative support for educational programs that meet accreditation standards, making accreditation an important issue to institutions of higher education. It is also important to students in choosing an institution. Institutions that are not accredited are not eligible for most federal assistance programs.

COPA was dealt a serious blow in 1993 when the six regional accrediting agencies announced plans to abandon the umbrella agency and start their own (Leatherman, 1993). Among the criticisms of COPA was that the wide diversity of

accreditors represented by the council made for such different and competing interests that the council could not effectively represent any of them. Regional accreditors also have complained that the benefits of COPA do not match its costs and that it has not slowed the proliferation of groups that accredit specific programs.

For purposes of college and university institutional accreditation, the nation is divided into regions. Examples of regional accrediting associations recognized by the Department of Education are the Southern Association for Colleges and Schools and the Middle States Association. Although it seldom evaluates actual teaching and learning, institutional accreditation has been a useful tool in evaluating certain aspects of an institution's performance. Therefore, though the formats may change, institutional accreditation is here to stay.

National Council on Accreditation of Teacher Education

NCATE is a specialized accrediting body for teacher education programs. NCATE standards recently have been redesigned (National Council for Accreditation of Teacher Education, 1985). Burch (1991) stated,

> The redesign of NCATE was fully intended to achieve a national evaluation, based on standards of performance which are agreed upon and acclaimed by professionals as representing high quality. The redesign efforts spanned nearly a decade, and the ultimately derived standards and criteria were developed through participation and consensus from all of the shareholders in the professional community for teacher education.

The ultimate meaning is that NCATE is shaping modern teacher education curricula. Institutions applying for NCATE evaluation under the new standards have reported a good deal of change in their elementary and secondary programs. Perhaps the most important of these changes have resulted from efforts to address the "knowledge base" standard (National Council for Accreditation of Teacher Education, 1987). Programs must demonstrate how they articulate "essential knowledge, established and current research findings, and sound professional practice" throughout the curriculum (National Council for Accreditation of Teacher Education, 1985). Better teacher assessment is one of the reasons for the requirement of improved articulation of the knowledge base standard. Thus, NCATE clearly is flexing its muscles and exerting considerable leverage over individual institutions. As with institutional accreditation, students seeking to major in a teacher education program, including that for school health education, may wish to determine if their choice has NCATE accreditation.

NCATE exerts substantial influence directly on school health education programs. In the absence of specific standards for health education performance, NCATE contracts with the Association for the Advancement of Health Education (AAHE), a division of the American Alliance for Health, Physical Education, Recreation, and Dance (AAHPERD) to review the portfolios of institutional departments of health education. The review, composed largely of examination of syllabi of required courses, is based on the Role Delineation Curriculum Project Framework (National Task Force in the Preparation and Practice of Health Educators, 1985).

Although NCATE accreditation is technically "voluntary," the prestige of a teacher education program is enhanced greatly by this recognition. In the future, the influence of NCATE on colleges and universities will continue to grow. It also will enforce a sense of similarity and conformity on colleges and departments of teacher education.

CHANGING ISSUES IN PROFESSIONAL PREPARATION

As society changes, so must the preparation health educators receive. Courses that illustrate

and clarify the many ethical considerations facing the profession and the society will be needed. Many of these courses will be interdisciplinary. Current ethical considerations related to euthanasia and assisted suicide, uses of prenatal tests such as amniocentesis, rationing of health care, surrogate parenthood, in vitro fertilization, genetic engineering, and chemical abortion have not been resolved and may not be settled for generations. Professional organizations and individual educators, however, may have to take a stand on these issues that require philosophic reflection.

The sexual revolution of the 1960s and 1970s changed behavior patterns and values regarding sexuality. It has been condemned for destroying traditional values, marriage, and family life. As society reeled from the sexual revolution, on its heels came aftershocks in the form of the women's liberation movement and the gay liberation movement. Any revolution brings changing conditions and some degree of chaos. Some obvious changes resulting from these sexual uprisings were more sexually explicit language and behavior portrayed in movies, television, and other media; open cohabitation on a large scale; explosion of the production and sale of pornographic materials; increase in child abuse and child pornography; more single-parent homes; and a breakdown of parent-child and grandparent-grandchild bonds. All of these changes have an impact on the total school as well as on school and community health education. Schools and communities must adjust to these changes and design creative ways to reverse some of their negative effects.

Tomorrow's health educators will need skills in developing programs that respond to rapid changes in family and social issues. They must be able to work with practitioners from other disciplines to solve social and health problems. "Turf guarding," or preserving resources and programs for our own departmentalized goals, must be replaced by an attitude of cooperation and willingness to utilize expertise from all campus and community sources.

The issue of institutional and professional accountability will continue to haunt education. With the increasing competition for resources, we will need to more accurately demonstrate program effectiveness regardless of the setting. Evaluative strategies will become more critical to program continuation. Sophisticated assessment tools must be designed and implemented to monitor program success. Constructing objectives, in terms of measurable outcomes applicable to specific populations, will become more important than ever.

CHANGING CONSUMER POPULATIONS

As has been pointed out repeatedly in this book, health and education are interrelated. Children whose lives are impeded by depression, physical abuse, substance abuse, or hunger are not healthy children. Children who are not healthy are impaired as learners. It is a reciprocal relationship. Education can contribute to health and, conversely, a child's health status is a major determinant of educational achievement. To improve the academic achievement of children, schools and other institutions must devote more attention to health concerns through health services and health education.

Traditionally, society's responsibility for educating children began as they entered school. In the future, more emphasis will be placed on the welfare of preschool children. The increasing body of knowledge of child development requires society to place far more emphasis on early development of the child before he or she enters school, if for no reason other than to ensure that children are prepared for school.

The National Education Goals Panel (1991) made this point:

> *Goal 1:* By the year 2000, all children in America will start school ready to learn.
> Objectives: . . . Children will receive the nutrition and health care needed to arrive at school with healthy minds and healthy bodies.

No matter how much money we spend or how many facilities we build, we must attend to the critical needs of young children. If we do not concern ourselves with the nutrition, health care, emotional development, and family life of infants and preschoolers, it may be too late for many children before they reach school age.

Improving the health of American children requires a wide range of interventions. Many of these already are in place and functioning. Head Start is an example of a successful program that provides many services to young children. Health screening, nutrition education, and healthy diets are just three examples. Head Start has a wonderful record of assisting at-risk children to develop readiness for school. Currently, Head Start is constituted to limit access primarily to those in low-income families. In the future,

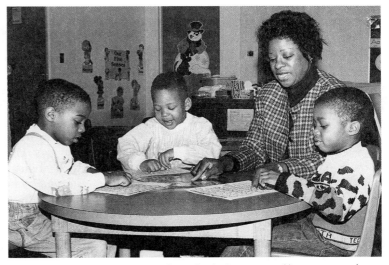

Head Start is a successful program of preschool education. Health screening and nutrition education are provided for at-risk children in this government-sponsored program.

programs similar to Head Start may be available to all children. This program has demonstrated the practicality of early health services and health education.

Daycare facilities offer a tremendous opportunity to provide health education and to help young children develop the skills of coping, decision making, and valuing. In the future, licensed daycare centers may be forced to prove that they provide a range of educational experiences that meet criteria for skill development and health education.

Community organizations such as the YMCA also will play a larger role in the education of preschool children. Opportunities will increase for health educators in these agencies.

The population at the other end of the age scale also will be a larger target for health education. The percentage of Americans over age 65 is growing rapidly. Many older Americans are in excellent health and need information and services to maintain their health. Others are in need of services and information about chronic diseases and the limitations accompanying them.

We are only beginning to explore the opportunities for health education of elderly people. Nursing homes, senior citizen centers, schools, recreation centers, clubs, health maintenance organizations, and hospitals have a chance to offer much needed education about issues such as safe exercise, changing nutritional needs, compliance with medical advice, proper use of medications, and availability of services. Health educators will be a vital part of programming of services and education for the elderly population.

CHANGING TECHNOLOGY OF EDUCATION

Changing technology does not apply to medical technology here. Rather, it refers to educational technology. Just as today's technology was yesterday's dream, tomorrow's educational technology is today's dream. The dreams will continue to unfold.

Most institutions of higher education have implemented some sort of computer literacy policy. These policies frequently require a single course. Obviously, this is insufficient to prepare future teachers for technological competence. Technology is improving so rapidly that by the time students graduate from college, their technological skill is usually obsolete. Therefore, we should teach the flexibility to see beyond today and not be overcome by new and even revolutionary methodology. We need programs that will train teachers to assess technology, including software, as it is developed.

Today, through fiberoptics and satellite communication, classes can be conducted across the campus, across the country, or around the globe. Some institutions award degrees through satellite-delivered courses so the student never sets foot on the campus. This is only the beginning of what the college of tomorrow will be. The system will be more open and less centralized, with less institutional control over the where, when, and how of learning. Educators will prepare lessons and courses to be delivered to students in their homes thousands of miles away. These skills do not come about intuitively; they must be developed by colleges and universities, many of which are far behind in current technology.

Technology, such as interactive videodiscs, is now the state of the art. Who can predict what the state of the art will be in 15 years? All we can say is that it will be advanced. Many of today's educators have not kept up with technological innovations. Those who remain in this rut will find themselves to be antiquated and of little real service to their students. Classroom teachers of the future will not be evaluated on their ability to prepare and deliver a lecture but, instead, in how effective they are at utilizing and developing computer programs and applications to allow students to progress at their own pace.

Most practitioners of the future probably will develop much of their own educational software and will be able to evaluate existing programs on their own. Moreover, they will be able to judge the educational utility of existing programs and

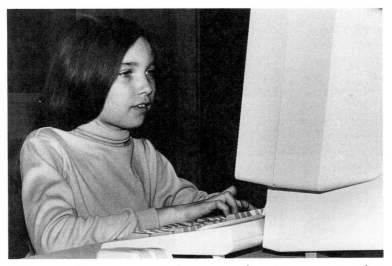

Children seated at computer terminals are a more frequent occurrence in today's schools. Improved software will make it even more common in the future.

POLITICAL ACTIVISM

Many of the issues mentioned previously are political in nature. Others, such as government support for the tobacco industry, preservation of environmental resources, location of medical treatment facilities, and safety modifications on motor vehicles, have distinctly political implications. Certainly, as citizens, health educators should be involved in the process by which these issues are addressed.

O'Rourke (1989) foresaw a climate of shifting emphasis. He predicted that health educators will be involved less with changing individual behavior and more with alleviating the causes of social and health problems. He believes our arsenal of health-promoting strategies should contain not only those directed toward self-help and self-care but also those directed toward promotion of a healthful environment, a safer workplace, and a caring medical system; promotion of public participation; development of healthful public policy, a community approach to health status improvement, a caring and sharing philosophy, and a focus that is not overly reliant on individual effort.

An example of such a generic effort is, while encouraging individuals to stop smoking, to implement supportive government policies regarding smoking in the workplace, tobacco marketing addressed to young people, and eliminating government subsidies of the tobacco industry. Of course, health educators have been involved in many of these kinds of efforts for years, and these more general approaches to health are compatible with promoting individual responsibility.

This macro level of activity, which recognizes health education as a political function as well as an education activity, seeks to create public

apply those that meet their standards and needs with astonishing efficiency. The ability to tailor programs to individual needs also will be a major requirement of future educational programs, calling for more technological proficiency among health educators (Akah, 1989).

The "methods and materials" courses of tomorrow will be much different from those of today. Many present courses are not current at all. Today's and tomorrow's college students should have the spirit of adventurers where educational technology is concerned. The more they experiment, the more skills they develop. The more they explore, the more they learn. Teachers must be prepared to sustain the adventuresome spirit in their students. The future holds an explosion of new information, which will be delivered in thousands of scientific papers and new and expanded journals, many of them electronic. Much of this information likely will be delivered not in printed form but through computers with access to on-line services. This will allow the capacity to correlate and cross-index information to reveal interrelationships that are more difficult to establish today.

understanding of the political issues involved in public health problems. It adopts a broadened perspective incorporating the simple realization that individuals, communities, and societies are related to one another.

As professionals, the need to become politically active will become even more critical on the local level. The development of health education curricula, especially elements addressing human sexuality, is already political. The relatively recent development of school-based health clinics has faced extensive political debate. Most districts that implement school-based health clinics face considerable opposition. Supporters for these and other health services must become involved in the political process.

The use of lobbyists, as well as personal involvement, will increase because of greater competition with other professional entities for shrinking governmental subsidies. Deficits will reduce the overall amount of funding available, increasing the need for political expertise and activism.

A general understanding of the political process is called for. Becoming involved in it does not necessarily mean running for public office, although that is one effective way. Forming coalitions, writing legislation, writing letters, and lobbying by professional organizations are effective ways to affect public policy through the political system. Innovative practicum experiences designed to examine the politics of health and education is an idea that designers of future college requirements should consider.

ENTREPRENEURSHIP

More health educators of the future will opt for self-employment. Worksite health promotion has provided an opportunity that will continue to grow. Health educators will offer consultation, program planning, and evaluation to businesses and health care facilities. An individual might be under contract with several businesses at one time, leading to considerable financial opportunity.

Many health educators already are selling their services as consultants during the summer months, a practice that will continue and expand. With the more efficient technological innovations implemented by college professors, they will be free to do more consulting. This could become a part of the faculty member's workload, providing significant income to the institution.

FUNDING REALIGNMENT

As Akah (1989) pointed out, by the beginning of the next century, governments could be so much in debt that most informed health educators will not expect governments to allocate funds voluntarily for health education projects. Consequently, to secure funds for projects, health educators will raise them through voluntary health agencies, individual philanthropists, foundations, or actively lobbying governments.

This realignment of funding will require greater accountability. Educators will have to develop more and more realistic goals and objectives, well-planned programs, and strenuous evaluation protocols.

MARKETING HEALTH EDUCATION/ PROMOTION

Educators frequently avoid issues that they consider to be associated with business and profit. Recognition of the value of marketing health education and health promotion, however, can be a key to a successful program. In the future, health educators and promoters will come to this realization or run the risk of continuing to miss out on a large segment of their audience.

A definition of the term *marketing* illustrates its importance to health promotion and indeed its similarities to the profession of health education and promotion. Marketing is (Kotler, 1975):

> The analysis, planning, implementation and control of carefully formulated programs designed to bring about voluntary exchanges of values with target markets for the purpose of achieving organizational objectives.

Bonaguro and Miaoulis (1983) pointed out several similarities between health promotion and marketing. Both disciplines:

— strive to motivate the consumer to behaviors.

— identify target populations.

— attract and hold the attention of consumers if they are to be successful.

— convey information and possess something of value to the consumer.

— involve an exchange of some sort.

— give the consumer the choice of accepting or rejecting the action.

To believe the marketing approaches of laundry detergents and car companies can be easily and completely transferred to health promotion and disease prevention would be a mistake (Novelli, 1991). The health promoter/ educator attempts to convince the consumer to adopt a lifestyle or undertake a recommended behavior. To do this efficiently, we must identify a target population. This process, *needs assessment*, is similar to the market research that sellers of tangible products utilize, in that both depend heavily on demographic information and analysis of the possible benefits to the consumer of undertaking the behavior.

Health promoters/educators also must attract and hold the consumer's attention to a similar extent that the purveyor of products utilizes advertisements to attract and hold attention. This is a major problem for educators. We must eliminate the perception in our own minds that we are above using some of the same principles that marketers of products use to attract and retain consumers. One of the reasons educators

frequently feel uncomfortable utilizing marketing strategies is the perception, sometimes accurate, that sellers of products do not present truthful information or present it in misleading ways. We in health education must present our product in a positive rather than a negative way, and we must convey accurate information. We also must recognize that a change in behavior requires an exchange. In buying and selling merchandise, money is the exchange. In health, the benefits are intangible effects such as confidence and self-efficacy, feelings of satisfaction, value for health, or a feeling of well-being, as well as more measurable effects such as fewer illnesses and longer life span.

The issue in the consumer's mind is whether the cost of the action is equal to the benefits. The challenge to the health educator/promoter is to advocate the exchange of lifestyle for intangible benefits. In the end, the consumer must make the decision. A good salesperson knows this just as a health educator knows it. Perhaps it would be more palatable for many educators to accept Kotler's (1982) definition of *social marketing* as "the design, implementation, and control of programs seeking to increase the acceptability of a social idea or practice."

Many avenues of communication are available to health educators who wish to market their programs and services. Many nonprofit organizations depend solely on public service announcements. This type of advertising, however, is quite limited in availability. Billboards, announcements in church bulletins, and bits of information in local professional newsletters provide opportunities for advertising programs.

Public relations tactics can communicate longer, more in-depth messages than advertising, and they provide more credibility. Strategies such as writing columns in the op-ed pages of newspapers, alerting the press to outstanding program events, placing spokespersons on television and radio news and talk shows—all are good at getting a program or philosophy before the public. Public relations also can be of the nonmedia variety, such as classroom materials, conferences, speaker placement, and special events such as auctions and health screenings.

Face-to-face communication is the most direct and dynamic way to deliver information and to persuade (Novelli, 1991). It allows for messages tailored for the audience and for feedback from the audience.

Over the past few decades the trend in health education, physical education, dance education, and recreation has been for each discipline to be more and more independent of the others. Recently, however, professionals have come to realize that, in their emphasis on wellness, the disciplines overlap to a certain extent. This has led to an attempt at group advocacy, a cooperative attempt among the disciplines to promote the benefits of them all. This is seen generally as a positive movement.

Health educators and health promoters are in a marketplace. We cannot expect people to come pounding on our doors begging for our services. Whether it be a school health classroom with a captive audience or a community health organization with a broad and varied public, we must employ marketing techniques and advocacy efforts to attract consumers, hold their attention, and produce motivation for them to act.

SUMMARY

The changing present and the sometime unpredictable future require health educators to develop certain skills for our profession to flourish. The ability to adapt to change is one of the most important of these skills. Many educators will opt for self-employment.

Credentialing is taking place on a number of levels. The progress of national credentialing of health educators and health education programs may have profound impact on the profession. Most of this impact will result in improvement of the profession, although some

forms of credentialing may thwart diversity in professional preparation programs and place the practice of health education in some settings above those of other settings.

Professional preparation programs in the future must face the many ethical issues tied to health-related behavior. Rapid societal changes require rapid development of programs to address their impact on the individual, the family, and the community. In addition, the issue of professional accountability will not go away. As we make claims as to our intent, we must carefully evaluate our performance.

Health education will expand in the future from the traditional settings and target populations. Programs will develop at both ends of the age scale. Growth of the elderly population will require creative programs to meet the need of aging individuals. Expansion of programs for preschool children will explore opportunities that have been touched only minimally. Community organizations will develop into community health education programs.

The technology of education will continue to change. The individual health educator must remain current in new teaching/learning strategies. Professional preparation programs must adjust much more quickly to change in teaching methodologies.

The politics of education is increasingly focused in health education. Controversial issues must be dealt with. Funding fights must be fought in state legislatures.

A different view of funding must be developed. Even as we demonstrate our worth in terms of cost-effectiveness, we risk losing financial support from the states. We must learn to market our product to attract consumers and to attract funding from nontraditional sources.

The future holds a great deal of promise for health educators. We must run to greet tomorrow with the zeal that has brought the profession to its current standing. New skills and new approaches, coupled with demonstrated success, will build an even stronger foundation for health education.

REFERENCES

Akah, R. M. A portrait of health educators in 2001. *Health Education, 20* (April/May 1989): 33–35.

Beaudry, M. L. Post-Carnegie developments affecting teacher education: The struggle for professionalism. *Journal of Teacher Education, 41* (January/February 1990): 63–70.

Bonaguro, J. A., and Miaoulis, G. Marketing: A tool for health education planning. *Health Education, 14* (January/February 1983) 6–11.

Burch, B. G. *A brief review of NCATE standards as shapers of teacher education curriculum.* Presented at annual meeting of American Association of Colleges for Teacher Education, Atlanta, GA, 1991.

Campbell, D. Theory into practice. In J. W. Butzow, editor. *Toward a Model of Post-Baccalaureate Teacher Education.* Harrisburg, PA: Pennsylvania Academy for the Profession of Teaching, 1990. (monograph)

Cleary, M. J. Restructured schools: Challenges and opportunity for school health education *Journal of School Health,* 61 (April 1991): 172–175.

Cleary, M. J. Is board certification necessary for school health educators? *Journal of School Health,* 62 (April 1992): 121–125.

Gold, R. S. Credentialing and the future of health education. *Wellness Perspectives, 6* (Fall 1989): 49–54.

Green, L. W. Letter to the editor. *Health Education Quarterly,* 18 (Winter 1991): 525–527.

Kotler, P. *Marketing for Nonprofit Organization.* Englewood Cliffs, NJ: Prentice-Hall, 1975.

Kotler, P. *Marketing for Nonprofit Organizations.* Englewood Cliffs, NJ: Prentice-Hall, 1982.

Laws, B. B. Why teachers must play a role in setting national standards. *Educational Leadership, 49* (November 1991): 37–38.

Leatherman, C. 6 regional groups say they'll drop out of Council on Postsecondary Accreditation. *Chronicle of Higher Education, 39* (February 10, 1993), A15+.

Murphy, J. Helping teachers prepare to work in restructured schools. *Journal of Teacher Education, 41* (September/October 1990): 50–56.

National Board for Professional Teaching Standards. *Toward High and Rigorous Standards for the Teaching Profession: Initial Policies and Procedures of the National Board for Professional Teaching Standards.* Washington, DC: National Board of Professional Standards, June 1991.

National Commission for Health Education Credentialing. *Application Handbook: 1991 Certification Examination for Health Education Specialists.* New York: NCHES, 1991.

National Council for Accreditation of Teacher Education. *NCATE Redesign.* Washington, DC: NCATE, 1985.

National Council for Accreditation of Teacher Education. *Standards, Procedures, and Policies for the Accreditation of Professional Units.* Washington, DC: NCATE, 1987.

National Education Goals Panel. *Building a Nation of Learners: The National Education Goals Report.* Washington, DC: National Education Goals Panel, 1991.

National Task Force in the Preparation and Practice of Health Educators. *Framework for the Development of Competency-Based Curricula for the Entry Level Health Educators.* New York: National Center for Health Education, 1985.

Needham, N. R. The fad that failed. *NEA Today, 6* (May 1987): 3.

Novelli, W. D. Applying social marketing to health promotion and disease prevention. In K. Glanz, F. M. Lewis, and B. K. Rimer, editors, *Health Behavior and Health Education: Theory, Research and Practice.* San Francisco: Jossey-Bass Publishers, 1991.

O'Rourke, T. Reflections on directions in health education: Implications for policy and practice (AAHE Scholar Presentation). *Health Education, 20* (October/November 1989): 4–14.

Smith, G. P., M. C. Miller, and J. Joy. A case study of the impact of performance-based testing on the supply of minority teachers. *Journal of Teacher Education, 39* (July/ August 1988): 45–53.

U. S. Department of Health and Human Services. *Initial Role Delineation for Health Education: Final Report.* Public Health Service, Publication No. (HRA) 80–44). Washington, DC: Government Printing Office, 1980.

APPENDIX

RESPONSIBILITIES AND COMPETENCIES FOR ENTRY-LEVEL HEALTH EDUCATORS

RESPONSIBILITY I:
ASSESSING INDIVIDUAL AND COMMUNITY NEEDS FOR HEALTH EDUCATION

Competency A: Obtain health-related data about social and cultural environments, growth and development factors, needs, and interests.

Subcompetencies:

1. Select valid sources of information about health needs and interests.
2. Utilize computerized sources of health-related information.
3. Employ or develop appropriate data-gathering instruments.
4. Apply survey techniques to acquire health data.

Competency B: Distinguish between behaviors that foster, and those that hinder, well-being.

Subcompetencies:

1. Investigate physical, social, emotional, and intellectual factors influencing health behaviors.
2. Identify behaviors that tend to promote or compromise health.
3. Recognize the role of learning and affective experience in shaping patterns of health behavior.

Competency C: Infer needs for health education on the basis of obtained data.

Subcompetencies:

1. Analyze needs assessment data.
2. Determine priority areas of need for health education.

RESPONSIBILITY II: PLANNING EFFECTIVE HEALTH EDUCATION PROGRAMS

Competency A: Recruit community organizations, resource people, and potential participants for support and assistance in program planning.

Subcompetencies:

1. Communicate the need for the program to those who will be involved.
2. Obtain commitments from personnel and decision makers who will be involved in the program.
3. Seek ideas and opinions of those who will affect, or be affected by, the program.
4. Incorporate feasible ideas and recommendations into the planning process.

Competency B: Develop a logical scope and sequence plan for a health education program.

Subcompetencies:

1. Determine the range of health information requisite to a given program of instruction.
2. Organize the subject areas comprising the scope of a program in logical sequence.

Competency C: Formulate appropriate and measurable program objectives.

1. Infer educational objectives that facilitate achievement of specified competencies.
2. Develop a framework of broadly stated, operational objectives relevant to a proposed health education program.

Competency D: Design educational programs consistent with specified program objectives.

Subcompetencies:

1. Match proposed learning activities with those implicit in the stated objectives.
2. Formulate a wide variety of alternative educational methods.
3. Select strategies best suited to implementation of educational objectives in a given setting.

4. Plan a sequence of learning opportunities building upon, and reinforcing mastery of, preceding objectives.

RESPONSIBILITY III: IMPLEMENTING HEALTH EDUCATION PROGRAMS

Competency A: Exhibit competence in carrying out planned educational programs.

Subcompetencies:

1. Employ a wide range of educational methods and techniques.
2. Apply individual or group process methods as appropriate to given learning situations.
3. Utilize instructional equipment and other instructional media effectively.
4. Select methods that best facilitate practice of program objectives.

Competency B: Infer enabling objectives as needed to implement instructional programs in specified settings.

Subcompetencies:

1. Pretest learners to ascertain present abilities and knowledge relative to proposed program objectives.
2. Develop subordinate measurable objectives as needed for instruction.

Competency C: Select methods and media best suited to implement program plans for specific learners.

Subcompetencies:

1. Analyze learner characteristics, legal aspects, feasibility, and other considerations influencing choices among methods.
2. Evaluate the efficacy of alternative methods and techniques capable of facilitating program objectives.

3. Determine the availability of information, personnel, time, and equipment needed to implement the program for a given audience.

Competency D: Monitor educational programs, adjusting objectives and activities as necessary.

1. Compare actual program activities with the stated objectives.
2. Assess the relevance of existing program objectives to current needs.
3. Revise program activities and objectives as necessitated by changes in learner needs.
4. Appraise applicability of resources and materials relative to given educational objectives.

Subcompetencies:

1. Apply criteria of effectiveness to results obtained from a program.
2. Translate evaluation results into terms easily understood by others.
3. Report effectiveness of educational programs in achieving proposed objectives.

Competency D: Infer implications from findings for future program planning.

Subcompetencies:

1. Explore possible explanations for important evaluation findings.
2. Recommend strategies for implementing results of evaluation.

RESPONSIBILITY IV: EVALUATING EFFECTIVENESS OF HEALTH EDUCATION PROGRAMS

Competency A: Develop plans to assess achievement of program objectives.

Subcompetencies:

1. Determine standards of performance to be applied as criteria of effectiveness.
2. Establish a realistic scope of evaluation efforts.
3. Develop an inventory of existing valid and reliable tests and survey instruments.
4. Select appropriate methods for evaluating program effectiveness.

Competency B: Carry out evaluation plans.

Subcompetencies:

1. Facilitate administration of the tests and activities specified in the plan.
2. Utilize data-collecting methods appropriate to the objectives.
3. Analyze resulting evaluation data.

Competency C: Interpret results of program evaluation.

RESPONSIBILITY V: COORDINATING PROVISION OF HEALTH EDUCATION SERVICES

Competency A: Develop a plan for coordinating health education services.

Subcompetencies:

1. Determine the extent of available health education services.
2. Match health education services to proposed program activities.
3. Identify gaps and overlaps in the provision of collaborative health services.

Competency B: Facilitate cooperation between and among levels of program personnel.

Subcompetencies:

1. Promote cooperation and feedback among personnel related to the program.
2. Apply various methods of conflict reduction as needed.
3. Analyze the role of health educator as liaison between program staff and outside groups and organizations.

Competency C: Formulate practical modes of collaboration among health agencies and organizations.

Subcompetencies:

1. Stimulate cooperation among personnel responsible for community health education programs.
2. Suggest approaches for integrating health education within existing health programs.
3. Develop plans for promoting collaborative efforts among health agencies and organizations with mutual interests.

Competency D: Organize in-service training programs for teachers, volunteers, and other interested personnel.

Subcompetencies:

1. Plan an operational, competency-oriented training program.
2. Utilize instructional resources that meet a variety of in-service training needs.
3. Demonstrate a wide range of strategies for conducting in-service training programs.

RESPONSIBILITY VI:
ACTING AS A RESOURCE PERSON
IN HEALTH EDUCATION

Competency A: Utilize computerized health information retrieval systems effectively.

Subcompetencies:

1. Match an information need with the appropriate retrieval system.
2. Access principal on-line and other database health information resources.

Competency B: Establish effective consultative relationships with those requesting assistance in solving health-related problems.

Subcompetencies:

1. Analyze parameters of effective consultative relationships.
2. Describe special skills and abilities health educators need for consultation activities.
3. Formulate a plan for providing consultation to other health professionals.
4. Explain the process of marketing health education consultative services.

Competency C: Interpret and respond to requests for health information.

Subcompetencies:

1. Analyze general processes for identifying the information needed to satisfy a request.
2. Employ a wide range of approaches in referring requesters to valid sources of health information.

Competency D: Select effective educational resource materials for dissemination.

Subcompetencies:

1. Assemble educational material of value to the health of individuals and community groups.
2. Evaluate the worth and applicability of resource materials for given audiences.
3. Apply various processes in the acquisition of resource materials.
4. Compare different methods for distributing educational materials.

RESPONSIBILITY VII:
COMMUNICATING HEALTH AND HEALTH
EDUCATION NEEDS, CONCERNS, AND RESOURCES

Competency A: Interpret concepts, purposes, and theories of health education.

Subcompetencies:

1. Evaluate the state of the art of health education.

2. Analyze the foundations of the discipline of health education.

3. Describe major responsibilities of the health educator in the practice of health education.

Competency B: Predict the impact of societal value systems on health education programs.

Subcompetencies:

1. Investigate social forces causing opposing viewpoints regarding health education needs and concerns.

2. Employ a wide range of strategies for dealing with controversial health issues.

Competency C: Select a variety of communication methods and techniques in providing health information.

Subcompetencies:

1. Utilize a wide range of techniques for communicating health and health education information and education.

2. Demonstrate proficiency in communicating health information and health education needs.

Competency D: Foster communication between health care providers and consumers.

Subcompetencies:

1. Interpret the significance and implication of health care providers' messages to consumers.

2. Act as liaison between consumer groups and individuals and health care provider organizations.

Source: National Task Force on the Preparation and Practice of Health Educators, A Framework for the Development of Competency-Based Curricula for Entry-Level Health Educators (New York: National Task Force on the Preparation and Practice of Health Educators, 1985). Reprinted by permission of the National Commission for Health Education Credentialing, Inc.

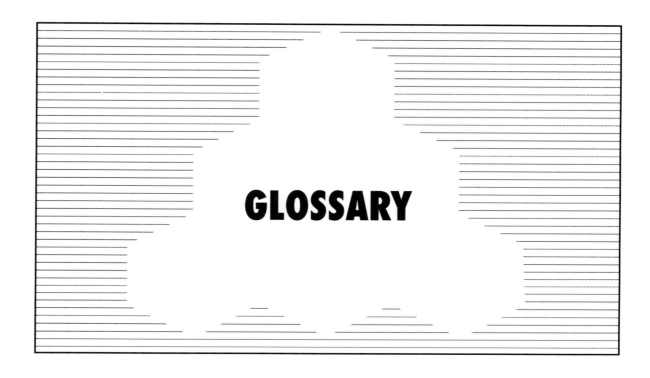

GLOSSARY

Administrability: a quality a measurement instrument possesses when it meets time and resource requirements.

Community health education: the application of a variety of methods that result in the education and mobilization of community members in actions for resolving health issues and problems that affect the community.

Comprehensive school health education: organized, planned programs designed to protect and promote the health and well-being of students by delivering health services and health instruction in a healthful environment in an integrated, coordinated, and sequential way from kindergarten through grade 12.

Diagnostic evaluation: the type of evaluation done for the purpose of analyzing health problems and issues to determine which groups or individuals most need knowledge, attitude change, behavior change, or skill development.

Discrimination: the characteristic of measurement instruments that accurately provides different scores between those who possess the quality being measured and those who do not.

Epidemic: occurrence of a disease in numbers that are above those that normally would be expected.

Evaluation: comparison of some object to a preset standard.

Family life education: a multiphasic curriculum component that includes aspects of managing family finances, human sexuality, decision-making skills, coping skills, parenting skills, and other related subjects.

Generalizability: the quality of a sample such that conclusions drawn from the sample can be applied to the population at large.

Hardiness: an optimistic and committed approach to life, viewing problems, including disease, as challenges that can be handled.

Health promotion: a combination of educational, organizational, political, social, and economic interventions that have as their purpose adaptations and adjustments that will improve or protect the health of individuals who already have a high level of health.

Health science education: the teaching and acquisition of health facts, their relation to each other, and how these relationships can establish health principles.

Impact evaluation: comparison of the immediate result of a program on knowledge, attitudes, and behavior to a preset standard.

Incidence: the number of new occurrences of a disease or condition in a prescribed time period.

Learning: change in behavior brought about by experience, insight, perception, or a combination of the three, which causes the individual to approach future situations differently.

Maturation: a developmental process within which a person manifests increasingly sophisticated traits.

Measurement: determination of quantity or quality of an object of interest.

Meta evaluation: a secondary analysis of one or more empirical summative evaluations that has the power to yield generalizations from the original (primary) evaluations.

Needs assessment: the process of identifying the needs of a target population.

Objectivity: the capacity of a measurement instrument to yield similar scores on successive administrations and when administered by different persons.

Optimal health: the highest level of health possible for an individual under the current set of environmental conditions and capacity of the organism.

Outcome evaluation: comparison of the long-term effects of a program to standards set prior to initiation of the program.

Pandemic: widespread epidemic, frequently affecting more than one nation.

Planning: making decisions in the present in light of their consequences in the future.

Prevalence: the number of existing cases of a disease or condition at a specified time.

Primary prevention: interventions to prevent disease, illness, or deterioration of health before it occurs.

Process evaluation: comparison of professional practice to a preset standard.

Qualitative information: statements describing processes or experiences that result from exposure to a program or an activity.

Quantitative information: numerical values about an entity or group of entities, such as the number of pounds a person weighs or the number of questions answered correctly on an examination.

Reliability: indication that a measurement instrument or test will yield similar results on successive administrations to the same people.

Representative: having the characteristics of the population at large.

Sample: the portion of the population that is characteristic of the population and is utilized to measure some trait and to draw some conclusion.

School health services: all of the procedures the school carries out to promote, appraise, and protect the pupils' health.

Screening: low-cost health appraisal technique for identifying health problems that indicate referral to trained specialists.

Secondary prevention: activities intended to identify diseases at their earliest stages and to apply treatment that will limit the consequences and severity of the diseases and their prevalence.

Self-efficacy: confidence a person feels about his or her ability to perform an action or to control his or her own life.

Sensitivity: quality a measurement instrument has when it reflects changes in the state or amount of the phenomenon being measured.

Tertiary prevention: interventions to assist diseased or disabled people in limiting the effects of their diseases or disabilities or activities to prevent recurrence of a disease.

Type A personality: an aggressive, competitive, hard-driving, impatient personality that is prone to heart disease.

Validity: indication that a measurement instrument or test measures or tests what it purports to measure or test.

Worksite health promotion program: a combination of educational, organizational, and environmental activities carried out in the workplace that have as their purpose the development and support of behavior conducive to employees' health.

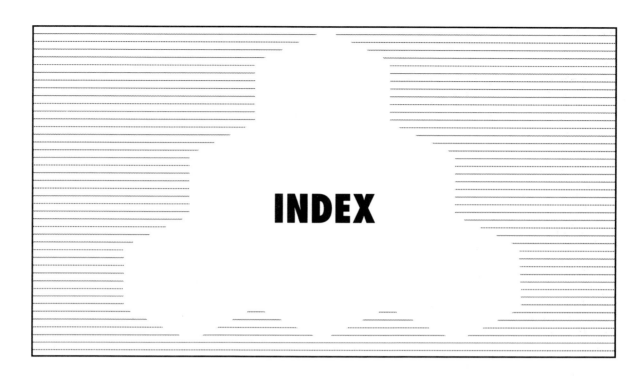

INDEX